W0042706

Breast Cancer 1
Advances in Research and Treatment

Current Approaches to Therapy

Breast Cancer
Advances in Research and Treatment

Edited by **WILLIAM L. McGUIRE, M.D.**

Volume 1 • **CURRENT APPROACHES TO THERAPY**

A Continuation Order Plan is available for this series. A continuation order will bring delivery of each new volume immediately upon publication. Volumes are billed only upon actual shipment. For further information please contact the publisher.

Breast Cancer 1
Advances in Research and Treatment

Current Approaches to Therapy

Edited by
William L. McGuire, M. D.
University of Texas Health Science Center
San Antonio, Texas

Springer Science+Business Media, LLC

Library of Congress Cataloging in Publication Data

Main entry under title:

Breast cancer.

Includes bibliographical references and index.
CONTENTS: v. 1. Current approaches to therapy, edited by W.L. McGuire.
1. Breast–Cancer. [DNLM: 1. Breast neoplasms. 2. Breast neoplasms–Therapy.
WP870 B8245]
RC280.B8B673   616.9′94′49   77-23505
ISBN 978-1-4757-0482-2   ISBN 978-1-4757-0480-8 (eBook)
DOI 10.1007/978-1-4757-0480-8

© 1977 Springer Science+Business Media New York
Originally published by Plenum US in 1977.

Softcover reprint of the hardcover 1st edition 1977

All rights reserved

No part of this book may be reproduced, stored in a retrieval system, or transmitted,
in any form or by any means, electronic, mechanical, photocopying, microfilming,
recording, or otherwise, without written permission from the Publisher

Contributors

George Blumenschein, Department of Medicine, The University of Texas System Cancer Center, M. D. Anderson Hospital and Tumor Institute, Houston, Texas

Paul P. Carbone, National Cancer Institute, Bethesda, Maryland. Present address: Division of Clinical Oncology, Wisconsin Clinical Cancer Center, University of Wisconsin, Madison, Wisconsin

Bernard Fisher, Department of Surgery, University of Pittsburgh, Pittsburgh, Pennsylvania

Edwin R. Fisher, Institute of Pathology, Shadyside Hospital, and Department of Pathology, University of Pittsburgh, Pittsburgh, Pennsylvania

Jordan U. Gutterman, Department of Developmental Therapeutics, The University of Texas System Cancer Center, M. D. Anderson Hospital and Tumor Institute, Houston, Texas

Evan M. Hersh, Department of Developmental Therapeutics, The University of Texas System Cancer Center, M. D. Anderson Hospital and Tumor Institute, Houston, Texas

Gabriel Hortobagyi, Department of Medicine, The University of Texas System Cancer Center, M. D. Anderson Hospital and Tumor Institute, Houston, Texas

Henry M. Keys, Division of Radiation Oncology, Strong Memorial Hospital, Rochester, New York

Giora M. Mavligit, Department of Developmental Therapeutics, The University of Texas System Cancer Center, M. D. Anderson Hospital and Tumor Institute, Houston, Texas

William Leo McGuire, Department of Medicine, University of Texas Health Science Center, San Antonio, Texas

Philip Rubin, Division of Radiation Oncology, Strong Memorial Hospital, Rochester, New York

Douglass C. Tormey, National Cancer Institute, Bethesda, Maryland. Present address: Division of Clinical Oncology, Wisconsin Clinical Cancer Center, University of Wisconsin, Madison, Wisconsin

Norman Wolmark, Department of Surgery, University of Pittsburgh, Pittsburgh, Pennsylvania

Preface

The enormous impact of both clinical and basic research on the field of breast cancer can now be readily appreciated. It is the purpose of this new series of books to bring together the recent major advances in our understanding of the disease. The first volume is devoted exclusively to treatment. It is written by scholars who are actually investigating the biological principles which underlie our current approaches to therapy.

For example, countless articles have appeared proposing some advantage for one surgical approach to primary breast cancer compared with another. The new message is that these arguments for the superiority of one surgical approach over another are valid only in that *minority* of patients whose disease is absolutely confined to the primary tumor site. It is far less important which surgical approach is selected for the larger group of patients who present with occult distant metastases.

The whole subject of adjuvant therapy is still in its infancy. We have progressed from single-agent adjuvant chemotherapy to combined modality regimens consisting of combination chemotherapy plus immunotherapy, plus radiotherapy, plus endocrine therapy. It will undoubtedly take many years to sort out the proper use of these agents. The important point is that we are no longer at the stage of considering whether systemic therapies should be given to high-risk breast cancer patients, but rather what agents, how much, and for how long. Despite our impatience, there is no short cut to these answers. They will come only from well-designed prospective randomized trials in fully informed patients. Such studies are discussed in detail in this book.

Therapy for advanced disease can often be discouraging, since therapeutic achievements are only temporary. Nevertheless, remarkable improvements in remission rates, survival figures, and the quality of life have been achieved. New information regarding pharmacology and cell kinetics has led to innovative strategies. Current efforts are focusing on better methods for selecting combinations of cytotoxic agents for the individual patient. A reasonable outlook for chemotherapy trials in patients with advanced disease is to determine the most effective agents and to combine or sequence them for maximum effect based upon measurements of the particular tumor sensitivity as well as other host factors. The next logical step will be to apply these principles to the high-risk patient with occult metastases. It is in this group with low tumor burden where cure should be the goal.

The importance of the endocrine system in breast cancer has long been appreciated. But only very recently have we begun to understand exactly how individual hormones stimulate breast tumor growth. This information has led to biochemical measurements in breast tumors which remarkably correlate with the response of the tumor to endocrine therapies. Now the oncologist can select or reject endocrine therapies with considerably more confidence than in the past. In addition, basic investigations of hormonal pathways have led to the discovery of hormone antagonists, for example, antiestrogens, which are now being used to treat breast cancer patients. This whole topic is discussed in detail in this volume.

In summary, the present volume provides a scholarly, in-depth, critical analysis of current therapies for breast cancer as well as a clear indication of unresolved problems and a focus for future investigation. Because of its emphasis on sound biological principles underlying therapy, it should be an important reference for the student and investigator as well as for the clinican caring for breast cancer patients.

William L. McGuire

February, 1977

Contents

3. **Systemic Adjuvant (Combined Modality) Therapy in the Treatment of Primary Breast Cancer**

Bernard Fisher and Norman Wolmark

5. Physiological Principles Underlying Endocrine Therapy of Breast Cancer

William Leo McGuire

6. The Changing Role of Radiation Therapy in Breast Cancer: A Study in Therapeutic Controversy

Henry M. Keys and Philip Rubin

7. Immunology and Immunotherapy of Human Breast Cancer: Recent Developments and Prospects for the Future

Jordan U. Gutterman, Giora M. Mavligit, Evan M. Hersh, Gabriel Hortobagyi, and George Blumenschein

1

Surgery of Primary Breast Cancer

BERNARD FISHER

1. Principles of Breast Cancer Surgery: From Halsted to the Present

Whereas for almost 100 years radical mastectomy was virtually unchallenged and accepted as standard therapy for clinically curable female breast cancer, there presently exists great controversy and actual confusion regarding the management of that disease. Women with breast cancers may have surgical procedures ranging from extended radical mastectomy with internal mammary node dissection to "lumpectomy," depending entirely upon the *belief* of the surgeon. Unfortunately, more often than not the decision regarding which operation to employ has been based upon information obtained from poorly carried out retrospective analyses of heterogeneous groups of case records (the comparison of data which are worthless because they were acquired from divergent series of patients); peer pressure; emotionalism; and an outmoded concept of tumor biology. It is the latter which this reviewer considers the most significant factor responsible for the present period of clinical uncertainty.

Breast (and all) cancer surgery has been and still is based almost entirely upon anatomic principles and upon the concept that a tumor remains as a local phenomenon for a finite period of time, whereupon it spreads to regional nodes and resides there for another interval prior to systemic dissemination. Moreover, as a result of a theory first formulated by Virchow in 1860, there has existed the belief that lymph nodes provide an effective barrier to the passage of tumor cells.[1] Con-

BERNARD FISHER · Department of Surgery, University of Pittsburgh, Pittsburgh, Pennsylvania.

sequently, cure has long been considered to be the result of a carefully executed surgical procedure in which *all* local and regional disease was eliminated. There thus arose the practice of *en bloc* dissection for cancer surgery—i.e., removal of the primary tumor in continuity with regional lymph nodes and all intervening and contiguous tissue. Failure to cure patients has been associated with the assumption that either the disease had extended beyond the confines of the surgical dissection, or an inadequate operation had been performed. Since it was supposed that there was a certain "orderliness" about tumor spread and that clinically recognizable cancer was in many instances a locoregional disease, it was considered to be more curable if the surgeon would be more *expansive* in his interpretation of what constituted the "region" and if, above all, he utilized better technique so that he could eradicate the last cancer cell. Locoregional recurrences were more often than not considered to be the result of inadequate application of surgical skill, rather than a manifestation of systemic disease. The hope was held high that "one more lymph node dissection would cure more cancers."

No one was more influential in conditioning the minds of generations of surgeons relative to the management of patients with neoplasms than was the American surgeon, William S. Halsted. His concept of the biology of cancer, which was in keeping with the knowledge of his time (circa 1890), provided the principles (outlined above) for present-day cancer surgery. He apparently placed little significance on the bloodstream as a mechanism for the development of metastases, as is indicated by his publication of 1907,[2] in which he stated, "Although it undoubtedly occurs, I am not sure that I have observed from breast cancer, metastasis which seemed definitely to have been conveyed by way of the blood vessels. . . ." Moreover, he was strongly influenced by the thinking of W. Sampson Handley, who opposed the concept of tumor dissemination via emboli, when he (Halsted) stated, "We believe with Handley that cancer of the breast in spreading centrifugally preserves in the main continuity with the original growth and before involving the viscera may become widely diffused along surface planes."

In keeping with such thinking, it was Halsted's belief that bone metastases in cases of breast cancer occurred very rarely in areas not actually invaded by subcutaneous nodules, and that "it [tumor] permeates to the bone rather than metastasizes to it, and this via the lymphatics along fascial planes."

Halsted's understanding of tumor dissemination is best summarized thus: "There is then a definite more or less interrupted or quite uninterrupted connection between the original focus and all the outlying deposits of cancer ... the centrifugal spread annexing by continuity a very large area in some cases. Thus, the liver may be invaded by way of the deep fascia, the linea alba and the round ligament, the brain by the lymphatics accompanying the middle meningeal artery."

The following quote from Halsted's publication concerning breast cancer is presented because it so clearly set the stage for an era of surgery which must be viewed as incredible both in terms of its longevity and in its freedom from criticism. It thus deserves careful consideration.

> Though the area of disease extended from cranium to knee, breast cancer in the broad sense is a local affection, and there comes to the surgeon an encouragement to greater endeavor with the cognition that the metastases to bone, to pleura, to liver, are probably parts of the whole, and that the involvements are almost invariably by process of lymphatic permeation and not embolic by way of the blood. Extension, the most rapid, taking place beneath the skin along the fascial planes, we must remove not only a very large amount of skin and a much larger area of subcutaneous fat and fascia, but also strip the sheaths from the upper part of the rectus, the serratus magnus, the subscapularis, and at times from parts of the latissimus dorsi and the teres major. Both pectoral muscles are, of course, removed.
>
> A part of the chest wall should, I believe, be excised in certain cases, the surgeon bearing in mind always that he is dealing with lymphatic and not blood metastases and that the slightest inattention to detail, or attempts to hasten convalescence by such plastic operations as are feasible only when a restricted amount of skin is removed, may sacrifice his patient.
>
> It must be our endeavor to trace more definitely the routes traveled in the metastases to bone, particularly to the humerus, for it is even possible in case of involvement of this bone that amputation of the shoulder joint plus a proper removal of the soft parts might eradicate the disease. So, too, it is conceivable that ultimately when our knowledge of the lymphatics traversed in cases of femur involvement becomes sufficiently exact, amputation at the hip joint may seem indicated.

Due to the utilization of those Halstedian principles, noteworthy gains in terms of patient survival and disease-free life have, during the past 30 or 40 years, eluded the surgeon, despite extraordinary technical skill. To the contrary, much physical and mental trauma has been inflicted without those dividends. Partially as a result of disappointment with results obtained and, more significantly, as a consequence of conceptual changes that have resulted from emerging information concerning tumor biology, a new basis for cancer surgery is undergoing synthesis. What considerations are leading to a redefinition of the role of operation in the treatment of breast cancer? The following section comments upon some of those which seem most pertinent to this reviewer.

Table I
Treatment Failures Five and Ten Years Following
Radical Mastectomy

Nodal status[a]	Five years (%)	Ten years (%)
Positive and negative (all patients)	40	50
Negative	18	24
Positive	65	76
1–3	50	65
≥4	79	86

[a]Histologic.

2. Factors Prompting Redefinition of the Basis for Breast Cancer Surgery

2.1. Breast Cancer as a Systemic Disease

Increasing information indicates that by the time a clinical diagnosis of breast cancer is established, most, if not all, patients have disseminated disease. Data recently reported by us[3] regarding the percent of treatment failures and survival ten years following radical mastectomy for what were considered to be clinically "curable" breast cancers strikingly emphasize the systemic nature of that cancer (Tables I and II). The finding that three of four patients with positive axillary nodal involvement and almost nine of ten with four or more of such nodes containing tumor at surgery become treatment failures lends confirmation to such a contention. That one of four patients without lymph node involvement develops metastases is also supportive. Because some patients fail to ever develop metastases is no indication that the operation has elimi-

Table II
Survival Five and Ten Years Following Radical
Mastectomy

Nodal status[a]	Five years (%)	Ten years (%)
Positive and negative (all patients)	64	46
Negative	78	65
Positive	47	25
1–3	62	38
4	32	13

[a]Histologic.

nated every cancer cell, that the disease was completely locoregional in extent, and that dissemination had not taken place. The residual cell burden following tumor removal may have been sufficiently minimal for its eradication by host factors that play a significant role in the success or failure of the operative procedure. It is impossible to estimate the number of micrometastases which may have been so aborted by removal of a primary tumor. Such a concept is at present still too discordant for general acceptance by surgeons.

It is not surprising that breast cancer is so frequently a systemic disease at the time of diagnosis when it is appreciated that a 1-cm tumor, which is usually the minimal size capable of physical diagnosis and which is looked upon as an "early" tumor, has already progressed through 30 of the 40 doublings that are lethal to a patient. Considering that relatively few tumors are detected when they are less than 1 cm, it is appropriate that they may be considered "advanced" at the time of diagnosis.

Correlating information concerning the fate of patients having breast cancer with that which is known about growth rates and other features regarding the kinetics of cells from such tumors, and employing certain assumptions, Skipper[4] has provided estimates of the residual tumor-cell burden that might be expected to be present in a host following primary tumor removal, i.e., the number of viable cancer cells that are beyond the reach of surgery (Fig. 1). Zero viable tumor cells refers to none above some relatively small number with which host immune

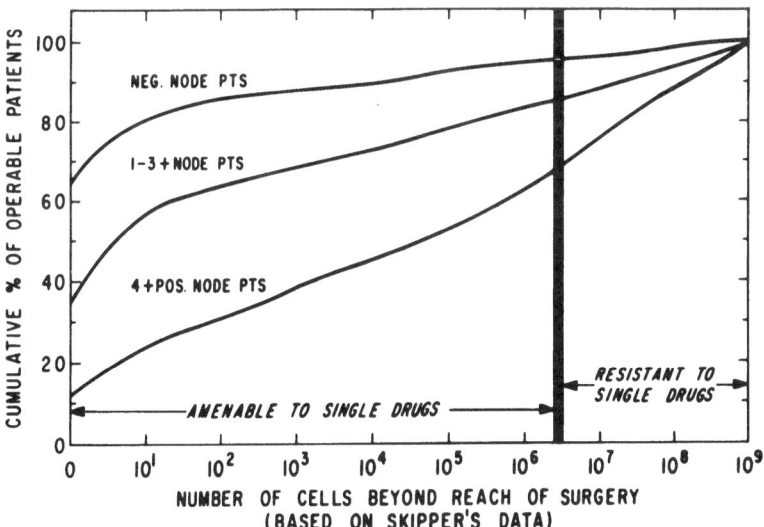

Fig. 1. Residual tumor burden in breast cancer patients following operation.

mechanisms may be able to cope. As a result of such "modeling," there arises some insight into the prevalence of cancer as a systemic disease at diagnosis and the numbers of cells which need to be eradicated by systemic therapy to enhance the curability of surgery.

2.2. Effects of Primary Tumor Removal

That removal of a primary breast tumor is not equivalent to the removal of a "foreign body" is becoming more apparent by the increasing number of reports describing a variety of changes in the host and in residual tumor cells after tumor removal. Not only are host immunological mechanisms affected by a growing tumor, but its removal may further alter those host functions so as to influence the course of a patient. The consequences of both the tumor removal and the surgical procedure itself seem important in that regard. In addition, there is evidence to indicate that removal of a primary tumor may alter the growth pattern of micrometastases.

2.2.1. Relative to Host Immunity

Removal of a primary tumor has been shown to have a diversity of effects on various aspects of the host immune response. Serum from patients with a variety of tumor types has been shown to be capable of interfering with the cytotoxic effects of lymphocytes. Whatever the mechanism(s) responsible—i.e., "blocking antibody" hindering lymphocyte/tumor-cell interaction by coating the latter, antigen—antibody complexes in the serum interfering with cell-mediated responses, or antigen released from tumor cells interfering with lymphocyte action by binding to their surface—evidence has accumulated to indicate that surgical removal of a tumor diminishes the inhibitory activity of serum directed toward cellular immunity. [5-8]

Removal of a primary tumor has also been observed to affect cells involved in the immune process in a variety of ways. Both impaired lymphocyte transformation [9] and tuberculin response [10,11] have returned to normal following tumor removal. Circulating antitumor antibodies have been detected only after surgical removal of a tumor. [12-14]

While extensive removal of a tumor mass may reduce the residual tumor burden to a level which might be eradicated by host mechanisms, the surgery employed could nonspecifically interfere with such defense mechanisms. Thus, the benefit of putting the residual tumor burden within the "rejection potential" of the patient may be negated.

Little information exists concerning the nonspecific effects of surgery and of anesthesia on systemic immunity in tumor and non-tumor-bearing hosts. There is evidence to suggest that cell-mediated, but not necessarily humoral, antibody responses may be altered by those modalities. Several investigators[15,16] have observed that following a variety of surgical operations, human lymphocyte transformation in response to phytohemagglutinin (PHA) stimulation was significantly depressed. Similarly, the number of antibody-producing cells in experimental animals was lessened by surgical trauma and anesthesia under some circumstances and was enhanced in others. It has also been found that surgery *per se* could serve as a stimulus for cell-mediated immunity in tumor-bearing hosts. Other effects of operation on host defense are depression of the activity of the reticuloendothelial system and phagocytosis as well as of circulating opsonin.

2.2.2. Residual (Metastatic) Tumor Cell Kinetics

Numerous studies[17-20] have demonstrated that as tumors increase in mass there is a slowing of their growth rate. This growth pattern of solid tumors has been described mathematically by means of the Gompertzian equation which expresses the rate of tumor growth and the effect of a retarding factor that fits the decreasing rate of growth as the tumor increases in size. Thus, solid tumor growth has been characterized as "Gompertzian." A variety of explanations have been utilized to account for the decreasing growth rate. Inadequacy of local blood supply,[19] immunological factors,[18,19] competition for nutrition,[19] and others[20] have all received consideration. Whatever the mechanism(s), of prime importance is how the presence or removal of a primary tumor influences the kinetics of metastatic tumor cells, for such information has direct therapeutic implication. According to Schabel,[21] when tumors increase in size the growth fraction of the viable tumor cells in the cell division cycle decreases. Large tumors are apt to contain a preponderance of resting tumor cells, i.e., those with a prolonged G_1 time. DeWys[20] has reported a synchronous slowing of the rate of growth of an implanted tumor as well as of its metastases, even though the latter were microscopic in size. With removal of the primary tumor, the slowing of metastatic tumor growth was reversed. Thus, a significant reduction of a large viable tumor cell population by operation or radiation or subcurative chemotherapy probably results in an increase in the growth fraction and shortening of the tumor-cell generation time in the metastases. Temporarily nondividing or noncycling cells comprising metastatic foci may once again become actively cycling and dividing and thus become more vulnerable to chemotherapeutic agents.[22] In a study by

Simpson-Herren and associates,[23] it was shown that small cell populations in distant metastases have a higher growth fraction than do those in the primary tumor from which they originated. In the Lewis lung tumor system, the metastatic tumors had a shorter doubling time than did primary tumors except in those surviving well past the median time of death. The cell cycle and S phase were shorter and the labeling index was higher in the metastatic tumors. Such findings again have important therapeutic implications. They suggest that metastases may display greater sensitivity than a primary tumor to chemotherapeutic agents and that the use of a large primary tumor as an index of drug effectiveness may be misleading. Further information correlating the growth characteristics of a primary tumor with its metastases is urgently needed.

2.3. Redefinition of the Role of Lymphatics and Lymph Nodes

There has been renewed concern with the role of lymph, lymph nodes, and the lymph vascular system in the biology of malignancy.[24] Old beliefs and considerations regarding the lymphatic system which had given rise to surgical concepts for almost a century are continuing to undergo revision. It is fully appreciated that tumor cells on gaining access to lymphatics may be carried as emboli directly to a lymph node. Likewise, it is accepted that cells may traverse collateral or alternative lymphatic pathways to lodge in more distant than proximal nodes, even when the latter are not involved. This phenomenon of skip metastases is related to direct lymphatic communication and the dynamics of lymph flow. Such bypasses can explain the noninvolvement of individual lymph nodes and atypical distribution of lymphogenous metastases. It has been established that in addition to being carried to regional lymph nodes, tumor-cell emboli may bypass such nodes to enter directly into the blood vascular system. Controversy has existed concerning the magnitude and significance of lymphaticovenous pathways throughout the body—particularly relative to their presence in lymph nodes and the part they play in the entry of tumor cells into the bloodstream. Studies are available to support the existence and possible importance of such communications in tumor-cell dissemination.

The concept that lymph nodes act as an effective barrier to tumor-cell dissemination has been challenged. Data obtained support the conclusion that the lymph node is not as effective a barrier to tumor cells as had been formerly believed.[25-27] The majority of tumor cells entering the node may fail to maintain permanent residence. While there is evidence to indicate that tumor cells that are primarily lymph-borne reach the blood vascular system, through·which they become further dispersed, only recently has it been demonstrated that tumor cells circulating in the blood vascular system may likewise find their way into the lymphatics, the thoracic duct, and back into the bloodstream.[28] Thus, the two vascular systems may be so unified insofar as tumor-cell dissemination is concerned that it is no longer realistic to consider them independently as routes of neoplastic dissemination.

Evidence implicating immunologic mechanisms in the fate of tumors provokes other considerations. Should a human neoplasm contain tumor antigens that evoke a host immune response, cells from that tumor disseminated via lymphatics may be destroyed by immune nodes. Experimental evidence in support of the tumor-cell destructive properties of sensitized lymphocytes supports such a possibility.

As a result of these considerations, it is unlikely that negative lymph nodes are indicative only of the fact that a given tumor has been removed *prior* to its lymphatic dissemination. Nor is the significance of the positive lymph node merely related to the supplying of evidence indicating that tumor cells have, prior to operation, disseminated via lymphatics. The positive node may indicate (a) that the number of disseminated tumor cells exceeded the capability of the node for cell destruction, (b) a reduction of the immune response of the host (node), and/or (c) a change in the biologic nature of the tumor cell.

Recent investigations[29] utilizing regional lymph nodes (RLN) from patients with operable breast cancers support the possibility that the reason why some nodes in a group harbor metastatic tumor and others do not is that such metastases are more likely to be related to biological differences between nodes than to anatomic happenstance (i.e., transport of tumor cells to some nodes but not to others), as is conventionally believed. Those studies indicated that cells of RLNs continue to possess immunological capabilities, despite the presence of growing tumors. There was, however, a singificant variation in lymphocyte transformation and thymidine uptake of cells derived from different RLNs within the same patient as well as among patients.

Thus, the significance of the positive or negative lymph node may not be that it serves to indicate whether lymphatic tumor-cell dissemination *has* or *has not* taken place. Such dissemination may have occurred in all patients. In those with negative nodes immune competence may be entirely adequate to eliminate disseminated tumor cells in nodes and elsewhere throughout the body; thus, the more favorable prognosis in negative-node patients. The positive lymph node may denote that these host and tumor factors which permit tumor cells to grow in nodes permit their developing metastases elsewhere; thus, the less favorable prognosis in positive-node patients.

2.4. The Significance of Multicentricity

That cancers of some organs and tissues may be multicentric in origin has long been recognized.[30] Particular attention has recently been directed toward the multicentricity of breast cancer, which has been shown to occur not only in humans[31-33] but in certain animals as well.[34,35] The impetus for such concern has been the consideration that segmental resections of the breast with or without radiation may be equally as effective in terms of curability, and cosmetically more acceptable than a more radical procedure. One of the major deterrents to the acceptability of such a limited resection is the realization that such an excision may ignore clinically and pathologically undetected *de novo* cancers at sites within the breast remote from the dominant mass.

Similarly, there has appeared evidence to indicate that the incidence of cancer in the contralateral breast may be *much* greater than had been previously supposed.[36,37] The disturbing fact is that despite the significant incidence of multifocal lesions in both breasts of a woman with a primary breast cancer, only extremely rarely will there be evidence of two or more clinically overt primary cancers in the same breast. Similarly, the presence of synchronous bilateral tumors is uncommon and the incidence of a second asynchronous primary tumor in the involved breast fails to approach the incidence of occult lesions detected by random biopsy or autopsy.[38] For example, Kramer and Rush[39] noted the incidence of clinically latent intraductal carcinomas in breasts of women over the age of 70 who died from causes other than mammary carcinoma to be 19 times greater than the reported incidence of clinical breast cancer. Such findings are highly suggestive that all cancers do not progress to overt lesions or may even undergo regression. That such a possibility is not remote comes from the knowledge that neuroblastomas of the adrenal in children, thyroid carcinomas, and carcinomas of the prostate are found more frequently in random pathologic material examined than they are found clinically in comparable populations.[40]

It is of the utmost urgency that the clinical significance of occult multicentric cancers be ascertained in order to define correct surgical strategies relative to them. At present, it is difficult for surgeons resorting to orthodox principles of cancer management to accept the possibility that "a cancer may not be a cancer"! From a basic biological point of view it seems to this reviewer that there is need for information relating the kinetics of growth of such tumor foci to those of the primary tumor. Does the presence or absence of a primary tumor influence their growth? Are their kinetics similar to those of distant metastatic foci? Will they become more susceptible to destruction by anti-tumor agents following removal of the primary?

3. A Biologic Basis for Cancer Surgery

As a result of the foregoing, it would seem that if patient curability was dependent upon the surgical removal of "every last cancer cell," the outlook would indeed be bleak and operative intervention could at best only be looked upon as a palliative procedure. The primary aim of oncologic surgery at present seems to this reviewer to be directed toward reducing the tumor burden of the patient to a number of viable cells that are entirely destroyable (a) by most immunological (and others) factors alone, (b) by systemically administered anticancer agents, or (c) by a combination of both. The increasing evidence indicating that primary tumor removal may result in a variety of beneficial host changes and may, by increasing the growth fraction of residual tumor cells, make them more susceptible to anticancer agents is of profound importance and provides a rational basis for cancer surgery. Most certainly, operation no longer employs the distinction of being an "only child" in the "family" of modalities available for the treatment of primary breast cancer. Until it is decided how these modalities may be best employed in concert, the present period of clinical uncertainty is bound to persist. Whatever proves to be the ultimate role of surgery in the treatment of breast cancer, it is certain that its position will be defined by biologic considerations and that the anatomic, mechanistic basis for cancer surgery is no longer appropriate.

4. An Overview of Presently Employed Operations

Not so long ago, to have suggested that there might be an alternative to the Halsted radical mastectomy led to ridicule and censure by one's peers and superiors. To have actually treated a patient with an alternative procedure was considered a flirtation with malpractice. In the past, much of the basis for criticism of radical mastectomy as a method of treatment was related primarily to dissatisfaction with results obtained, rather than to the acquisition of new clinical or biologic information which would justify such an attitude. Consequently, a dogmatic condemnation of criticism at that time can only be partially scorned. At present, however, evidence has accumulated from many sources which, while not absolute, is suggestive enough to allow for the possibility— and even the likelihood—that equivalent results may be obtained by surgical procedures other than Halsted mastectomy. Consequently, there can no longer be justification for the tolerance of those who would suppress and disparage such a consideration.

The following provides information that supports or denies the worth of the various alternatives available for the surgical treatment of primary breast cancer. It is not intended as an exhaustive review, but is presented to place the present surgical controversy in historical perspective.

4.1. Radical Mastectomy

After three-quarters of a century, radical mastectomy is probably still the most commonly employed surgical procedure in the United States for the treatment of primary operable carcinoma of the breast. To present, information from the plethora of reports that have accumulated over the years concerning the experiences of individual surgeons or institutions with that operation is not very meaningful. One surgeon who over several decades has influenced the course of breast cancer surgery in this country and who deserves special consideration—not only for his rigid defense of the radical mastectomy—is Haagensen.[41-43] Impressed with the futility of that operation in many of the cases in which it was performed, he and Stout began to define and refine the criteria of operability for breast cancer—a contribution of considerable importance. They categorized those clinical signs which they considered truly indicative of incurability, and they introduced the "triple biopsy" procedure as an attempt to further eliminate those cases which were not favorable for radical mastectomy. The latter consists of biopsy not only of the tumor, but also of the internal mammary lymph nodes in the first, second, and third intercostal spaces, and of the lymph nodes at the apex of the axilla. The biopsies are done as preliminary and separate operative procedures. Should the internal mammary or the highest apical nodes be involved with tumor, radical mastectomy (according to Haagensen) is not performed; the patients are treated with irradiation only. If nodes are free of tumor, radical mastectomy is carried out several days after biopsy. As a result of his criteria of operability, Haagensen formulated the Columbia Clinical Classification (CCC) to define the various clinical stages of breast cancer and to permit more valid comparison of data from one institution to another. Even though his criteria of operability have not received universal acceptance, and his "triple biopsy" technique is not commonly employed, and staging as it exists does not ensure that different series are comparable, Haagensen has influenced the course of breast cancer surgery. He has pointed out the futility of radical mastectomy in many of the cases in which it was previously performed and has shown that the operability of cancer—at least for the present—is dependent on more than ability to extirpate the primary lesion.

The information most accurately reflecting what, in general, has been accomplished by radical mastectomy in the United States during the past decade is that from the National Surgical Adjuvant Breast Project (NSABP). [44,45] This group was organized in 1957 under the auspices of the National Institutes of Health to evaluate the worth of several therapeutic modalities employed as adjuvants to radical mastectomy. Over the years, approximately 45 medical schools or cancer centers have, utilizing common protocols, contributed data from patients entered into the various studies. Since all data were recorded as they were accumulated in a central data-processing center, most of the vagaries and inaccuracies that exist in retrospective data accumulation were eliminated. Moreover, aside from accumulating patients more rapidly than would be possible by single or even multiple investigators working at one institution, such a cooperative effort has an advantage over that from a single institution in that it has a basis for internal verification.

A patient was eligible for inclusion in those studies only if (a) her tumor was confined to the breast or breast and axilla; (b) the tumor was movable in relation to the chest wall without extensive skin involvement or ulceration; (c) axillary nodes, when present, were movable in relation to the chest wall and blood vessels and there was no evidence of edema of the arm; (d) there was histologic evidence of malignancy; and (e) a radical mastectomy removing breast, pectoral muscles, and axillary contents *en bloc* had been performed. These criteria were essentially, but not exactly, comparable to the well-known Clinical Stages I and II patients, or the CCC Stages A and B patients. It becomes obvious from recurrence and survival rates obtained from such patients five and ten years after operation (Tables I and II) that conventional radical operation for the treatment of so-called curable breast cancer is a less than satisfactory form of therapy. The finding that 65% of those patients having any number of positive axillary lymph nodes at operation, and 79% of those with four or more nodes involved, demonstrated tumor recurrence within five years of operation attests to the inadequacy of therapy in such patients. Even women having the smallest size tumors removed (1.0–1.9 cm), but with four or more positive axillary nodes, had a 65% five-year tumor recurrence rate. [46] When tumors removed were 3.0 cm or greater in this four-plus positive-node group, the recurrence rate was between 81% and 94%, despite the fact that such patients met generally recognized criteria of operability. That nearly one of every four patients having negative axillary nodes at the time of her operation developed tumor recurrences within ten years should prevent satisfaction with such therapy.

In 1970, this reviewer wrote: "Since it has not been demonstrated that radical mastectomy has cured all patients with breast cancer no matter what the stage of the disease—the ultimate aim of cancer control short of prevention—the procedure serves only as a temporary control against which another promising therapeutic modality may be compared. When another therapy *has* been found to excel radical mastectomy, then *it* should serve as the 'baseline' for comparison. Only by such an orderly sequence of trials will progress be made in a reasonable period."

Subsequently (1971), an NSABP clinical trial was begun to compare (1) radical mastectomy with total mastectomy, with and without postoperative radiation, in patients with Clinical Stage I breast cancers, and (2) total mastectomy and postoperative radiation with radical mastectomy in those having Clinical Stage II disease. Patients with Clinical Stage I breast cancers treated with total mastectomy only and who subsequently develop axillary node involvement have an axillary dissection. This study, involving almost 1700 women, should answer important biological questions as well as indicate whether lesser procedures are equivalent to radical mastectomy.

The morbidity associated with radical mastectomy in terms of arm swelling, deformity, and problems with wound healing is not insignificant. Those problems are all the more unacceptable when they occur in women who have failed to be cured of their disease by the procedure.

4.2. Extended Radical Mastectomy

If the removal of the entire lymphatic drainage area in every cancer operation is of paramount importance, then the so-called radical operation for cancer of the breast may be considered inadequate, for the evidence is substantial that lymph nodes other than those in the axilla frequently are involved with tumor.

Turner-Warwick,[47] using dye and colloidal gold injection, demonstrated that about 75% of the lymph leaving the breast goes to the ipsilateral axillary nodes and the remainder drains mostly into the ipsilateral internal mammary chain, with a small amount going to the posterior intercostal lymph nodes. Of more importance were his findings that both the axilla and the internal mammary chain receive lymph from all quadrants of the breast and that there is no striking tendency for any particular quadrant to drain in one direction. While such a finding may have validity insofar as *lymph* is concerned, it is hazardous to conclude from such information that tumor cells behave similarly in their peregrinations. That they probably do so, however, is suggested by numerous observations. In 1946, Handley and Thackray began to do biopsies on internal mammary lymph nodes of consecutive cases undergoing radical mastectomy. Involvement of internal mammary nodes was observed in 31% of patients having inner-quadrant tumors.[48] When tumors were outer-quadrant or central, such nodes were involved in 19% and 47% of patients, respectively. Of women having axillary node involvement, those with inner-quadrant, outer-quadrant, or central lesions had internal mammary node involvement in 51%, 28%, and 59%, respectively. Such findings forced Handley to conclude that the classic radical operation is "not radical at all and will fail in its object in at least 25% of operable cases."

Others have also observed frequent involvement of the internal mammary chain. Dahl-Iversen[49] noted involvement of the parasternal lymph nodes in 30% of medial-half lesions and in only 12% of lateral breast cancers. Of cases in which he performed the conventional radical operation accompanied by extirpation of the parasternal nodes in the upper three intercostal spaces, positive lymph nodes were found in 24%. In an earlier report, Andreassen and Dahl-Iversen[50] reported that in a series of patients with positive axillary nodes, a supraclavicular dissection revealed microscopic evidence of tumor in 33% of instances. Later, Andreassen and associates[51] reported that in 100 patients, 41% had axillary node metastases, 17% internal mammary node involvement, and 3% supraclavicular involvement. More recently, Caceres[52] demonstrated the incidence of metastases in the internal mammary chain, as determined by its removal along with the breast and contents of the axilla, in 600 consecutive cases. In his series, inner-half lesions of the breast resulted in internal mammary node involvement in 28% of patients; tumors centrally located, 21%; and outer-half lesions, 13%. When there was no axillary involvement, the possibility of internal mammary chain involvement was 7%, and when axillary nodes contained tumor, 29% of the internal mammary chain did likewise. Analyzing the latter finding (positive axillary node) according to the location of the tumor, he found that when the tumor was located in the inner half, the incidence of metastases was 44%, and when located in the central portion, 33%. The incidence dropped to 19% when tumors were in the outer half of the breast.

With accumulation of such evidence, it was only reasonable that surgeons who believed that "one more lymph node dissection would cure more cancer" should extend their operative dissections. Over the years, the extended radical operation has been employed, utilizing almost as many techniques as the surgeons who have reported their experiences. Some believed that the procedure was advantageous. Margottini was the first to resect the internal mammary nodes as a routine therapeutic attack on breast cancer, beginning in 1948.[53] In 1963, he and his associates reported five- and ten-year findings with 900 patients treated, and compared them with those obtained from patients undergoing radical mastectomies.[54] Results were distinctly better for patients treated by extended radical mastectomy. For example, the percentage of patients alive and clinically free of recurrence at five years was 55%, versus 26% following radical mastectomy. In patients with lymph node metastases (axillary and/or internal mammary), the survival after extended radical mastectomy was 48% and after radical mastectomy, 24%. In cancers of the inner quadrants of the breast, the more radical procedure achieved a 31% five-year cure rate, in comparison to 17% with the standard operation. Margottini concluded that as long as radical mastectomy is still used as the main method of cure, it seems logical to perform the operation that follows the fundamental rules of cancer surgery. His findings certainly could have led him to no other rational conclusion. It must be pointed out, however, that his data gave no assurance that the case material compared was indeed equivalent.

Urban has been the prime advocate of such surgery in the United States. Beginning in 1951, he performed radical mastectomy *en bloc* with resection of the internal mammary lymph node chain, and over the years has repeatedly reported his findings with this procedure.[55-60] In a review, he summarized his experience with extended mastectomy in early breast cancer.[59] The extended radical mastectomy was carried out primarily in patients with a high risk of internal mammary spread—those having infiltrating breast cancers in the medial and central portions of the breast. In this series, he operated on 236 patients with Clinical Stage I cancers. These were defined by Urban as "an early lesion confined to the breast with no clinically suspicious axillary lymph nodes and no distant metastases suspected." In such patients, tissue examination revealed that 20% had internal mammary node metastases and 25% had axillary node involvement. Of those with no histologically demonstrable axillary involvement, 12% had internal mammary node metastases. In the entire group without axillary node metastases treated by superradical mastectomy, the incidence of five-year freedom from disease was 75%. Of those patients *with* positive internal mammary nodes and negative axillary nodes, 56% were clinically free of disease at five years—about the same percentage as occurs in those having only axillary node involvement. Because of the high risk of internal mammary spread, Urban concluded from these data that extended radical mastectomy is especially indicated for Stage I infiltrating cancers that occur in the medial and central portions of the breast. This conclusion remained essentially unchanged from that of his original paper 15 years previously, in which he emphasized that he believed the procedure was particularly indicated for Stage I and early Stage II medially located breast cancers. Of interest in this regard is the observation by the NSABP that 77% of patients with inner and central lesions of the breast and no axillary involvement were free of disease at five years, having been treated with the conventional radical mastectomy only.

In the 60 patients (25%) of Urban's series having axillary node involvement as determined by pathologic examination, internal mammary node metastases occurred in 40%. Of this group, 62% were reported clinically free of disease at five years following extended radical mastectomy. How this group compares with similar patients treated by radical mastectomy alone is the crux of the whole issue concerning the merits of the procedure. Unfortunately, no definite conclusion can be reached in this regard. Since 18% of Urban's patients with positive nodes received supervoltage X-ray therapy, comparison with other data is useless. Moreover, whether the Stage I cancers in his series are equivalent to Stage I cancers in other series would, at best, be only conjectural. Of interest is the notation by Urban in another report that 40% of patients with both axillary and internal node involvement treated by extended radical mastectomy were clinically free of disease at five years.[60] This result is almost identical to that found by the NSABP (38%) for patients with positive axillary nodes treated by conventional radical mastectomy and for whom no knowledge of the status of the internal mammary nodes was available.

Another American surgeon, Sugarbaker,[61] expressed his enthusiasm for extended radical mastectomy by stating in 1964 that "every responsible surgeon who treats breast cancer should add the *en bloc* removal of the internal mammary node chain to his technique." This was the result of his finding that the five-year survival rate for 940 patients in Jefferson City, Missouri, having conventional radical mastectomies between 1947 and 1950 was 57%, whereas for 151 patients having extended radical mastectomies between 1951 and 1957, the five-year survival rate was 70%. The author concluded that his series of patients were comparable because both groups had an equal number of positive- and negative-node patients. It is now appreciated that one positive node in a specimen is not, for example, equivalent to five with tumor. It is conceivable that more positive-node patients in the second series could have had fewer involved nodes than did such patients in the first group. This information is not available. Consequently, whether his patient material in the two groups was similar is only conjectural, and again points out the necessity that series of patients be accumulated simultaneously by randomization.

Aside from these few advocates of extended surgery for breast cancer, the findings of others have been more restrained. Veronesi,[62] after carrying out 700 extended mastectomies at the National Cancer Institute of Milan, and Lacour,[63] after performing 500 internal mammary node dissections at the Gustave Roussy Institute in Paris, were unwilling to acknowledge the absolute worth of the procedure and they called for coordinated clinical trials. In 1963, Dahl-Iversen reported on his extensive experience with such operations beginning in 1951.[64] He concluded that "as far as I can see, the results following extended radical operation and classical mastectomy are practically idential." Moreover, no difference in results was found when his patients were randomized between extended radical mastectomy and simple mastectomy with ir- radiation, as advocated by McWhirter.[65] According to Lacour, as a re- sult of this study, Dahl-Iversen abandoned extended operations for breast cancer.[63] It should be pointed out, however, that Andreassen, Dahl-Iversen, and Sorensen,[66] as early as 1954, had concluded that the prophylactic removal of the supraclavicular lymph nodes together with a radical mastectomy could not improve the five-year freedom from recur- rence. Abrao and Gentil,[67] in São Paulo, performed monobloc excision of the internal mammary chain as well as the supraclavicular contents along with radical mastectomy, and could report that only one patient in their series with supraclavicular node metastases survived five years after operation. In 1964, Gould[68] reported his experience with the ex- tended radical procedure. He compared results from 98 patients having cancer of the medial half of the breast treated with radical mastectomy and 75 who had extended radical mastectomy. There was no significant difference in the overall five-year survival rate between the two groups (66% in the former and 65% in the latter). Local recurrence rates were identical (8%). Because of these findings and the increased morbidity associated with its use, he challenged the further employment of the more radical operation. In 1967, Caceres[52] reported on his series of 600 cases treated at the National Cancer Institute in Lima, Peru, with the extended radical operation. No significant difference was found in sur- vival between those treated with extended or conventional radical mas- tectomy, there being an absolute five-year survival of 61% and 58%, respectively. Likewise, ten-year survival rates (42% and 44%) were not significantly different. More recently, Donegan[69] was unable to discern from his series of cases a superior survival or reduced incidence of chest wall recurrences after the extended operation. He concluded that "de- spite its feasibility and its logical appeal, the extended mastectomy has not rewarded its users with uniformly superior results."

Conceptually, the extended radical mastectomy is in keeping with present-day thinking concerning cancer surgery, and if those thoughts are valid, then such operations should be rewarding. From a thoroughly objective and unbiased analysis of the above reports and of others[70-75] there seems to be no evidence to substantiate the worth of the extended operation, despite its protracted employment.

4.3. Modified Radical Mastectomy

Twenty-five years after its description, an operation for breast cancer that was all but ignored in the United States is being employed with increasing frequency and is rapidly supplanting radical mastectomy. Patey and Dyson, influenced by anatomic studies[76] which demonstrated that "the deep fascia is a plane devoid of or very poor in lymphatics and hence not an important potential plane of spread," began to perform an operation that left the pectoralis major intact but removed the breast, pectoralis minor, and the axillary contents. In 1948, they reported their early experiences with this technique and concluded that this modified radical operation, with preservation of the pectoralis major, showed results as good as those of the standard radical operation.[77] Consequently, removal of this muscle was deemed not to add to the value of surgical treatment. Perhaps the most outstanding advocate of the Patey operation has been Handley, of the Middlesex Hospital in London. In 1965, he reported his observations with 200 such procedures.[78] Employing the Columbia Clinical Classification, he noted that 76% of 117 Stage A patients were alive at five years, although six had recurrent disease. Fifty-seven percent of 75 Stage B patients were alive at that time, but 11 had recurrent disease. From his findings, he concluded that "at this time of doubt and confusion, it appears that conservative radical mastectomy is a very reasonable compromise. It secures the advantages which Halsted first pointed out, without the deformity which sacrifice of the pectoralis major entails."

Others have left both pectoral muscles intact when performing this operation. While this reviewer believes that modified radical mastectomy provides results equivalent to those following radical mastectomy when employed in equivalent patients, it is to be pointed out that no properly conducted comparison of the two has ever been undertaken.

4.4. Total (Simple) Mastectomy

Throughout this review, the term "simple" mastectomy has been employed because of its general use in the literature and the universal familiarity with it. It has been our contention, however, that further usage of the adjective "simple" is not advisable, since its precise meaning is ambiguous. One suspects that many of the operations described as simple mastectomies are indeed no more than partial mastectomies. To carry out a total mastectomy, the resection must extend from the clavicle to the costal margin and from the midline to the latissimus dorsi. The entire axillary tail and the pectoral fascia must be completely removed. Moreover, adequate skin must be excised and the skin flaps should be similar in thickness to those in a radical mastectomy. Such an operation should be referred to as a "total" mastectomy.

In 1948, McWhirter, of the Royal Infirmary of Edinburgh, began a controversy that has not been properly resolved almost 30 years later. At that time and subsequently, he suggested that simple mastectomy combined with postoperative radiotherapy might be a better modality to employ in the treatment of breast cancer.[79-84] He reached this conclusion following analysis of results obtained from patients at the Royal Infirmary between 1941 and 1945 whose main method of treatment was simple mastectomy followed by X-ray therapy. These findings were compared with those in women who were treated at the same institution between 1930 and 1934 with radical mastectomy alone and with those treated between 1935 and 1940 when radical operation followed by postoperative irradiation was the therapy of choice. The five-year survival rate for all "operable" cases in the period 1930–1934 was 35.6%; for those between 1935 and 1940, 44.0%; and for those operated on between 1941 and 1945, when simple mastectomy and postoperative radiotherapy was employed, 55.9%. Subsequently, McWhirter redefined "operability" to conform to more usual criteria (Stages I and II only and not Stage III, as previously). With such classification, he noted a 62.1% five-year survival rate after simple mastectomy and irradiation, as compared to 50.1% for patients treated with radical mastectomy and postoperative radiotherapy.

McWhirter's primary rationale for the adoption of this "new" therapeutic regimen was related to his concern that radical operations failed to get rid of all tumor tissue in the operative area and that "at the time of operation tissues actually invaded by tumor must often be divided." It was his opinion that, as a result of this trauma, malignant cells would have an increased tendency to disseminate to other sites and, should this occur before the application of radiotherapy, its later use would be ineffective in saving the life of the patient. Although he appreciated the possibility that such cells could still be liberated from the area of operation when a simple mastectomy was performed, he was of the opinion that, in contrast to the situation following radical mastectomy, they would be trapped by the intact barrier of the axilla. Moreover, he believed that since wound healing was likely to take place more rapidly after simple mastectomy than after radical mastectomy, radiotherapy could be applied with less delay, thus reducing the interval during which cells could be disseminated to distant sites. Such views possessed rationality only in that they were in keeping with the usual simplistic, mechanistic approach toward both tumor dissemination and eradication.

Other considerations by McWhirter that led him to support simple mastectomy and irradiation were that (a) when the disease is confined to the breast, dissection of the axilla is unnecessary; (b) when the tumor has spread to the axillary nodes, radical mastectomy must frequently fail because occult metastases may be present in the supraclavicular nodes that are beyond the surgical dissection but which can be eradicated by radiation therapy; (c) radical mastectomy alone cannot influence the course of the disease in patients in whom metastases to the internal mammary nodes have already developed; (d) dissection of the axilla might desseminate the disease; and (e) edema of the arm would not be as frequent following the less radical procedure. These considerations, when taken as presented, defy strenuous opposition.

During the past twenty-five years, much has been written both in support of and against the merits of simple mastectomy as compared with radical mastectomy for the primary treatment of "curable" breast cancer. An attempt to catalogue information concerning results achieved with that operation is futile. The plethora of statistics and information achieved from retrospective analyses of the experiences of individual surgeons or single institutions with the procedure defies interpretation. The inclusion of dissimilar cases and circumstances in most series demands the impossible—comparison of the incomparable. Some of the studies do, however, merit comment.

As a result of a retrospective analysis of the results obtained from 1044 patients, Williams et al.[85] concluded in 1953 that where efficient radiotherapy is available, radical mastectomy should be abandoned in favor of limited procedures. The results in terms of survival were claimed by them to be no better with radical mastectomy. Moreover, edema of the arm occurred three times more often after radical mastectomy than after simple mastectomy. Radical operation did, however, reduce the incidence of local recurrence.

In a retrospective analysis of simple and radical mastectomy carried out at the same institution at the same time, Den Besten and Ziffren[86] were unable to demonstrate any statistical difference in five-year survival between patients undergoing simple mastectomy and those undergoing radical mastectomy, whether or not clinically detectable nodes were present. Similar conclusions were reached by Devitt and Beattie.[87]

One of the better studies carried out to determine the worth of McWhirter's method of treatment of breast cancer is that reported by Kaae and Johansen,[65] of the Radium Center in Copenhagen. Beginning in 1951, all new patients with breast cancer admitted to that institution were randomly assigned to two groups. Operable patients were treated by either simple mastectomy and postoperative irradiation or extended radical mastectomy with dissection of the lymph nodes in the supraclavicular region and the second to fourth intercostal spaces by the method of Dahl-Iversen. No postoperative irradiation was given the latter group. Staging of tumors was according to international clinical staging and, in part, according to that proposed by Haagensen. Results demonstrated in a similar five-year recurrence-free survival for both groups.[88] The ten-year results, likewise, demonstrated no differences.[89] Moreover, there was approximately the same incidence of local and regional recurrences in patients after each of the two methods of treatment.

No one in the United States has been more of a champion of simple mastectomy than Crile. Consequently, his contributions merit consideration. In a series of publications beginning in 1961 and continuing to the present, he has upheld the merits of this treatment for breast cancer. His first report in 1961 concluded that (a) in Clinical Stage I cancer of the breast, simple mastectomy without prophylactic irradiation appeared to be at least as effective as radical mastectomy with or without irradiation; (b) in those patients with Clinical Stage I cancer who were treated by simple mastectomy without irradiation and whose disease later reappeared in the axillary nodes and then was removed by axillary dissection, the chances of survival did not seem to be any less than if the axilla had been treated prophylactically by radical mastectomy; and (c) in favorable Clinical Stage II cancers, modified radical mastectomy without irradiation was as effective as any other treatment or combination of treatment. The greatest contribution of this study was, as Crile says, "that as a result of it and others, the success of simple treatments is well enough established so that controlled clinical studies can now be done without fear of doing an injustice to the patients receiving the simpler treatments."

In 1968, he reported that the five-year survival rate of patients whose axillae contained no palpably involved nodes at the time of operation was 13% higher when the nodes were left in place and not irradiated than when they were removed with the breast.[90] Once again, he cogently advised that "although both clinical and laboratory evidence indicates that uninvolved regional nodes contribute to the host's immunological resistance to systemic metastases, a large randomized study of patients with operative Stage I breast cancers will have to be done before it can be stated with certainty that removal of uninvolved nodes promotes metastases."

Because of the urgent need to evaluate total mastectomy, the NSABP, after almost a decade of planning, implemented a prospective clinical trial to determine the relative merits of conventional Halsted radical mastectomy and total (simple) mastectomy. As a result of the highly suggestive evidence that the two procedures might be equivalent, it was decided that it was more justifiable to carry out such a trial than

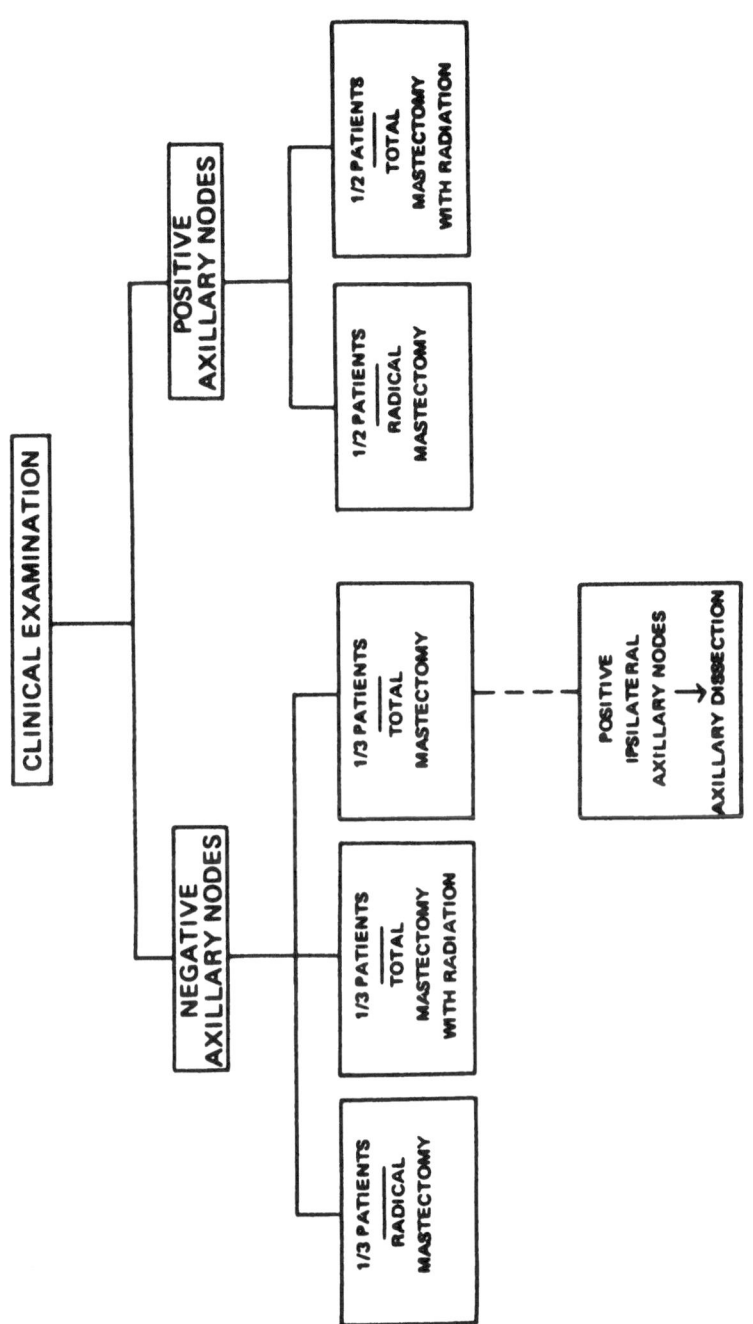

Fig. 2. Schema of protocol to evaluate total mastectomy.

not to do so. Late in August, 1971, the first patients were admitted to the trial (Fig. 2) in order to test the hypotheses (1) that in patients without clinical axillary node involvement, total mastectomy is as effective for breast cancer as is radical mastectomy—if those patients having total mastectomy who subsequently develop significant palpable nodes have them treated, and (2) that total mastectomy and immediate regional irradiation is as effective for breast cancer as is radical mastectomy or total mastectomy with postponement of treatment until significant palpable nodes occur. In patients with clinical axillary node involvement, the hypothesis to be tested is that radical mastectomy and total mastectomy with regional radiation are equivalent procedures.

Patients with potentially curable breast cancer who have clinically negative axillary nodes were randomized into three therapy groups: radical mastectomy, total mastectomy, and total mastectomy with regional irradiation. Those patients with clinically positive axillary nodes were randomly assigned to radical mastectomy or total mastectomy with regional irradiation. If axillary metastases in the absence of manifestations of other disease develop in patients following total mastectomy alone, such patients are treated by axillary dissection. This is not considered a treatment failure unless effective dissection cannot be accomplished.

Radiation therapy was begun six weeks following mastectomy. In general, the plan was to deliver 5000 rads to the chest wall, 4500 rads to the internal mammary nodes, 5000 rads to the midplane of the axilla, and 4500 rads to the supraclavicular area in five weeks.

In August, 1974, when almost 1700 patients had been entered, patient accession was discontinued. Follow-up is progressing and in about a year a definitive report of findings will be forthcoming.

4.5. Segmental Mastectomy

The spectrum of surgical modalities to be considered is completed by segmental mastectomy, which is aimed at preserving the breast and which has been improperly referred to as local excision, lumpectomy, or tylectomy. As with total mastectomy, there are numerous reports that offer suggestive evidence that partial mastectomy with and without irradiation can be an effective procedure under certain circumstances.

In 1954, Mustakallio of Finland first reported[91] that merely removing the tumor, sparing the breast, and roentgen therapy is a satisfactory method of treatment when lymph nodes cannot be palpated in the axilla or the supraclavicular fossa and the primary tumor is no larger than a "hen's egg." By this treatment, reliance was on X ray to control occult axillary metastases. Of 127 patients followed for at least five years, 84%

were alive. In 1972,[92] the same investigator presented survival figures for a series of 702 cases. For patients under 50 years of age, the five-year survival rate was 90% and the ten-year survival rate, 81%, whereas the corresponding rates for patients over 65 were 83% and 58%.

In 1964, Porritt reported his results with "segmental mastectomy."[93] The five-year survival rate for 74 patients subjected to segmental mastectomy was 65%, and for 109 patients treated with radical mastectomy, 50%. Porritt acknowledged that the factor of case selection makes it difficult to assess the significance of the results.

Peters has provided information[94] to support her conclusion that wedge resection and irradiation are as effective as any other treatment in Stages I and II breast cancer. In her retrospective study involving 825 patients, data were derived from 200 who had excisional biopsies and received radiotherapy as their first or only major treatment following biopsy either because they refused to accept mastectomy or because there was a delay of from two to ten weeks after excision, prompting the decision to irradiate instead of advising operation. She has reported on four groups of patients. The first two groups received radical irradiation at some interval following excisional biopsy. In one of these groups, a mastectomy was performed at a later date. In a third group, radical operation performed more than a day following excisional biopsy was the first major treatment. The last group had radical operation immediately after biopsy. The five-year survival rates were comparable in each of the four groups of patients, ranging from 71% to 76%.

In recent years, Crile has repeatedly reported[95-97] his results with local excision of breast cancer and has been a strong advocate of that procedure in selected cases. He noted[96] that in a series of 465 patients with operable Stages I and II carcinoma of the breast, 57 were treated by local excision of the tumor, "in most instances without either axillary dissection or postoperative radiation." The five-year survival rates of the two groups were almost identical: 67% and 68%, respectively. The incidence of local recurrence in both groups was 5% in patients with Stage I cancer. In those treated by local excision, no recurrent tumors were found in homolateral breast tissue.

Atkins and associates have recently reported[98] results of a trial carried out at Guy's Hospital, London, in which 370 patients aged 50 and over were randomized into two treatment groups. Approximately half the patients had radical mastectomy and postoperative radiation (2500–2700 rads, orthovoltage) to axilla, supraclavicular triangle, and internal mammary chain, and three doses of thio-TEPA (triethylenethiophosphoramide). The other half had an "extended tylectomy" (local excision) and postoperative radiation (2500–2700 rads) to the axilla and supraclavicular triangle as well as 3500–3800 rads to the breast via a linear accelerator, and three doses of thio-TEPA. Life-table analysis revealed no difference in survival of Stage I patients up to ten years after treatment. In patients with Stage II tumors, those subjected to radical mastectomy were reported to have a significantly better ten-year, but not five-year, survival than did those having extended tylectomy. In that study, however, most of the treatment failures occurred in the inadequately irradiated axillary nodes. Consequently, it has been considered that that trial of segmental mastectomy in positive-node patients has not provided an adequate test. The presently proposed trial that will employ axillary dissection should eliminate the frequency of axillary recurrence.

When all of the reports are considered *in toto* there would seem to be evidence to suggest that segmental mastectomy might have a place in the management of a certain group of patients having primary breast cancer and that a clinical trial to confirm or repudiate that contention is mandatory.

As a consequence, the NSABP will shortly implement a clinical trial in which patients who have potentially curable breast cancers amenable to segmental mastectomy will be randomized as indicated in the schema

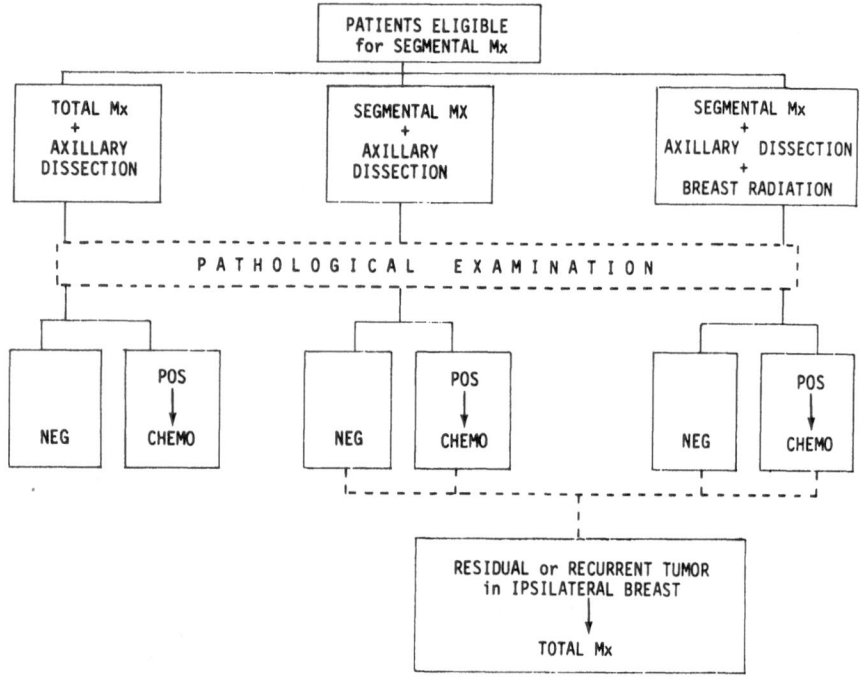

Fig. 3. Schema for a segmental mastectomy protocol.

(Fig. 3): All patients, whether treated by segmental mastectomy with or without radiation of the breast or by total mastectomy, will have an axillary dissection. Patients in all groups with positive axillary nodes will receive systemic chemotherapy. Such a trial, in addition to determining whether better cosmesis can be obtained with no additional risk to the patient, will also provide information regarding the clinical significance of the multicentricity of breast cancers—a theoretical objection to this procedure.

It is to be pointed out that segmental mastectomy can be applicable to only a portion of patients with breast cancer: those with small lesions located in the periphery of the breast and who have ample breasts so that a good cosmetic result may be achieved.

5. Considerations Regarding Special Surgical Problems

A variety of problems require separate comment. Equal or more confusion concerns the management of most of them than exists for treatment of the ordinary invasive duct carcinoma. Since they occur with less frequency, there are even fewer data comparing therapeutic options.

5.1. Paget's Disease

It has been suggested that the approach to treatment of this condition may be related to whether or not a mass is palpable in the breast. Nance et al.[99] observed that none of 16 patients without a mass had axillary metastases, whereas axillary metastases were present in 50% when a mass was present. Moreover, none of 21 patients without a mass died of cancer, whereas 18 of 32 with a mass died of cancer within five years. While a tumor was difficult to find when no mass was present, it was identified in 20 of 21 patients. In 17, the lesion was noninvasive intraductal carcinoma. Consequently, radical mastectomy was recommended for patients with masses and simple mastectomy for those without. On the other hand, Maier et al.[100] reported that eight of 56 patients without a mass had positive axillary nodes. Consequently, he advocated radical mastectomy in all patients. In all probability, mastectomy and axillary dissection is the present surgical treatment of Paget's disease—particularly if a mass is present.

5.2. Inflammatory Carcinoma

Operation plays no role in the management of this condition. Radiotherapy has been used as the treatment of choice. Despite local and systemic treatment, the average survival is less than two years.

5.3. Management of Noninvasive Breast Cancer

5.3.1. Lobular Carcinoma In Situ

In 1941, Foote and Stewart described a type of carcinoma arising in lobules and terminal ducts of the breast[101] which has attracted considerable attention. When such a lesion is confined to its site of origin without evidence of invasion, it is designated as lobular carcinoma *in situ*. That which infiltrates beyond the boundary of the lobule or terminal duct from which it arises is recognized as invasive lobular carcinoma. Only recently has sufficient information become available concerning the nature of such a lesion to permit several investigators to formulate a plan for its management.

The true incidence of such tumors is uncertain. Of 285 consecutive malignancies of the breast encountered by Warner,[102] *in situ* lobular carcinomas comprised 2.8% and invasive lobular carcinomas, 2.5%, of all the lesions. Similarly, Newman[103] observed that 40 of 1436 carcinomas of the female breast (2.8%) observed between 1948 and 1965 were *in situ* lobular carcinomas. Hutter and Foote[104] have reported that lobular carcinoma *in situ* represents about 6% of the breast cancers seen in the pathology laboratory of Memorial Hospital each year, "both in consultation and hospital material." When considered as a percentage of all noninvasive breast cancers, the frequency of lobular carcinoma *in situ* is higher. Of 403 noninfiltrating mammary cancers at Memorial Hospital, New York, between 1949 and 1965, almost 50% were lobular carcinomas *in situ*.[105] It must be emphasized, however, that all the noninvasive mammary carcinomas (intraductal or comedocarcinomas, papillary carcinomas, and lobular carcinomas *in situ*) probably comprise about 5% of all of the neoplastic lesions of the female breast.

The diagnosis of lobular carcinoma *in situ* is, for the most part, made during the course of the microscopic examination of a surgical specimen which has been removed because of the presence of an unrelated lesion—most frequently of a benign nature. They have also been found with great regularity in association with specimens removed because of infiltrating lobular carcinomas. It has been concluded that *in situ* lobular carcinoma is but a stage in the development of infiltrating lobular carcinoma, the two forming a continuum. In a number of series, however, there have been a substantial number of patients who have received no treatment aside from biopsy and local excision and who have failed to develop invasive breast cancer even after prolonged follow-up.[106–108]

It is virtually impossible to make a diagnosis of this lesion by clinical examination, and careful gross inspection of the surgical specimen is usually nonrevealing. Other diagnostic aids such as mammography or cytology have likewise not usually been helpful. Snyder, however, has stressed the value of mammography in aiding in the diagnosis.[109]

Of importance is information to indicate that such tumors are both multicentric and bilateral. Numerous authors have reported the finding of residual foci of lobular carcinoma *in situ* in mastectomy specimens removed after the diagnosis had been established by biopsy, and have stressed the multicentricity of the lesion[101,105,106,108,110,111] With what frequency bilateral involvement occurs is less than certain. An incidence of from 35 to 59% has been reported.

The use of the frozen section for establishing a diagnosis of *in situ* lobular carcinoma has been repeatedly denounced as "hazardous and unreliable,"[102,105,106,108,112,113] and there is unanimity that the diagnosis should be entertained only after the examination of multiple sections from fixed tissue, for then it is less likely that evidence of a focus of tumor invasion will be overlooked. Moreover, such delay will, on occasion, prevent the overdiagnosis of such lesions by permitting the pathologist to differentiate them from lobular hyperplasia, sclerosing adenosis, and periductal mastitis.[108]

As a result of the aforementioned considerations relative to the nature of lobular carcinoma *in situ,* several investigators have offered plans for the treatment of patients with such lesions. Consideration of management provokes two questions: What surgical procedures should be employed in the treatment of the involved breast? What, if anything, should be done about the uninvolved opposite breast? It was proposed by one investigator that once the diagnosis of lobular carcinoma *in situ* has been made from permanent sections, simple mastectomy should be carried out and the upper outer quadrant of the opposite breast biopsied. If the removed breast reveals invasive tumor, a standard radical mastectomy should be performed, since the prognosis of invasive lobular carcinoma may actually be worse than that of infiltrating ductal carcinoma.[106] If the biopsy of the opposite breast reveals *in situ* lobular carcinoma, then a second simple mastectomy is advised. While he has not so designated, it is presumed that should the second breast be found after simple mastectomy to have invasive tumor, he would recommend a radical mastectomy. Such a course of action leads to a variety of permutations which could conceivably result in a patient having four or five operations before completing her definitive therapy. Later,[114] he slightly revised his recommendations. While still advocating simple mastectomy for the involved breast, he encouraged simple mastectomy for the contralateral breast without preliminary biopsy. Such a mastectomy may, thus, be considered "prophylactic" if it contains no tumor. If the contralateral mastectomy is refused by the patient and mammography is unrevealing, then he has recommended random biopsy of the upper outer quadrant of that breast. If mammography demonstrates a suspicious area at another site, it is removed and X-ray examination performed to be sure that it corresponds to the area in question. When contralateral simple mastectomy has been refused, he has urged that such patients be examined and subjected to mamograms at periodic intervals for the remainder of their lives. A repeat biopsy or simple mastectomy is to be carried out if mammograms or physical examinations become "suspicious."

Others have recommended a different approach. Lewison and Finney[115] have decided that because lobular carcinoma *in situ* is probably a progressive disease in some patients, and because of its multicentricity, simple mastectomy is the procedure of choice. Their management of the opposite breast reflects a more conservative approach: "mammography and biopsy of the opposite breast if indicated, as well as careful follow-up examination, is absolutely mandatory."

Newman[103] and Farrow[105] have recommended a different approach for management of the involved breast. The former has advocated a "modified simple mastectomy" plus a random biopsy of the upper outer quadrant of the opposite breast at the time of mastectomy. The latter carries out a "modified radical mastectomy" on the involved breast and makes no specific recommendation relative to the other breast.

A difference of opinion thus exists concerning the extent of surgery required for management of a breast containing lobular carcinoma *in situ*. Unfortunately, as is the case with breast cancer management in general, there is little firm data to permit comparison of treatment modalities. While it would seem that the "treatment of consensus" at present would be total mastectomy, because of the possibility that residual *in situ* lobular tumor may progress to the invasive variety after an indefinite (prolonged) period of time, segmental mastectomy, in this reviewer's opinion, may be entirely adequate. In either situation, should invasive tumor (lobular or otherwise) be demonstrated, the treatment would be that employed for any other invasive breast cancer.

Insofar as treatment of the contralateral breast is concerned, this reviewer prefers to biopsy only those breasts designated as "suspicious" by mammography or by clinical examination. I do not subscribe to prophylactic mastectomy, but would prefer to maintain interval follow-up of such patients utilizing mammography and clinical examination.

5.3.2. Other Noninvasive Tumors

Management of noninvasive tumors other than lobular carcinoma *in situ* warrants brief comment. Such tumors comprise mainly papillary carcinomas confined to the ducts and intraductal or comedocarcinomas without stromal invasion. Like *in situ* lobular cancer, they are relatively uncommon, have a tendency to be multicentric, and can best be diagnosed from fixed tissue; and there is little information of substance available to indicate how they can best be treated. What has been said relative to the management of lobular carcinomas *in situ* also applies to these tumors. Once they are found to be invasive, their treatment should be that which is usually employed for all other invasive breast cancers—whatever that may be.

While total mastectomy may be employed for those preinvasive lesions, wide local excision may be entirely adequate. It seems unlikely that definite answers will or can ever be forthcoming relative to the correct method of treatment for such low-incidence lesions unless there is a pooling of patient material so that proper comparisons can be made. If, of course, it is demonstrated that segmental mastectomy, with or without radiation, is adequate treatment for invasive breast cancer, then the employment of that treatment regimen for noninvasive tumors would follow.

5.4. Management of the Uninvolved Breast

Another facet of the uncertainty that exists today relative to the proper treatment of clinically curable female breast cancer is that concerned with the management of the contralateral breast that does not simultaneously contain a clinically recognizable neoplasm. As far back as 1921, Kilgore[116] estimated that 7 to 10% of women who survive the removal of a first cancer will develop another in their other breast. Over the years, numerous investigators have reported their experiences in that regard. The incidence of asynchronous contralateral breast cancers was found by many[110,117–120] to be similar to Kilgore's estimation. The risk of developing a cancer in the second breast has been reported[120–123] as being between four and seven times greater than would be the risk of an initial cancer by an equivalent segment of the general population. In a prospective study of primary cancer in the opposite breast, Robbins and Berg[120] showed that following mastectomy there was almost a 1% chance per year that a woman would develop a new cancer in the remaining breast. Results from other sources, however, indicate a lower incidence. Lewison[118] found that only 1.5% of his own private patients developed a second nonsimultaneous primary breast cancer during their lifetime. He refers to a similar experience (1.5%) at the Leningrad Postgraduate Institute (2027 patients). Observations of NSABP patients demonstrated the incidence of such tumors to be only 1.9% in six years following mastectomy.

There has, however, appeared evidence to indicate that the incidence of cancer in the contralateral breast may be *much* greater than previously supposed. A review of available data in that regard relative to lobular carcinoma *in situ* has been presented elsewhere in this report. One report cited has indicated that almost 60% of patients with such lesions may demonstrate bilaterality. Several of Urban's more recent publications[36,37,60] have aroused more interest concerning this problem than has any other factor. In one of his papers,[37] he noted that of 337 women who had undergone biopsy of both breasts (either at time of first mastectomy or during treatment of a second lesion), 20% of those with all types of infiltrating carcinomas as well as noninfiltrating intraductal carcinomas had bilateral tumors. Bilaterality was present in 54% of patients with *in situ* lobular carcinoma. If there exists such a high risk of breast cancer in the opposite breast, it is difficult not to advocate that a prophylactic total mastectomy be carried out simultaneously or shortly after mastectomy on the involved side, as Leis and associates have recommended.[110] At least there would seem to be ample reason for generous random biopsy of the unsuspicious contralateral breast, as Urban has proposed, with treatment then determined after noting the microscopic findings. Although such a procedure seems appealing, at the present time, I advocate a more conservative attitude toward management of the opposite breast. As does Lewison,[118] I find it difficult to explain the dichotomy between the high incidence of tumors found by random biopsy and the number of patients who develop overt cancers in their contralateral breasts. If Urban's findings can be reiterated from other sources, then the findings may be highly suggestive that all cancers do not progress to overt lesions—they may undergo regression. Just as was mentioned regarding the multicentricity of breast cancer (see Section 2.4), other cancers are found much more frequently in pathologic examination than ever become clinically significant.

As discussed elsewhere regarding the management of noninvasive breast cancers (Section 5.3), this reviewer does not subscribe to the performance of prophylactic total mastectomy nor to random biopsy of the unsuspicious breast. Lewison's advice that "aggressiveness would be better applied to follow-up than at the operating table" is heeded.

6. Surgery in Conjunction with Other Therapeutic Modalities

Elsewhere in this volume, the use of systemic therapy in conjunction with operation is fully discussed. This section will concern itself with the use of postoperative radiation, another modality directed toward locoregional disease control—i.e., the destruction of residual tumor cells that remain at the operative site or in adjacent lymphatics that are beyond surgical reach. Just as after almost three-quarters of a century there is indecision concerning the type of operation that is best for the treatment of breast cancer, so, until recently, has there been uncertainty concerning the merits of radiotherapy as an adjunct to operation. Little can be said about the value of preoperative radiotherapy because of the paucity of studies in this regard. As a result of experimental evidence that tumor cells damaged by irradiation are less prone to implantation and that damaged cells are less likely to produce distant metastases when released into the bloodstream at the time of the surgical procedure, such therapy would seem reasonable. Unfortunately, however, it really has not been demonstrated that cells disseminated at operation are of significance. One of the few reports is that by White et al.,[124] who used preoperative irradiation followed by radical mastectomy when the primary lesion and the breast had been grossly disturbed by a previous incision for biopsy, or in cases having borderline criteria of operability. In 68 patients with axillary nodal metastases so treated, there was a local recurrence rate of 8.8%, as compared with 19.2% in nonirradiated cases. Five-year survival of patients was, however, not influenced by treatment. At present, there seems to be no justification for the use of preoperative radiotherapy in the treatment of breast cancer.

Emil Grubbe[125] is believed to have first treated breast cancer with radiotherapy in 1896. As Collins[126] appropriately pointed out in 1960, "Now 64 years and perhaps a million patients later, it is established custom to offer prophylactic radiotherapy in combination with radical mastectomy. While continuing the custom, the question is repeatedly raised whether this improves the results over surgery alone." Certainly the rationale for its use is reasonable. Irradiation should destroy occult cancer cells remaining at the operative site or in the adjacent lymphatic drainage that is beyond the reach of surgical dissection. Thus, local recurrence and dissemination to more distant sites should be deterred by its use. In reality, what has actually been accomplished with the use of this modality?

Over the years, a large number of papers have appeared which have presented results of personal experience with the use of that modality. Unfortunately, none has provided the quality of data necessary for making definitive conclusions regarding its worth.

One of the most often-quoted studies is that by Paterson and Russel.[127] These investigators analyzed the results obtained from 1461 cases of breast cancer treated with radical mastectomy at the Christie Hospital in Manchester, England, between 1949 and 1955. During that period, two different types of radiotherapy were administered. Between 1949 and 1952, treatment was by the "quadrate" technique, which aimed at treating the whole of the breast flap and the apex of the axilla in continuity. No attempt was made to treat the supraclavicular fossa. The goal was to administer a tumor dose of 3500 rads in three weeks at 250 kV. From 1952 to 1955, the "peripheral" technique of treatment was employed. Here, approximately the same amount of irradiation as was administered by the "quadrate" technique was given to the apex of the axilla and the infraclavicular and supraclavicular fossae. The homolateral parasternal area was also treated (4250 rads in three weeks). The flap area was not treated. One part of each series (720 patients) was treated with immediate postoperative irradiation following radical mastectomy, and the rest (741 patients) were watched and treated only if and when the need arose. Consequently, it is to be emphasized that this study was not to evaluate the results of prophylactic radiotherapy and of no radiotherapy, but was to compare the effects of radiotherapy immediately after operation and of radiotherapy when recurrences appeared. No statistically significant overall differences in crude mortality rates were observed between the groups. In the "quadrate"-treated cases, 54.6% of patients receiving immediate irradiation were dead at seven years, as were 52% of those in the "watched" group. In the "peripheral"-treated series, 52% of the immediately treated and 49% of the "watched" group were dead at seven years. No advantage was observed for immediate irradiation whether lymph nodes were or were not involved. A slightly minor advantage seemed to have been demonstrated for the Stage I cases and for younger women who were "watched." Although prophylactic irradiation seemed effective in the treated areas, this advantage was evened out by subsequent treatment. Paterson concluded that irradiation did what was expected of it—it prevented recurrences in the irradiated areas, but if treatment was delayed until recurrences appeared, they could substantially be as well controlled. A possible increase in the incidence of liver metastases in the prophylactically irradiated cases was commented on. Since only one-third of the "watched" patients required treatment at a later time for local recurrences or metastases, two-thirds of the patients avoided unnecessary treatment.

Faced with the need to resolve this clinical dilemma, the NSABP began a randomized prospective trial in 1961 to determine the worth of postoperative radiotherapy. Patients received radiotherapy to their parasternal, axillary, and supraclavicular regions immediately following radical mastectomy. The study design, methodology, and results have been published elsewhere.[128] In brief, it was observed that there was no significant difference in disease status between all patients receiving radiotherapy and those serving as controls at three, four, or five years following surgery. Examination of these data relative to axillary nodal (positive or negative), menopausal, or nodal *and* menopausal status failed to demonstrate a superiority for the radiotherapy group. Subdivision of positive-node patients into those having from one to three and four or more involved, with or without regard for menopausal status, likewise revealed no statistically significant difference between controls and those subjected to postoperative irradiation.

It was observed that in patients receiving postoperative irradiation, regional recurrences were significantly decreased when compared with controls. The incidence of distant metastases was slightly greater following irradiation that in controls.

Survival was determined three, four, or five years following operation in the various groups of patients. At each of these times, the survival rate of patients receiving irradiation was slightly less than that observed in the controls.

Life-table plots of disease status and survival were made, utilizing *all* patients with follow-up data. When such curves were prepared according to menopausal and/or nodal status of patients, in no instance was there found to be any significant difference between the irradiated and control groups.

As a result of this study, there seems to be no justification for the use of radiation as an adjunct to radical mastectomy in the *primary* treatment of breast cancer. There is no disagreement that postoperative irradiation—a local form of therapy—when added to another local therapy—operation—can decrease the regional involvement. But it would seem that such local control, although obviously desirable and to be encouraged, is not the factor that determines the ultimate fate of the patient.

It has been claimed that a justification for the use of postoperative radiation is that it is much easier to prevent locoregional recurrences than to eradicate them once they have occurred. If such metastases extensively involve the chest wall and/or node areas, perhaps this may be so, but with diligent follow-up and treatment at the first sign of recurrence, effective control has been obtained in this reviewer's experience.

Finally, findings relative to the use of systemic adjuvant therapy raise an important question: Is such therapy equally as effective as radiation therapy alone in preventing local and regional recurrences? It is extremely likely that effective postoperative systemic therapy will be as meritorious as postoperative radiation in that regard.

7. Comments and Prospects for the Future

There are two aims in the management of patients with breast cancer. In order of importance, the first is related to achieving a disease-free life, and the second is directed toward attaining the best cosmesis and quality of life possible without compromising the patient's chance for cure. Until the present, arguments concerned with the merits of less radical operative procedures have been directed toward testing the null hypothesis, i.e., that such procedures are as good as but no better than more extensive operations relative to survival. Operations such as segmental or total mastectomy for breast cancer, for example, have been advocated essentially for improvement of cosmesis, rather than the prolongation of disease-free survival. It has been hoped that the improvement in cosmesis could be achieved with a disease-free interval equal to that obtained by a more radical procedure, i.e., as good or as bad, depending upon one's satisfaction or dissatisfaction with results obtained by the radical operation.

As the worth of combined modality therapy, i.e., adjunctive chemo-, immuno-, and/or hormonal therapy, is demonstrated, all treatment (surgery and radiation) directed toward local and regional tumor control will require reappraisal. For example, the reported[129] worth of L-phenylalanine mustard (L-PAM) (or other chemotherapeutic regimens) when administered following radical mastectomy is related to its effect on systemic disease. That same systemic effect should be observed if L-PAM is given following total or segmental mastectomy. Moreover, the possibility exists that such systemic therapy may be equally effective against minimal residual local and/or regional disease. As a consequence, all modalities which have been considered for local and regional control must be evaluated and reevaluated in the light of findings indicating the effectiveness of a systemic agent. For example, even should total mastectomy not be as effective as radical mastectomy, the possibility remains that with effective systemic therapy, the procedures could produce equivalent results. Similarly, even if segmental mastectomy is at this time not as efficacious as total or radical mastectomy, the addition of chemotherapy could make it an equivalent procedure. As systemic therapy becomes more effective, the more likely it becomes that lesser operative procedures could be comparable. Consequently, increased disease control may be accomplished together with better cosmesis and quality of life. It is not unreasonable to anticipate that the use of systemic therapy will make more remote the chance that a lesser surgical procedure will be putting the patient at a disadvantage.

In conclusion, it is likely that at some time in the not too distant future, when diagnostic methodology has improved so that earlier cancers are detected, and when there is better understanding regarding the proper use of anticancer agents, in concert so as to obtain maximum effectiveness, surgery will play a subsidiary role in the management of solid tumors and may be entirely supplanted by other modalities.

8. References

1. R. Virchow, *Cellular Pathology*, J.B. Lippincott, Philadelphia (1863).
2. W.S. Halsted, The results of radical operations for the cure of carcinoma of the breast, *Ann. Surg.* **46**, 1–19 (1907).
3. B. Fisher, N. Slack, D.L. Katrych, and N. Wolmark, Ten year follow-up of breast cancer patients in a cooperative clinical trial evaluating surgical adjuvant chemotherapy, *Surg. Gynecol. Obstet.* **140**, 528–534 (1975).
4. H.E. Skipper, Combination Therapy, Booklet 13, Southern Research Institute, Birmingham, Alabama (December, 1974), p. 1.
5. I. Hellstrom, K.E. Hellstrom, and H.O. Sjogren, Serum mediated inhibition of cellular immunity to methylcholanthrene-induced murine sarcomas, *Cell. Immunol.* **1**, 18–30 (1970).
6. G.H. Heppner, *In vitro* studies on cell-mediated immunity following surgery in mice sensitized to syngeneic mammary tumors, *Int. J. Cancer* **9**, 119–125 (1972).
7. B. Fisher, Unpublished information.
8. G.A. Currie and C. Basham, Serum mediated inhibition of the immunological reactions of the patient to his own tumour. A possible role for circulating antigen, *Br. J. Cancer* **26**, 427–438 (1972).
9. S.M. Watkins, The effects of surgery on lymphocyte transformation in patients with cancer, *Clin. Exp. Immunol.* **14**, 69–76 (1973).
10. L.E. Hughes and W.D. McKay, Suppression of the tubercular response in malignant disease, *Br. Med. J.* **2**, 1346–1348 (1965).
11. L. Israel, J. Mugica, and P. Chahinian, Prognosis of early bronchogenic carcinoma. Survival curves of 451 patients after resection of lung cancer in relation to the results of the preoperative tuberculin skin test, *Biomedicine* **19**, 68–72 (1973).
12. Y.H. Pilch and R.S. Riggins, Antibodies to spontaneous and MC-induced tumors in inbred mice, *Cancer Res.* **26**, 871–875 (1966).
13. J.B. Graham and R.M. Graham, Antibodies elicited by cancer in patients, *Cancer* **8**, 409–416 (1955).
14. J.L. Odili and G. Taylor, Transience of immune responses to tumor antigens in man, *Br. Med. J.* **4**, 584–586 (1971).
15. P.R. Riddle, Disturbed immune reactions following surgery, *Br. J. Surg.* **54**, 882–886 (1967).
16. S.K. Park, J.I. Brody, H.A. Wallace, and W.S. Blakemore, Immunosuppressive effect of surgery, *Lancet* **1**, 53–55 (1971).
17. E. Frindel, E.P. Malaise, E. Alpen, and M. Tubiana, Kinetics of cell proliferation of an experimental tumor, *Cancer Res.* **27**, 1122–1131 (1967).
18. A.K. Laird, Dynamics of tumor growth, *Br. J. Cancer* **18**, 490–502 (1964).
19. J.A. McCredie, W.R. Inch, J. Druuv, and T.A. Watson, The rate of tumor growth in animals, *Growth* **29**, 331–347 (1965).
20. W.D. DeWys, Studies correlating the growth rate of a tumor and its metastases and providing evidence for tumor related systemic growth retarding factors, *Cancer Res.* **32**, 374–379 (1972).
21. F.M. Schabel, Jr., The use of tumor growth kinetics in planning "curative" chemotherapy of advanced solid tumors, *Cancer Res.* **29**, 2384–2389 (1969).
22. F.M. Schabel, Jr., Concepts for systemic treatment of micrometastases, *Cancer* **35**, 15–24 (1975).
23. L. Simpson-Herren, A.H. Sanford, and J.P. Holmquist, Cell population kinetics of transplanted and metastatic Lewis lung carcinoma, *Cell Tissue Kinet.* **7**, 349–362 (1974).

24. B. Fisher and E.R. Fisher, Role of the lymphatic system in dissemination of tumor, in: *Lymph and the Lymphatic System* (H.S. Mayerson, ed.), pp. 324–347, Charles C. Thomas, New York (1968).

25. B. Fisher and E.R. Fisher, Transmigration of lymph nodes by tumor cells, *Science* **152**, 1397–1398 (1966).

26. B. Fisher and E.R. Fisher, The barrier function of the lymph node to tumor cells and erythrocytes. I. Normal nodes, *Cancer* **20**, 1907–1914 (1967).

27. B. Fisher and E.R. Fisher, The barrier function of the lymph node to tumor cells and erythrocytes. II. Effect of x-ray, inflammation, sensitization and tumor growth, *Cancer* **20**, 1914–1919 (1967).

28. B. Fisher and E.R. Fisher, Interrelationship of hematogenous and lymphatic tumor cell dissemination, *Surg. Gynecol. Obstet.* **122**, 791–798 (1966).

29. B. Fisher, E.A. Saffer, and E.R. Fisher, Studies concerning the regional lymph node in cancer. III. Response of regional lymph node cells from breast and colon cancer patients to PHA stimulation, *Cancer* **30**, 1202–1215 (1972).

30. G.L. Cheatle and M. Cutler, *Tumours of the Breast—Their Pathology Symptoms and Diagnosis and Treatment*, J.B. Lippincott, Philadelphia (1931).

31. F.W. Foote and F.W. Stewart, Comparative studies of cancerous versus noncancerous breasts, *Ann. Surg.* **121**, 5–53 (1945).

32. H.S. Gallager and J.E. Martin, The study of mammary carcinoma by mammography and whole organ sectioning, *Cancer* **23**, 855–878 (1969).

33. G.W. Nicholson, Carcinoma of breast, *Br. J. Surg.* **8**, 527–528 (1921).

34. G.M. Bosner, Microscopical study of evolution of mouse mammary cancer—Effect of milk factor and comparison with human disease, *J. Pathol. Bacteriol.* **57**, 413–422 (1945).

35. R.A. Willis, *Pathology of Tumours*, 2nd Edition, Butterworths, London (1953).

36. J.A. Urban, Bilaterality of cancer of the breast. Biopsy of the opposite breast, *Cancer* **20**, 1867–1870 (1967).

37. J.A. Urban, Biopsy of the "normal" breast in treating breast cancer, *Surg. Clin. North Am.* **49**, 291–301 (1969).

38. N.H. Slack, E.J. Bross, T. Nemoto, and B. Fisher, Experience with bilateral primary carcinoma of the breast in a cooperative study, *Surg. Gynecol. Obstet.* **136**, 433–440 (1973).

39. W.M. Kramer and B.F. Rush, Mammary duct proliferation in the elderly—A histopathologic study, *Cancer* **31**, 130–137 (1973).

40. F.M. Burnet, Immunological aspects of malignant disease, *Lancet* **1**, 1171–1174 (1967).

41. C.D. Haagensen and A.P. Stout, Carcinoma of the breast. I. Results of treatment, *Ann. Surg.* **116**, 801–815 (1942).

42. C.D. Haagensen and A.P. Stout, Carcinoma of the breast. II. Criteria of operability, *Ann. Surg.* **118**, 859–870 and 1032–1051 (1943).

43. C.D. Haagensen and A.P. Stout, Carcinoma of the breast. III. Results of treatment, 1935–1942. *Ann. Surg.* **134**, 151–172 (1951).

44. B. Fisher, R.G. Ravdin, R.K. Ausman, N.H. Slack, G.E. Moore, R.J. Noer, and Cooperating Investigators, Surgical adjuvant chemotherapy in cancer of the breast: Results of a decade of cooperative investigation, *Ann. Surg.* **168**, 337–356 (1968).

45. B. Fisher, G.E. Moore, R.G. Ravdin, R.K. Ausman, N.H. Slack, R.J. Noer, and Cooperating Investigators, in: *Breast Cancer: Early and Late* (Thirteenth Annual Clinical Conference on Cancer, 1968, at The University of Texas M.D. Anderson Hospital and Tumor Institute), pp. 135–153, Year Book Medical Publishers, Inc., Chicago (1970).

46. B. Fisher, N.H. Slack, I.D.J. Bross, and Cooperating Investigators, Cancer of the breast: Size of neoplasm and prognosis, *Cancer* **24**, 1071–1080 (1969).

47. R.T. Turner-Warwick, The lymphatics of the breast, *Br. J. Surg.* **46**, 574–582 (1959).
48. R.S. Handley, The early spread of breast carcinoma and its bearing on operative treatment, *Br. J. Surg.* **51**, 206–208 (1964).
49. E. Dahl-Iversen, Recherches sur le métastases microscopiques des ganglions lymphatiques parasternaux dans le cancer du sein, *J. Int. Chir.* **11**, 492 (1951).
50. M. Andreassen and E. Dahl-Iversen, Recherches sur le métastases microscopiques des ganglions lymphatiques sus-clavicularis dous de cancer du sein, *J. Int. Chir.* **9**, 27 (1949).
51. M. Andreassen, E. Dahl-Iversen, and B. Sorensen, Glandular metastases in carcinoma of the breast: Results of a more radical operation, *Lancet* **1**, 176–182 (1954).
52. E. Caceres, An evaluation of radical mastectomy and extended radical mastectomy for cancer of the breast, *Surg. Gynecol. Obstet.* **125**, 337–341 (1967).
53. M. Margottini and P. Bucalossi, El metastasi lymphoghiandolari mammario interne nel cancro della mammella, *Boll. Oncol.* **23**, 79 (1949).
54. M. Margottini, G. Jacobelli, and M. Cau, The end results of enlarged radical mastectomy, *Acta Unio Int. Contra Cancrum* **19**, 1555–1559 (1963).
55. J.A. Urban, Discussion on radical mastectomy in breast cancer with supraclavicular and/or internal mammary node dissection, *Proc. Natl. Cancer Conf.* **2**, 243–246 (1952).
56. J.A. Urban, Radical mastecotmy with *en bloc* in-continuity resection of internal mammary lymph node chain, *Surg. Clin. North Am.* **36**, 1065–1082 (1956).
57. J.A. Urban, Clinical experience and results of excision of the internal mammary lymph node chain in primary operable breast cancer, *Cancer* **12**, 14–22 (1959).
58. J.A. Urban, Extended radical mastectomy for breast cancer, *Am. J. Surg.* **106**, 399–404 (1963).
59. J.A. Urban, What is the rationale for an extended radical procedure in early cases? *J. Am. Med. Assoc.* **199**, 742–743 (1967).
60. J.A. Urban, Primary operable breast cancer. Current status of treatment, *Rocky Mount. Med. J.* **65**, 39–46 (1968).
61. E.D. Sugarbaker, Extended radical mastectomy. Its superiority in the treatment of breast cancer, *J. Am. Med. Assoc.* **187**, 96–99 (1964).
62. U. Veronesi and L. Zingo, Extended mastectomy for cancer of the breast, *Cancer* **20**, 677–680 (1967).
63. J. Lacour, The place of the Halsted operation in treatment of breast cancer, *Int. Surg.* **47**, 282–287 (1967).
64. E. Dahl-Iversen and T. Tobiassen, Radical mastectomy with parasternal and supraclavicular dissection for mammary carcinoma, *Ann. Surg.* **157**, 170–175 (1963).
65. S. Kaae and H. Johansen, Breast cancer. A comparison of the results of simple mastectomy with postoperative roentgen irradiation by the McWhirter method with those of extended radical mastectomy, *Acta Radiol. Suppl.* **188**, 155–161 (1959).
66. M. Andreassen, E. Dahl-Iversen, and B. Sorensen, Extended exeresis of regional lymph nodes at operation for carcinoma of breast and result of 5-year follow-up of first 98 cases with removal of axillary as well as supraclavicular glands, *Acta Chir. Scand.* **107**, 206–213 (1954).
67. A. Abrao and F. Gentil, Mastectomia radical ampliada com esvaziamento ganglionar supraclavicular, axillar a da codlia mammaris interna em monobloco, *Rev. Paul. Med.* **46**, 217–226 (1955).
68. E.A. Gould, Prognosis of carcinoma involving the medial half of the breast, *Am. Surg.* **30**, 9–11 (1964).
69. W.L. Donegan, An experience with extended radical mastectomy for mammary carcinoma, *Mo. Med.* **65**, 109–112 (1968).
70. T.H. Ackland, Extended mastectomy, *Med. J. Aust.* **i**, 715–720 (1969).

71. P. Bucalossi and V. Veronesi, Long-term results of radical mastectomy with removal of internal mammary chain, *Acta Unio Int. Contra Cancrum* **15**, 1052–1055 (1959).

72. H.C. Chin, T.T. Chang, T.Y. Wang, P.C. Cheng, Y.Y. Li, and T.T. Huang, A comparison of results of radical mastectomy and that combined with resection of internal mammary lymph node chains, *Acta Unio Int. Contra Cancrum* **19**, 1572–1574 (1963).

73. S.A. Kholdin, Extended radical operations for mammary cancer, *Prog. Clin. Cancer* **1**, 438–449 (1965).

74. O.F. Noel, Extended operation for carcinoma of breast—surgical techniques, *Surgery* **38**, 423–431 (1955).

75. A. Prudente, L'amputation inter-scapulo-mammo-thoracique, *J. Chir.* **65**, 729–746 (1949).

76. H.J. Gray, Relation of the lymphatic vessels to the spread of cancer, *Br. J. Surg.* **26**, 462–495 (1939).

77. D.H. Patey and W.H. Dyson, The prognosis of carcinoma of the breast in relation to the type of operation performed, *Br. J. Cancer* **2**, 7–13 (1948).

78. R.S. Handley, The technic and results of conservative radical mastectomy (Patey's operation), *Prog. Clin. Cancer* **1**, 462–470 (1965).

79. R. McWhirter, The value of simple mastectomy and radiotherapy in the treatment of cancer of the breast, *Br. J. Radiol.* **21**, 599–610 (1948).

80. R. McWhirter, Discussion: The treatment of cancer of the breast, abridged, *Proc. R. Soc. Med.* **41**, 122–129 (1948).

81. R. McWhirter, Treatment of cancer of the breast by simple mastectomy and roentgenotherapy, *Arch. Surg.* **59**, 830–842 (1949).

82. R. McWhirter, The principles of treatment by radiotherapy in breast cancer, *Br. J. Cancer* **4**, 368–371 (1950).

83. R. McWhirter, Simple mastectomy and radiotherapy in the treatment of breast cancer, *Br. J. Radiol.* **28**, 128–139 (1955).

84. R. McWhirter, Should more radical treatment be attempted in breast cancer? Caldwell lecture, 1963, *Am. J. Roentgenol.* **92**, 3–13 (1964).

85. J.G. Williams, R.S. Murley, and M.P. Curwen, Carcinoma of the female breast: Conservative radical surgery, *Br. Med. J.* **2**, 787–796 (1953).

86. L. Den Besten and S.E. Ziffren, Simple and radical mastectomy: A comparison of survival, *Arch. Surg.* **90**, 755–759 (1965).

87. J.E. Devitt and W.G. Beattie, Rational treatment of carcinoma of the breast? *Ann. Surg.* **160**, 71–80 (1964).

88. S. Kaae and H. Johansen, Breast cancer. Five-year results: Two random series of simple mastectomy with postoperative irradiation versus extended radical mastectomy, *Am. J. Roentgenol.* **87**, 82–88 (1962).

89. S. Kaae and H. Johansen, Simple mastectomy plus postoperative irradiation by the method of McWhirter for mammary carcinoma, *Prog. Clin. Cancer* **1**, 453–454 (1965).

90. G. Crile, Jr., Results of simple mastectomy without irradiation in the treatment of operative stage I cancer of the breast, *Ann. Surg.* **168**, 330–336 (1968).

91. S. Mustakallio, Treatment of breast cancer by tumor extirpation and roentgen therapy instead of radical operation, *J. Fac. Radiol.* **6**, 23–26 (1954).

92. S. Mustakallio, Conservative treatment of breast carcinoma—review of 25 years follow-up, *Clin. Radiol.* **23**, 110–116 (1972).

93. A. Porritt, Early carcinoma of the breast, *Br. J. Surg.* **51**, 214–216 (1964).

94. V.M. Peters, Wedge resection and irradiation, an effective treatment in early breast cancer, *J. Am. Med. Assoc.* **200**, 134–135 (1967).

95. G. Crile, Jr., Treatment of breast cancer by local excision, *Am. J. Surg.* **109**, 400–403 (1965).

96. G. Crile, Jr. and S. O. Hoerr, Results of treatment of carcinoma of the breast by local excision, *Surg. Gynecol. Obstet.* **132**, 780–782 (1971).

97. G. Crile, Jr., The case for local excision of breast cancer in selected cases, *Lancet* **1**, 549–554 (1972).

98. H. Atkins, J.L. Hayward, D.L. Klugman, and A.B. Wayte, Treatment of breast cancer: A report after ten years of a clinical trial. *Br. Med. J.* **20**, 423–429 (1972).

99. F.C. Nance, D.H. DeLoach, R.A. Welsh, and W.F. Becker, Paget's disease of the breast, *Ann. Surg.* **171**, 864–874 (1970).

100. W.P. Maier, G.P. Rosemond, E.L. Harasym, T.I. Al Saleem, E.M. Tassoni, and S.S. Shor, Paget's disease in the female breast, *Surg. Gynecol. Obstet.* **128**, 1253–1263 (1969).

101. F.W. Foote, Jr. and F.W. Stewart, Lobular carcinoma *in situ:* Rare form of mammary cancer, *Am. J. Pathol.* **17**, 491–495 (1941).

102. N.E. Warner, Lobular carcinoma of the breast, *Cancer* **23**, 840–846 (1969).

103. W. Newman, Lobular carcinoma of the female breast: Report of 73 cases, *Ann. Surg.* **164**, 305–314 (1966).

104. R.V.P. Hutter and F.W. Foote, Jr., Lobular carcinoma *in situ.* Long term follow-up, *Cancer* **24**, 1081–1085 (1969).

105. J.H. Farrow, Clinical considerations and treatment of *in situ* lobular breast cancer, *Am. J. Roentgenol.* **102**, 652–656 (1968).

106. J.R. Benfield, M. Jacobson, and N.E. Warner, *In situ* lobular carcinoma of the breast, *Arch. Surg. (Chicago)* **91**, 130–135 (1965).

107. J.W. Berg and G.F. Robbins, 20 year follow-ups of breast cancer, *Acta Unio Int. Contra Cancrum* **19**, 1575–1577 (1963).

108. W. Newman, *In situ* lobular carcinoma of the breast: Report of 26 women with 32 cancers, *Ann. Surg.* **157**, 591–599 (1963).

109. R.E. Snyder, Mammography and lobular carcinoma *in situ, Surg. Gynecol. Obstet.* **122**, 255–260 (1966).

110. H.P. Leis, Jr., W.L. Mersheimer, M.M. Black, and A. de Chabon, The second breast, *N.Y. State J. Med.* **65**, 2460–2468 (1965).

111. R.W. McDivitt, R.V.P. Hutter, F.W. Foote, Jr., and F.W. Stewart, *In situ* lobular carcinoma. A prospective follow-up study indicating cumulative patient risks, *J. Am. Med. Assoc.* **201**, 82–86 (1967).

112. F.W. Foote, Jr. and F.W. Stewart, A histologic classification of carcinoma of the breast, *Surgery* **19**, 74–99 (1946).

113. F.W. Stewart, Tumors of the breast, in: *Atlas of Tumor Pathology,* Section IX, Fascicle 34, Armed Forces Institute of Pathology, Washington, D.C. (1950), pp. 7–13, 43–52.

114. F.R. Benfield, A.G. Fingerhut, and N.E. Warner, Lobular carcinoma of the breast— 1969. A therapeutic proposal, *Arch. Surg. (Chicago)* **99**, 129–131 (1969).

115. E.F. Lewison and G.G.Finney, Jr., Lobular carcinoma *in situ* of the breast, *Surg. Gynecol. Obstet.* **126**, 1280–1286 (1968).

116. A.R. Kilgore, The incidence of cancer in the second breast, *J. Am. Med. Assoc.* **77**, 454–457 (1921).

117. W.T. Fitts, Jr. and L.T. Patterson, The spread of mammary cancer, *Surg. Clin. North Am.* **35**, 1539–1551 (1955).

118. E.F. Lewison, The management of the contralateral breast, *Hosp. Pract.* **5**, 101–106 (1970).

119. G.T. Pack, Bilateral mastectomy, *Surgery* **29**, 929–931 (1951).

120. G.F. Robbins and J.W. Berg, Bilateral primary breast cancers. A prospective clinicopathological study, *Cancer* **17**, 1501–1527 (1964).

121. T.B. Hubbard, Jr., Nonsimultaneous bilateral carcinoma of the breast, *Surgery* **34**, 706–723 (1953).

122. A.R. Kilgore, H.G. Bell, and R.E. Ahlquist, Jr., Cancer in the second breast, *Am. J. Surg.* **92**, 156–161 (1956).
123. P. Mustacchi, A Pandolfi, and P. Bucalossi, Bilateral mammary cancer in Italian women, *J. Natl. Cancer Inst.* **19**, 1035–1042 (1957).
124. E.C. White, G.H. Fletcher, and R.L. Clark, Surgical experience with preoperative irradiation for carcinoma of the breast, *Ann. Surg.* **155**, 948–956 (1962).
125. E.H. Grubbe, *X-Ray Treatment, Its Origin, Birth, and Early History*, Bruce Publishing Company, St. Paul (1949).
126. V.P. Collins, Changing concepts of breast cancer and radiotherapy, *Proc. Natl. Cancer. Conf.* **4**, 239–250 (1960).
127. R. Paterson and M. H. Russell, Clinical trials in malignant disease, Part III. Evaluation of postoperative radiotherapy, *J. Fac. Radiol.* **10**, 175–180 (1959).
128. B. Fisher, N.H. Slack, P.J. Cavanaugh, B. Gardner, R.G. Ravdin, and Cooperating Investigators, Postoperative radiotherapy in the treatment of breast cancer: Results of the NSABP clinical trial, *Ann. Surg.* **172**, 711–732 (1970).
129. B. Fisher, P. Carbone, S. G. Economou, R. Frelick, A. Glass, H. Lerner, C. Redmond, M. Zelen, D.L. Katrych, N. Wolmark, P. Band, E. R. Fisher, and Other Cooperating Investigabors, L-Phenylalanine mustard (L-PAM) in the management of primary breast cancer: A report of early findings, *N. Engl. J. Med.* **292**, 117–122 (1975).

2

Pathology of Breast Cancer

1. Introduction

The literature contains several monographs and numerous reports dealing with the pathologic aspects of mammary carcinoma. Many are concerned with correlations of certain pathologic features of these lesions
with prognosis. Examples of such studies are those relating such so-
called pathologic discriminants of the tumor as nuclear and histologic
grades, lymphoid infiltrate, and reactions of regional lymph nodes, to
survival. There are a modest number of reports attesting to the favorable
clinical course of certain histologic types of mammary carcinoma,
namely, medullary, tubular, mucinous, and adenocystic types. Some
studies might be regarded as principally descriptive in nature. These
refer to features of mammary carcinoma which may be unappreciated by
routine staining techniques, such as their elastic or mucin content. Although perusal of many of these pathologic studies may reveal information relevant to the interrelationships among several pathologic and clinical parameters, only one comprehensive, systematic study of this nature has appeared.[1] It is noteworthy that the material utilized in the
latter, as well as in most other studies concerned with clinicopathologic
correlations, had been retrospectively selected. As a result, its uni-
formity is highly debatable and prevents meaningful comparisons of
results emanating from different institutions. Indeed, it is our impression that many of the divergent findings in the literature are, in large
part, attributable to defects inherent in retrospective analyses.

This presentation will be concerned with the various his-

EDWIN R. FISHER · Institute of Pathology, Shadyside Hospital, and Department of
Pathology, University of Pittsburgh, Pittsburgh, Pennsylvania.

topathologic, and in some instances, the electron microscopic, features of mammary cancer. Most of the histopathologic material has been obtained from patients with invasive, operable mammary cancer who are entered in the National Surgical Adjuvant Breast Project, Protocol No. 4. The details of the material and methods, as well as some of the results obtained, have been previously published.[2] The ultrastructural findings are based principally on tissues from my personal collection. The details of that aspect of this report also appear in another communication.[3]

2. Histologic Types of Breast Cancer

The prognostic significance of morphologic or histologic typing of breast cancer has been emphasized by a number of investigators.[4-9] A variety of classifications[10-14] have resulted from attempts to classify breast cancers on the basis of their histopathologic features. Most reveal either descriptive terminology for the various patterns of tumor growth or a numerical grade, the latter regarded as an index of malignancy. In some instances, the classifications appear to reflect both characteristics. Although all possess merit, we have found a simple listing of histopathologic type or types based principally on growth pattern and/or special histopathologic features to be highly practical, inclusive, and reproducible.

Although it is widely appreciated that a mammary carcinoma may exhibit histologic features common to several types, only a few of the classifications cited appear to consider this problem. This deficiency appears to be minimized by the simple descriptive designations of tumor types that may occur as "pure" or combination forms. No special credence has been given to oxyphilic or apocrine change or to squamous metaplasia in our system except to note their presence. Indeed, such changes may occur with tumors exhibiting a variety of different growth patterns. In this context, oxyphilic change in breast cancer is analogous to that encountered in thyroidal cancer. As concerns the latter, there is little merit in designating papillary carcinomas with epithelial oxyphilia as well as solid, nonpapillary forms with this cytologic change as Hurthle or oxyphil-cell tumors when their growth patterns, clinical features, and prognosis are totally divergent. A similar judgment may be made regarding the occurrence of squamous metaplasia, an alteration which may occur in a wide variety of malignant neoplasms. On the other hand, squamous-cell carcinoma would be regarded as a distinct entity in our scheme. Its occurrence in pure form in the breast is exceedingly rare (see Section 2.9.5). It is imperative to recognize that the descriptive designations utilized in this scheme of histologic typing are based upon the invasive component of the neoplasm. Qualitative and quantitative features of the histologically apparent noninvasive or intraductal elements are independently evaluated.

2.1. Infiltrating Ductal Carcinoma, Not Otherwise Specified (NOS)

The most common histologic type of mammary carcinoma, representing approximately 50% of all cases, appears as solid cords or groups of tumor cells varying in size and stromal content. These tumors are devoid of special features that are characteristic of the other types encountered (Fig. 1). Because of this, the designation NOS (not otherwise specified) is utilized. When compared with other tumor types, there is a greater likelihood that they will be histologic Grade 3; lymphatic invasion will be present, but necrosis slight. Mucin, if present, will be PAS (periodic acid Schiff)-positive; patients will be regarded as likely to have

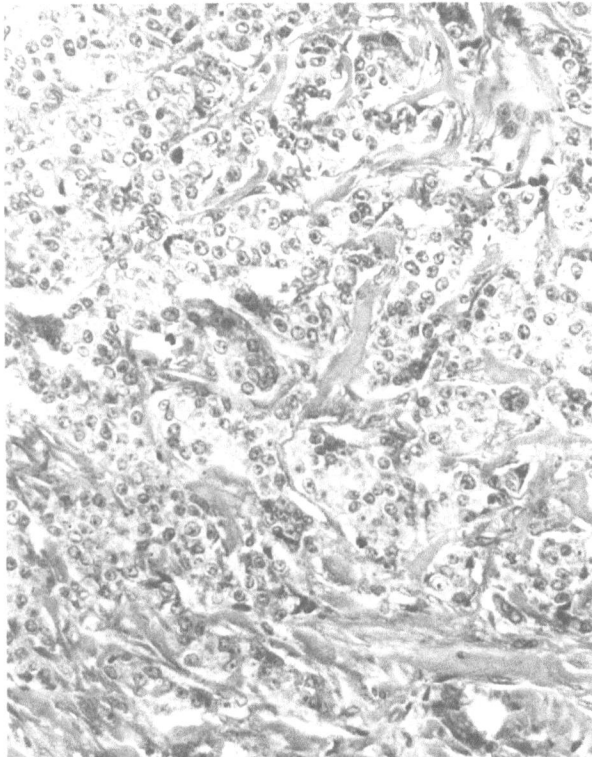

Fig. 1. Infiltrating ductal carcinoma of the NOS type characterized by nests of tumor cells in dense collagenous stroma. ×250.

clinically positive axillae. It is suspected that subsequent studies might reveal criteria allowing for further nosologic refinement of tumors of this group. Indeed, some of these have been observed in this study. Many small-cell or lymphomatoid cancers, as well as giant-cell forms, exhibit the basic growth pattern of the NOS as well as that of other types, particularly the lobular invasive in the former and medullary in the latter. Whether these represent distinct entities is not known at present. This has prompted us for the present to categorize such tumors as to their basic growth pattern. Another apparently distinctive type of carcinoma with the growth pattern of the infiltrating ductal NOS type is that form which we have arbitrarily designated as basaloid. In some respects, it also resembles a carcinoid tumor as encountered in other sites. However, attempts to demonstrate argentaffin granules in the cytoplasm of its tumor cells with appropriate stains have been unsuccessful.

A modest number of studies pertaining to the ultrastructural characteristics of infiltrating ductal carcinoma without special features have been recorded. Unfortunately, in many of these, it would appear that the designations "infiltrating ductal" and "scirrhous" carcinoma are used synonymously. Yet, it is our distinct impression that the scirrhous carcinoma of older terminology actually represents the infiltrating or invasive lobular type of cancer. This has led to some confusion concerning the ultrastructural characteristics, particularly the identification of cell types, of so-called infiltrating cancers of the breast. Most references to infiltrating cancers note the variation in appearance of the cells.[15-18] Cells replete with organelles may be in juxtaposition with others lacking such a complement of structures. Some have considered the latter cell type, often referred to as being analogous to the clear or B-cell type of the normal duct, to be predominant,[19] whereas others[15,18] apparently have not encountered such exclusivity. Glycogen, lysosomal bodies, and cytoplasmic filaments have been regarded as increased.[19-21] These latter structures may assume the configuration of tonofibrils in occasional cells, and have been considered as indicative of squamous metaplasia.[20,22] Several authors have been impressed with the rarity of desmosomal attachment plates,[23] and at least one has regarded this as evidence of the lack of cohesiveness of cancer cells.[23] Cell membranes may exhibit interdigitations or appear straight, but microvilli are often larger and more numerous than in the normal; this may also be encountered in so-called atypical hyperplasia (see below). Intracytoplasmic lumens, regarded as invaginations of the intercellular spaces, are often conspicuous. The nuclei are large, often irregular, with dense chromatin particles and large solitary or multiple nucleoli.

Much attention has been directed to the identification of cell types constituting invasive mammary cancer. This is not unexpected, when it is recalled that the myoepithelial cell traditionally has been considered, at least by light microscopy, to represent a *sine qua non* of benignancy in breast lesions. On the one hand, there are those who contend that the "scirrhous" carcinomas of the breast are comprised almost exclusively of myoepithelial elements or of cells of intermediate type, i.e., with features of both secretory and myoepithelial forms.[22,24] Others, as noted above, have been impressed with the preponderance of the clear or B form of secretory cells. A more compromising view has been expressed by most who indicate the occasional presence of myoepithelial cells among the cell population. Ahmed[25] has expressed the view that myoepithelial cells encountered in such tumors represent persistent, rather than neoplastic, elements. However, he raises the unique possibility that some of the stromal fibroblasts may actually represent transformed myoepithelium. Since, by his own admission, the techniques employed do not appear specific for the identification of myoepithelium, it is difficult to be certain about this suggestion. Although basal lamina material is generally absent about cancer cell clusters, it may be found about some apparently neoplastic cells or in some instances, even appear increased and festooned.[16,19] Collagen fibers of the stroma appear to be increased, as do fibroblasts, which often exhibit an increase in their coarse endoplasmic reticulum.[15,18] Elastic fibers appear variable. Busch[26] has described an increase in smooth muscle cells in the stroma.

Observations performed in our laboratory on 12 examples of the NOS tumor type were generally similar to those recounted above (Figs. 2 and 3). Variable numbers of dark and clear neoplastic cells were found in any one cancer. In addition, many tumors contained syncitial aggregates of tumor cells apparently lacking distinct cytoplasmic borders. Intracytoplasmic lumens were frequent (Fig. 4). Such structures might be interpreted as representing tubular differentiation. In this light, one might challenge the identity of the NOS variant and, as we shall see, cast some doubt on the validity of currently employed grading systems of mammary carcinoma which are based in large part upon tubule formation. Lipid droplets were not uncommon and Golgi structures were well developed; the coarse endoplasmic reticulum exhibited dilatation. Mitochondria were frequently large, irregular in shape, and vacuolated with attenuated cristae. Although cytoplasmic filaments could be discerned in some tumor cells, these never assumed the proportions of tonofibrils, at least as noted in the example of squamous-cell carcinoma, and only rarely were as conspicuous as in myoepithelial cells. Of course, the absence of tonofibrils might be explained by the lack of squamous

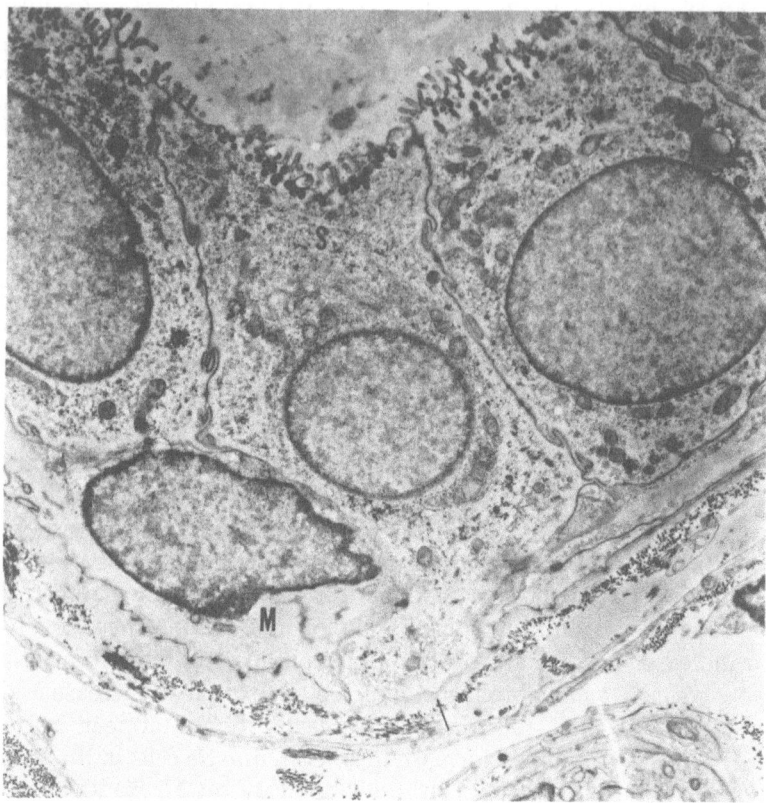

Fig. 2. Electron micrograph of a portion of a normal breast ductule revealing secretory (S) and myoepithelial (M) cells. The luminal surface of the former contains many microvilli subtended by dense secretory granules. The lamina basalis (arrow) is continuous and appears slightly thickened in some foci. ×9000. (From Fisher.[3]) (Reduced 35% for reproduction.)

metaplasia in the examples studied. Elastic fibers were variable within the stroma, without any consistent pattern or arrangement. No evidence was obtained to suggest that these fibers were derived from the epithelial elements of these neoplasms, as recently proposed by Shivas and Mackenzie.[27] Indeed, on the contrary, their intimate association with stromal fibroblasts suggested that the latter might be their possible source. It is of interest to note that histologically normal-appearing ducts in areas of NOS cancer appear ultrastructurally normal or with minimal alterations similar to those of fibrocystic disease.[3]

Although we did not have any tumors that appeared exclusively intraductal by histologic techniques, several areas in these otherwise infiltrating tumors which appeared to represent intraductal foci were ex-

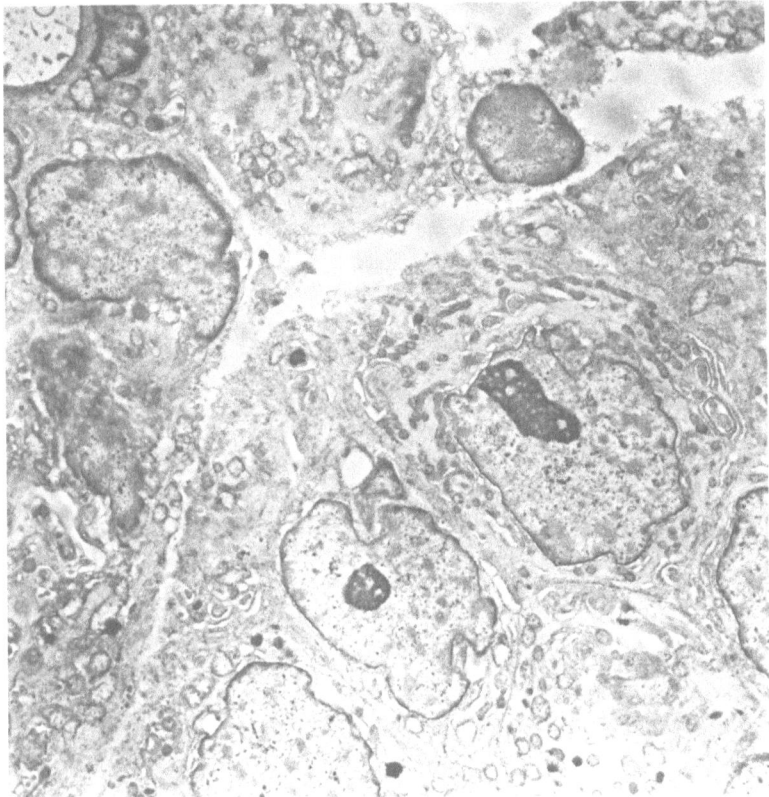

Fig. 3. Electron micrograph of cells comprising NOS carcinoma. The cells lie free without investment by lamina basalis. Their nuclei are irregular, with clumped chromatin and prominent nucleoli. Mitochondria are swollen. Cytoplasmic borders between some cells appear indistinct. Coarse endoplasmic reticulum is dilated and tortuous. A rare intracytoplasmic lumen is present. ×10,000. (Reduced 35% for reproduction.)

amined. Cells constituting these areas exhibited features similar to those of the infiltrating component. However, in these intraductal carcinomatous foci, gaps as well as loss of lamina basalis were observed. This alteration has been emphasized by Ozello[18] as occurring in those cancers regarded histologically as purely intraductal and, of course, provokes some degree of skepticism concerning the authenticity of a "true" intraductal carcinoma as an entity.

The combination of NOS with other tumor types is not infrequent, and actually represents the second most common histologic type of breast cancer. A comparison of the associations of the pure NOS and combination forms containing this element reveals a more frequent occurrence of lymphatic invasion, clinically positive axillae, more ma-

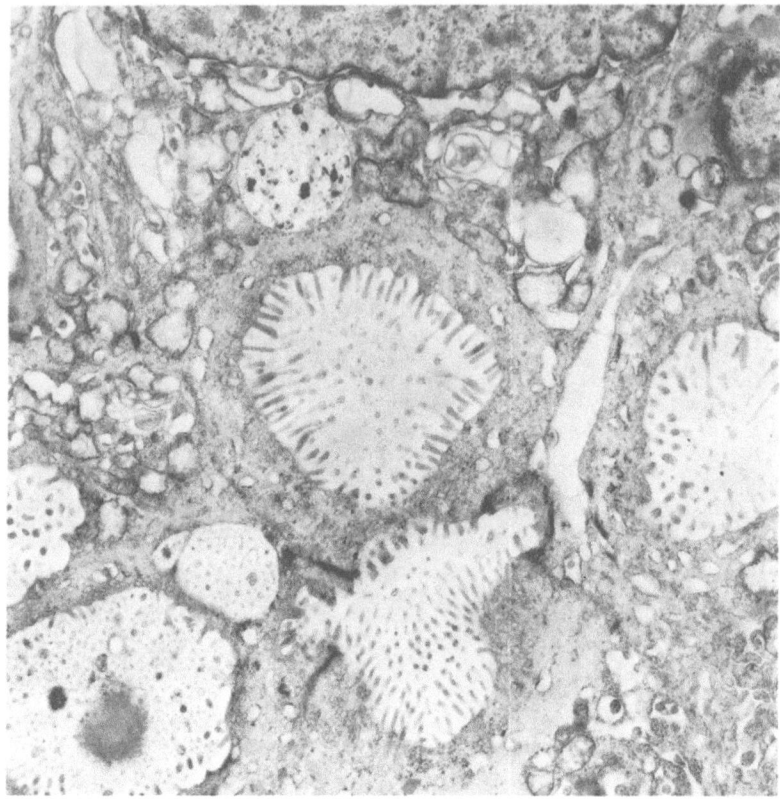

Fig. 4. Higher magnification of NOS tumor cells, revealing aberrations in mitochondria and endoplasmic reticulum. Many intracytoplasmic lumens are present, although these were not appreciated by light microscopy. ×6000. (Reduced 35% for reproduction.)

lignant histologic grade, and occurrence of noninvasive multicentric cancer in the pure form. On the other hand, NOS combination tumors exhibit a greater association with invasive multicentric cancers than do the pure type, as well as with other factors that apparently do not relate to their degree of malignancy. This information provokes the query whether it is truly appropriate to view those breast tumors with varied histologic structure according to their most poorly differentiated elements. In support of such practice, however, is the recognition of a lack of difference in relation to short-term treatment failure between the two groups.[2] Evidence provided by the results of longer follow-up studies should help resolve this problem.

2.2. Medullary Carcinoma

The significance of this tumor type was first clearly indicated by Moore and Foote in 1949,[28] although earlier reference to this form of mammary cancer was made by Geschickter.[29] Such tumors are often considered to be large, but grossly circumscribed. Histologically, they appear to be comprised of anastomosing cords and masses of large cells with vesicular, often pleomorphic, nuclei containing prominent nucleoli. Mitotic forms are frequent (Fig. 5). This constellation of features warrants a designation of nuclear Grade 1 (highest degree of anaplasia or atypia). Their fibrous stroma is scant, but a lymphoid infiltrate is striking. The latter feature has prompted the designation of this tumor type as a medullary carcinoma with lymphoid stroma. Such tumors are microscopically circumscribed. Despite the ominous cytologic features of

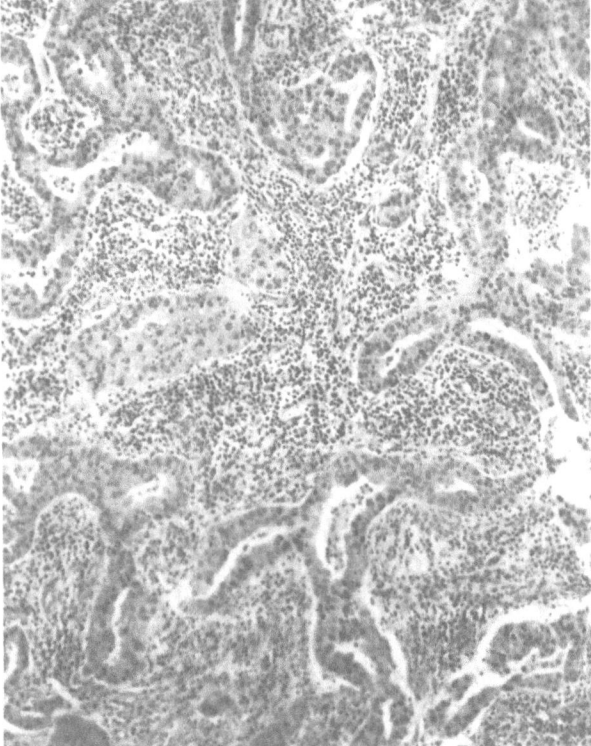

Fig. 5. Portion of medullary carcinoma revealing anastomosing cords of large tumor cells. The stroma contains an intense lymphoid infiltrate. ×100.

such tumors, their prognosis reportedly has been better than that observed with other tumors of the more usual NOS appearance, at least after radical mastectomy.[28,30,31] Some investigators have included papillary forms of carcinoma in their designations of the medullary variant. However, only those highly cellular nonpapillary tumors (1) that are histologically circumscribed, (2) that contain a moderate or marked lymphoid stroma with a scant fibrous component, and (3) whose nuclei are regarded as either Grade 1 or 2 should be regarded as medullary carcinomas. Some highly cellular tumors exhibit the general appearance of medullary carcinoma but are either devoid of lymphoid stroma or exhibit a stellate or infiltrating border—in essence, lacking one or the other of these two important diagnostic features. This provokes a dilemma whether to designate such aberrant forms as medullary carcinomas or as infiltrating ductal carcinomas, NOS type. By strict definition, they qualify as belonging to the latter group. The atypical medullary tumors possess certain clinical and pathologic associations that are significantly different from those encountered in the more classical form which might warrant their distinction. There is a significantly greater likelihood that the nodal status of patients with atypical medullary carcinoma, as compared to the classical form, will be clinically positive; pathologically, four or more nodes will be positive for metastases; tumor stroma will be variable and elastica within the tumor marked. The atypical medullary carcinoma will contain calcium and lymphatic extension, and noninvasive cancer in the vicinity of the dominant mass will be present. A comparison of NOS and atypical medullary tumors[2] revealed the latter to be more likely to have a severe cell reaction, gross and microscopic circumscription, and nuclear and histologic Grades of 1 and 3, respectively. This is not totally unexpected, since these are features that initially suggested their similarity to the classical form rather than to NOS tumors. In addition, the atypical medullary tumors are more frequently associated with clinically positive nodes than are the NOS type, whereas the latter occur more frequently in patients greater than 55 years of age, and their stroma have a greater likelihood of being moderate or marked. There is no difference between atypical medullary cancer and its classical form and NOS tumors in regard to short-term treatment failure (up to a period of 24 months).[2] The data collected thus far suggest that the atypical medullary tumors may be pathologically distinct from the classical form. Whether they are more appropriately regarded as a form of NOS tumor or a unique entity does not appear certain at this time. However, we have tentatively included them in the NOS group.

Previous electron microscopic studies of the medullary type of mammary cancer indicate the presence of pale and dark secretory cells. [22,32] Intracellular and occasionally true lumen formation, desmosomal attachment plates, and microvilli have been noted. Gould and associates [32] observed some cells at the periphery of the tumor to contain hemidesmosomes lying on a basal lamina which often exhibited focal discontinuities or reduplication. Apparently, these cells were not regarded as myoepithelial in nature and we have not observed such structures in the four examples of this tumor type in our material. Murad and Scarpelli [22] failed to mention such elements and indicated the total absence of basal lamina material. They did note the presence of dense cytoplasmic bodies, but only scant mitochondria and rare lipid droplets. The coarse endoplasmic reticulum appeared, for the most part, to be collapsed. Although both Gould [32] and Murad [22] and their associ-

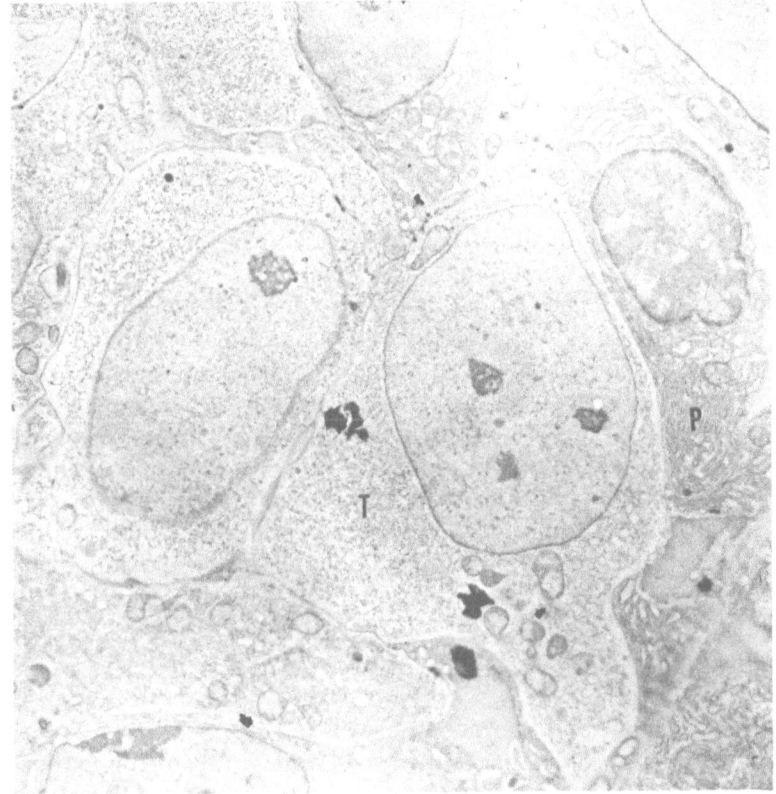

Fig. 6. Electron micrograph of cells of a portion of the medullary cancer depicted in Fig. 5. The tumor cells (T) are large and their cytoplasm contains few organelles, but many polyribosomes and free RNA and some lipid droplets. Portions of plasma cells (P) are noted in apposition to some of the tumor cells, but no evidence of degeneration of tumor cells is present. ×8200. (Reduced 35% for reproduction.)

ates noted the presence of lymphoid elements within the tumor-cell aggregates, they failed to make mention of possible alterations in the neoplastic cells in contact with them.

The tumor cells comprising medullary carcinomas in our material contained large round and oval nuclei with one or more relatively small nucleoli. Nuclear chromatin appeared dispersed evenly in a euchromatin pattern. The cells were large and their borders irregular. The paucity of mitochondria was conspicuous (Fig. 6); those that were present appeared large and somewhat irregular in shape. Narrow and rounded lacunae of coarse endoplasmic reticulum were variable, but almost all cells contained abundant polyribosomal aggregates. Despite the latter, the cells did impart a relatively clear appearance. Lipid droplets were present and were quite abundant in some cells, but secretory granules, cytofilaments, and Golgi structures were exceedingly rare. Apposition of tumor cells was, for the most part, linear with relatively few interdigitations or desmosomes. Lymphocytes and plasma cells, when present among the tumor cells, exhibited linear or slightly irregular apposition with them. In some instances, emperipolesis of lymphocytic elements by the tumor cells was evident. No perceptible ultrastructural differences were noted between tumor cells in such situations and those not associated with this inflammatory infiltrate. This experience is similar to that in our previous studies in experimental tumor systems, where such purported effector cells lacked any discernible effect on tumor cells.[33] No lamina basalis *per se* was evident among individual tumor cells or aggregates, although laminated bands and large accumulations of a moderately electron-dense amorphous material resembling that comprising lamina basalis were occasionally found. Relatively few collagen fibers were present. No intracytoplasmic lumens were noted, although rarely a true lumen with microvilli was present.

Electron microscopic study of three examples of atypical medullary cancers revealed their component tumor cells to be indistinguishable from those of the classical medullary type as described above.

2.3. Lobular Invasive Carcinoma

In 1941, Foote and Stewart,[34] as well as Muir,[35] called attention to an *in situ* form of carcinoma of the breast apparently arising within the end parts of the lobule, which they designated as lobular carcinoma *in situ*. Subsequent to their reports, as well as to those of others, it became recognized that *in situ* carcinoma may develop into, or at least be associated with, an infiltrating form—so-called lobular infiltrating or lobular invasive carcinoma. The frequency of such a development from *in situ* carcinoma is unknown; judgments indicating both its frequency as well as rarity in this regard have been made.[36-40] It is well recognized that both *in situ* as well as invasive lobular carcinomas may be found in the same tumor. However, the presence of the former is not essential for the diagnosis of the invasive type.[41] Despite the apparent derivation and association of this type of invasive cancer with its *in situ* analogue, retrospective studies have disclosed that this type of carcinoma is associated with a relatively poor prognosis.[42] There are several excellent accounts of the histopatholic features of lobular invasive carcinoma[37-40]; its appearance is usually sufficiently distinctive to allow for its recognition. Briefly, this consists of the dispersion of small, sometimes innocuous-appearing, neoplastic cells singly, or at most in small clusters, in an "Indian file" or targetoid pattern, often about nonneoplastic ducts (Fig. 7). The presence of "skip" areas in some instances atavistically signifies its lobular derivation. We suspect that most, if not all, scirrhous carcinomas of the older terminology represent examples of this

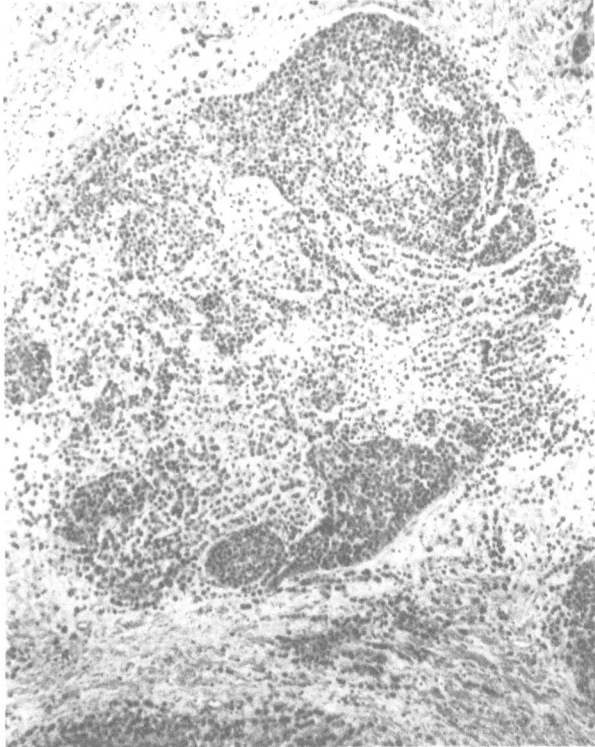

Fig. 7. Lobular invasive carcinoma appears as cords and individual tumor cells about, and apparently radiating from, larger foci of lobular carcinoma *in situ*. ×100.

type of invasive carcinoma. Examples of the lobular invasive type of cancer are quite frequently combined with other types of invasive carcinoma. In a few instances, this lobular, targetoid pattern was preserved but the neoplastic cells were arranged in tubules. In other instances, the individual cells, as well as small clusters, were of the signet-ring type containing mucin. It has been indicated that "small-cell" carcinomas of the breast may represent examples of this form of cancer. It has been emphasized that on occasion, the nodal metastases from an otherwise distinctive lobular invasive carcinoma may morphologically mimic lymphoma, particularly reticulum-cell sarcoma.[39] However, as we have noted above, "small-cell" carcinomas may exhibit other patterns of growth within the breast as well. It is of interest that despite the purported lethality of this tumor type, lymphatic invasion is usually absent. A high frequency of noninvasive cancer was found in the vicinity of the infiltrating lobular carcinomas, as might be expected from that which has been noted previously. However, it is somewhat surprising that there is no association between this tumor type and foci of cancer in quadrants of breast remote from that harboring the dominant tumor mass (multicentric cancers), since the *in situ* as well as invasive lobular forms have been regarded as having a high incidence of bilaterality.[36,39,40,43,44] On the other hand, the combination of NOS and lobular invasive cancer does show a greater frequency of invasive multicentric cancers and nipple involvement, as well as a greater likelihood of occurring in the 20–44-year-old age group, than do other tumor types. The combination of lobular invasive cancer with the tubular type is associated with features of both tumor types, as well as the occurrence of lymphatic invasion within the tumor, a feature not present in either type in its pure form.

There have been only a few reports concerning the ultrastructural features of lobular carcinoma, including its invasive and *in situ* forms.[19,45–48] As indicated previously, some of the ultrastructural descriptions of so-called infiltrating scirrhous carcinoma are suspected of being examples of this histologic type of breast cancer. Carter and associates[45] found the ultrastructural features of cells comprising *in situ* and infiltrating lobular carcinomas to be similar; both contained large numbers of cytoplasmic filaments similar to those found in myoepithelial cells. They offered the somewhat ambiguous conclusion that although the tumor cells contained myoepithelial characteristics, in no instance were normal myoepithelial cells noted. They also concluded that the abundance of these filaments allowed for the differentiation of lobular carcinomas from other infiltrating and noninfiltrating ductal as well as colloid (mucinous) and medullary forms of breast cancer. At least some of the examples of so-called scirrhous cancer recorded by Murad and Scarpelli[22] appear to represent instances of invasive lobular carcinoma. They considered such tumors to be derived from myoepithelial elements, a conclusion also reached by Kermarec and associates[49] in their report of a case which was designated as myoepithelial cancer. Yet, in another communication, Murad[46] called attention to the similarity between the cells of in situ and invasive lobular carcinoma (which he designated as ductular carcinoma) to those of ductules of the pregnant and involuting breast, which would presumably be of secretory type. Ozello[18,47] also noted the similarity between the cells comprising the in situ and invasive forms of lobular carcinoma. In addition, he, as well as Tobon and Price,[48] noted central lumens in the tumor-cell aggregates of the in situ form. This is of interest, since the cell collections of in situ lobular carcinoma are usually regarded histologically as being devoid of lumens. Ozello[18] was also impressed with the generally pale appearance and secretory nature of cells of both invasive as well as in situ forms. According to Tobon and Price,[48] myoepithelial cells, when present in in situ lobular carcinoma, were compressed and were regarded as residual rather than proliferating neoplastic elements. These investigators also noted the lamina basalis to be intact about the cell aggregates of lobular carcinoma in situ, although Ozello[18] emphasized the occurrence of gaps and, on rare occasions, cytoplasmic pseudopodal extensions into the surrounding stroma.

Our material contained three examples of lobular invasive carcinoma. Cells arranged in "Indian file" pattern imparted a pale appearance with very few cytoplasmic organelles. Occasional members, however, exhibited dilatation of their coarse endoplasmic reticulum. No lamina basalis material was present about the tumor cells, which abutted upon heavy bundles of mature collagen fibers. Cells arranged in clusters in this form of cancer also were, for the most part, pale, although darker forms were also present. In addition, some of the pale forms contained aggregates of cytoplasmic filaments, although these as well as other features of the cells did not allow for their absolute identification as myoepithelial elements (Fig. 8). Again, no lamina basalis material was present about these cell clusters. Foci of in situ carcinoma in these examples disclosed changes comparable to those described by Ozello[18] and Tobon and Price,[48] including true as well as intracytoplasmic lumens, occasional cytofilaments, and sparse organelles. In addition, many of the cells contained lipid droplets. The lamina basalis exhibited focal gaps. Normal-appearing myoepithelial cells were evident in basal portions of the ductules. These appeared to be quite distinct from the more obviously neoplastic elements and were decidedly compressed. As might be expected, those tumor cells of small-cell carcinomas exhibiting a pattern of lobular invasive carcinoma were ultrastructurally similar to

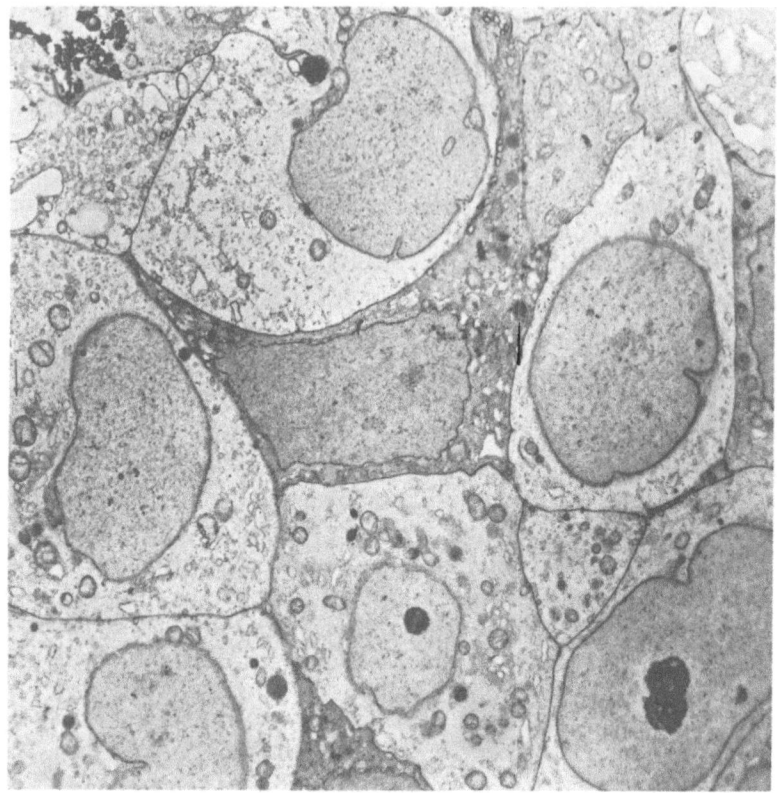

Fig. 8. Electron micrograph of cells comprising lobular invasive carcinoma. Light and dark forms are present. Some cells contain prominent cytoplasmic filaments (arrow), but other features of myoepithelial cells are not apparent. The simplified appearance of the cancer cells is evident. ×9000. (From Fisher.[3]) (Reduced 35% for reproduction.)

those of this type described above. On the other hand, those comprising more solid masses or the NOS pattern were somewhat different. Noteworthy in this regard was their arrangement in syncitial clusters with indistinct cell borders. The cell cytoplasm contained many vesicles and vacuoles as well as dilated coarse endoplasmic reticulum. No secretory droplets or cytoplasmic filaments were recognized, although Golgi structures and centriole bodies were occasionally conspicuous. Mitochondria were large and their matrices rather clear with attenuated cristae. Cytoplasmic lipid droplets were also frequent. Nuclei were large with irregular borders; they frequently exhibited invaginations of cytoplasmic material. Nucleoli were frequently large. Lymphocytes and rare plasma cells were often intermingled with the tumor cells, as were varying amounts of mature collagen fibers. The readily apparent difference in ultrastructural appearance between these cells and the tumor cells allowed for the conclusion that such small-cell tumors did not represent examples of malignant lymphoma of the breast. Again, whether these small-cell tumors represent a distinct entity is uncertain. Nevertheless, ultrastructurally they do appear to be a form of either lobular invasive or other infiltrating ductal carcinomas.

2.4. Mucinous Carcinoma

Mucinous carcinoma, also designated as mucoid, gelatinous, or colloid carcinoma, represents a distinct histopathologic type of mammary cancer. It may occur in pure form or in association with other types.[2,50,51] Its characteristics and associations with various pathologic parameters appear related to such a composition. Pure mucinous carcinomas have been observed to occur in older women with a relatively long duration of symptoms.[51] They are also associated with less-frequent axillary metastases and a pushing, rather than infiltrating, border.[51] The survival rate has been noted to be appreciably greater in patients with the pure rather than the mixed type or other infiltrating ductal carcinomas of the breast.[50–53] In addition, it has been noted that there is a greater likelihood for such tumors to be devoid of a cell reaction. Necrosis and lymphatic invasion within the tumor are absent and elastica is slight.[2]

The mucinous tumors are comprised of aggregates of cells, usually with well-differentiated features, including high nuclear grade, lying in pools of mucin (Fig. 9). All possible tinctorial reactions of the latter are present in sections stained by the alcian blue–PAS technique, and conform to views regarding breast mucin as non- or poorly sulfated acid mucopolysaccharide.[54,55] The cellular elements of these neoplasms may appear as solid masses or less commonly exhibit papillary projections, tubules, or an adenocystic configuration. Rarely, areas of some infiltrating duct cancers may mimic a mucinous focus because of the presence of clusters of cancer cells surrounded by a loose mucinous or edematous stroma. The presence of fibroblastic elements within the latter should be sufficient to allow for its distinction from mucinous carcinoma.

There have been only a few electron microscopic studies of examples of mucinous carcinoma.[18,56–58] Cells comprising the mucinous carcinomas available to us for study were noted to contain relatively large nuclei with only modest clumping of chromatin and occasional small nucleoli. The cytoplasm contained small, compact mitochondria which appeared to be slightly more numerous than in the normal cell. Noteworthy were the conspicuous stacks and whorls of narrow lacunae of coarse endoplasmic reticulum. An increase in smooth endoplasmic

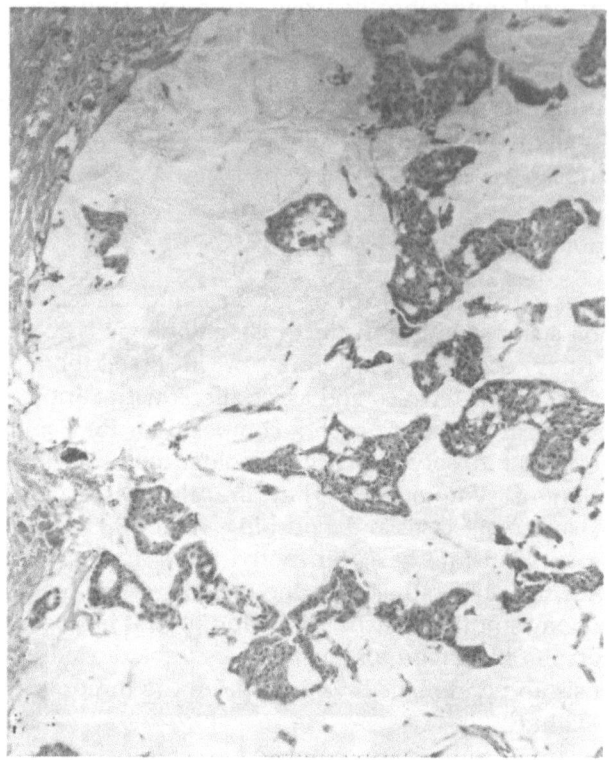

Fig. 9. Mucinous carcinoma characterized by islands and adenocystic configurations of tumor cells lying in mucinous pools. ×100.

reticulum represented by small vesicles and larger vacuoles—the latter occasionally containing rather homogeneous, moderately electron-dense material within their lumens which resembled the intracellular mucin secretion of intestinal cells—was also present[59] (Fig. 10). Free RNA particles and polyribosomes, prominent Golgi structures, and membrane-bound secretory droplets were also found. The latter were frequently observed within apical or juxtaluminal positions of cell cytoplasm. The extracellular mucin collections appeared as rather amorphous, slightly electron-dense material resembling that noted within the large cytoplasmic vacuoles. Neoplastic cells abutting upon stromal elements assumed an elongated, spindle form. Cell apposition was, for the most part, linear. Desmosomes were present, but infrequent. Other cell surfaces showed frequent, blunt microvillous processes. No myoepithelial cells were noted. No lamina basalis was discerned, and the fibroblasts adjacent to neoplastic aggregates and abundant collagen fibers exhibited

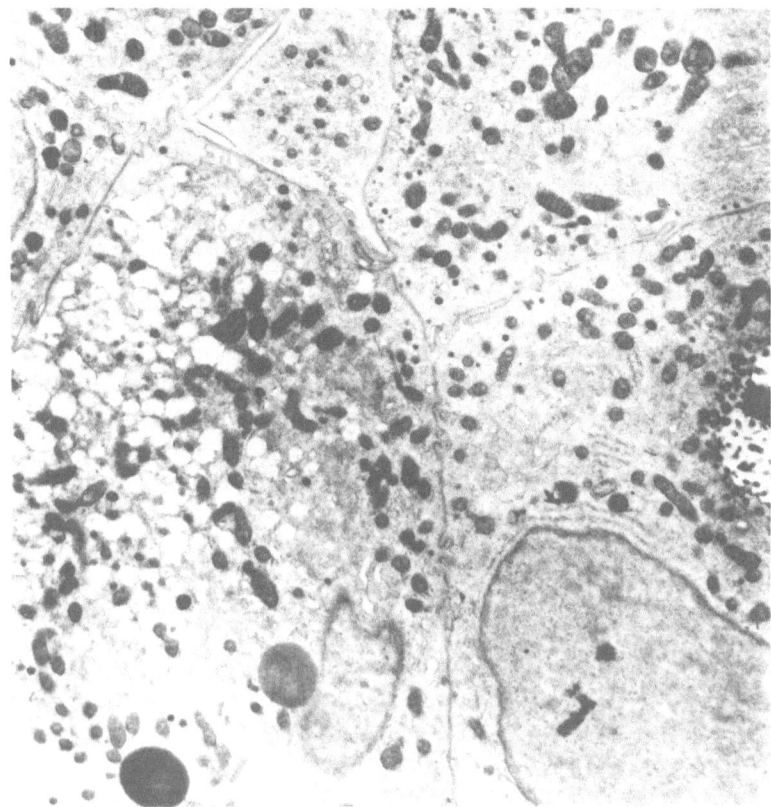

Fig. 10. Electron micrograph of tumor cells of mucinous carcinoma revealing lamination of coarse endoplasmic reticulum. Small, dense secretory granules, as well as larger mucinous spaces appearing as honeycombed vacuoles, are conspicuous in cells of this tumor type. ×10,000. (Reduced 35% for reproduction.)

a marked increase in coarse endoplasmic reticulum, Golgi structures, and other small vesicles.

The pronounced proliferation of endoplasmic reticulum of both the coarse and smooth variety, as well as abundant Golgi structures in the cells of the mucinous carcinoma, appear clearly related to the synthesis, storage, and secretion of mucin characteristic of this tumor type. It is of interest that in addition to evidence of this abnormal production of mucin, was the abundance of secretory granules qualitatively similar to those in normal ductal cells, suggesting that there is an increase in mucin production in these cancers by normal as well as abnormal pathways.

2.5. Tubular Carcinoma

Tubular carcinoma of the breast, also known as well-differentiated[60] or orderly carcinoma,[61] only recently has received attention. Prognosis in this form of carcinoma is regarded as excellent, as emphasized by the studies of Taylor and Norris[60] and Carstens and associates,[62] even though axillary metastases may be present.

Histologically, this form of cancer may superficially mimic sclerosing or blunt-end adenosis. It is comprised of tubular structures which are typically lined by a single layer of well-differentiated epithelium (Fig. 11). The luminal borders of the tumor cells frequently contain bulbous projections regarded by some as representing so-called "apocrine snouts."[62] The surrounding stroma is abundant and may exhibit the green fluorescence of amyloid after Congo red staining.[62] Illustrations in all reports also include tubular elements arranged in multiglandular, cribriform, or adenocystic configurations. We have chosen to designate the

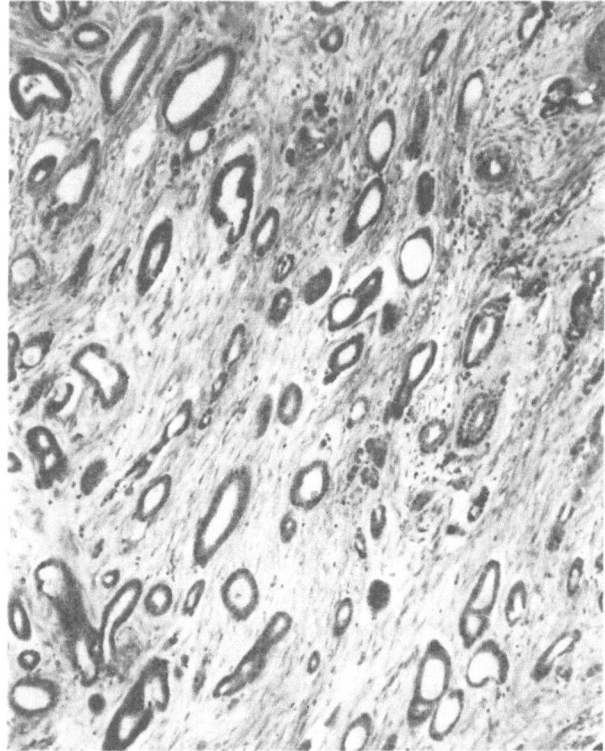

Fig. 11. Tubular carcinoma of the breast appears as somewhat banal-appearing ductal structures in a dense collagenous stroma. ×100.

presence of these latter foci as evidence of an adenocystic component (see Section 2.6), and have reserved the designation "tubular" for those tumors exhibiting only the more simple structure. That tubular elements may be found in association with other histopathologic types of cancer is well recognized. Indeed, the association of tubular and NOS carcinoma represented the second most frequent form of mammary carcinoma in our recent study.[2] Carstens and associates[62] noted such combinations in 80% of the 35 cases of tubular carcinoma they studied. According to them, this other element apparently had no effect on the favorable prognosis of tubular carcinoma.

It is of interest that this type of carcinoma should be associated with perineural extension, since the latter has been noted to occur with other features which, at least on the basis of putative evidence, might be considered to indicate a poor prognosis (see below). Consonant with the view relating adenocystic elements to tubular carcinoma is the recognition that an intraductal component, when present in tubular carcinoma, is most frequently of the adenocystic type. The low degree of pathologic malignancy, as reflected by histopathologic grade, and the presence of mucin and calcifications within these tumors have been observed.[60]

The ductal nature of tubular carcinoma appears well confirmed by the few ultrastructural studies of this mammary cancer.[32,63] Its component cells have been thought to simulate those of normal ducts or ductules, although their cytoplasm has been observed to contain greater numbers of tonofilaments and so-called intracytoplasmic lumens than that of normal cells. Desmosomes and terminal bars, which are considered to reflect its well-differentiated development, may also be appreciated near the tubular lumens. Myoepithelial cells have only been encountered occasionally, and apparently reveal no abnormalities of significance. Most importantly, lamina basalis surrounding the tubular aggregates is absent or, at best, incomplete, allowing for its distinction from the benign disorders that it may mimic. The stroma upon which the neoplastic cells abut is comprised of abundant collagen fibers with interspersed fibroblasts, reflecting the desmoplastic tumor stroma revealed by light microscopy in these neoplasms.

Two of the three tubular carcinomas in our material contained cells that were extremely well differentiated. Indeed, their tubules could be distinguished from normal tubules or those of fibrocystic disease only by the absence of lamina basalis. The third tumor was less differentiated in that the mitochondria were variable in size, shape, and density, and appeared to be clustered about the nuclei, which, for the most part, were large, scalloped, and contained heterochromatin masses and large nucleoli (Fig. 12). This feature, as well as prominent cytofilaments, suggested that many of the cells were of myoepithelial or at least of

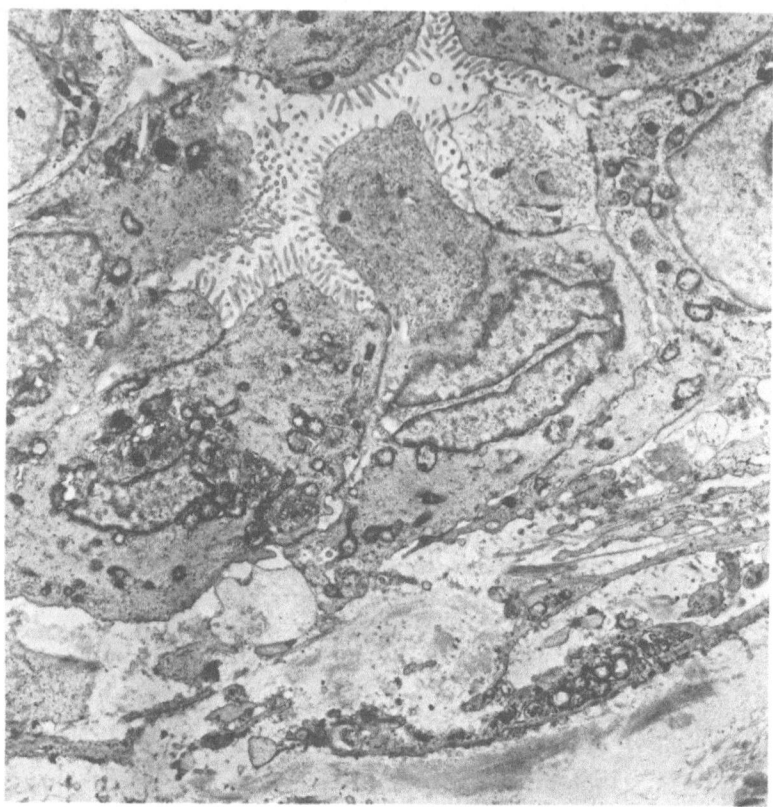

Fig. 12. Electron micrograph of a portion of tubular carcinoma. The cells in this area appear to be of intermediate type. The secretory characteristics are evident principally by the pronounced microvilli, whereas the clustering of organelles about the nucleus and cytofilaments are reminiscent of myoepithelial cells. Lamina basalis is absent and pseudopodal cytoplasmic extensions into the underlying stroma are evident. ×9000. (From Fisher.[3] (Reduced 35% for reproduction.)

so-called intermediate type. Cristae of mitochondria appeared condensed, imparting a paracrystalline appearance similar to that described by Ramos and Taylor[64] in so-called lipid-rich carcinoma. Coarse endoplasmic reticulum usually was comprised of short, narrow lacunae, although on occasion more tortuous forms were appreciated. A modest amount of RNA and glycogen particles was present. Golgi structures and lysosomal bodies, although present, were infrequent. Sites of cellular attachment were linear as well as moderately interdigitated, the latter resulting in intercellular spaces. The luminal surface of many of the tumor cells, including those designated as intermediate type, were replete with microvillous processes. The similarities in appearance of the cells comprising this tubular carcinoma to those of the NOS variant suggest that it represents advanced tubular or ductular differentiation of an NOS tumor, indicating that there may be at least two types of tubular carcinoma. Whether there is practical value in making such a distinction remains to be demonstrated. It would appear that the quantitative variability in mucin in these tumors noted by light microscopy after appropriate staining may be related to quantitative differences in their secretory and nonsecretory cells, perhaps representing another variation in cell differentiation. Basal portions of the neoplastic cells comprising the tubular structures in both tubular forms rested upon the underlying stromal collagen without any recognizable basal lamina. Many cells at such sites also exhibited pseudopodal extensions into the stromal collagen, which was quite dense and frequently appeared laminated, as did the fibroblasts in these foci. Coarse endoplasmic reticulum of many of the latter cells was prominent. Occasional clumps of elastic fibers were also noted.

2.6. Adenocystic Carcinoma

This is a rare form of mammary carcinoma. Less than 100 cases have been recorded. Most accounts[62,65-71] emphasize its favorable prognosis, which may be related to the paucity of axillary node involvement associated with it. Although distant metastases are likewise rare, some examples have been noted. Elsner[72] indicates that generally the follow-up observations of patients with this form of cancer that have been reported have been relatively short. He and others[73-75] have recorded instances in which metastases have developed after long periods of time in patients who might otherwise have been regarded as cured. Axillary metastases were observed in the case recorded by Verani and Van der Bel-Kahn.[76]

Histologically, the adenocystic carcinoma of the breast has been regarded as analogous in appearance to those tumors with similar appellation that occur in other sites, for example, the trachea and the salivary and lacrimal glands (Fig. 13) Why the latter have a less favorable prognosis than has been reported for those in the mammary gland is not apparent.

Some investigators[67,68,77] have emphasized the necessity of differentiating the adenocystic form of mammary carcinoma from the less-differentiated types of infiltrating carcinoma with a cribriform pattern. We have concluded from our observations in this study that there is insufficient evidence to warrant such a distinction. Some[67] have indicated that the presence of myoepithelial cells about the tubule-containing cell masses warrants an adenocystic designation. Others[68,77]

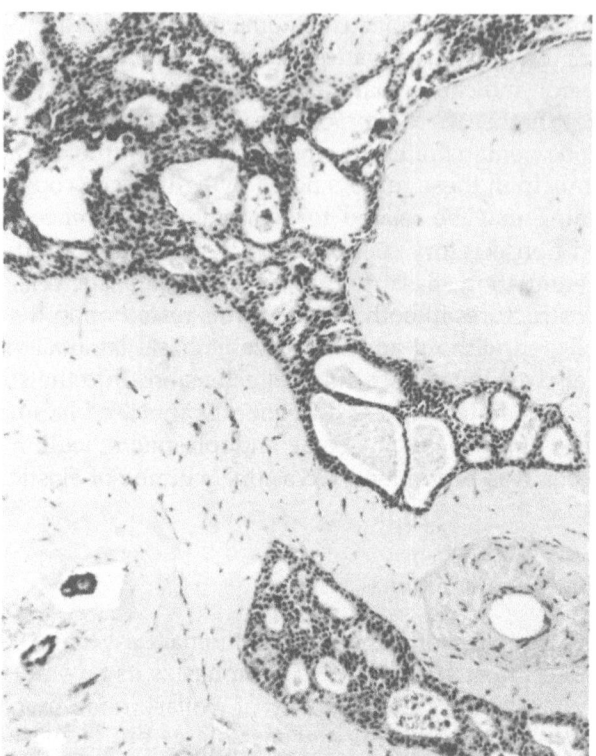

Fig. 13. Focus of adenocystic carcinoma of the breast resembling its counterpart in salivary glands and other tissues. ×100.

indicate that the presence of mucin within the tubular elements characterizes the adenocystic lesion, whereas necrosis in such foci represents a change indicative of cribriform ductal carcinoma. It is of interest that we have noted such necrosis in some well-differentiated tumors such as those of the tubular variety. Conversely, mucin may be encountered in lumens of structures which we feel would be universally accepted as cribriform foci of NOS carcinomas. A commonly applied criterion for the differentiation of true adenocystic carcinoma and cribriform foci of other cancers is the presence of well-differentiated nuclei in the former.[67,68,77] Yet, we have encountered some adenocystic carcinomas in which this feature was lacking, their nuclei appearing only moderately differentiated (nuclear Grade 2). On the other hand, some foci of other carcinomas which might be regarded as cribriform have well-differentiated nuclei. A similar statement may be made in regard to the predilection of myoepithelial cells for either the adenocystic or cribriform variant. Classical adenocystic foci not infrequently may be found in association with the tubular elements of so-called tubular carcinoma, a tumor also purported to be prognostically favorable, as noted above. Most interesting in this regard is the recognition that such proponents of histologic grading as Bloom[78] and Tough et al. [79] depict adenocystic formations as an example of one type of tubule formation in mammary cancers indicating advanced differentiation. Although this information is perhaps not relevant to the problem of distinguishing cribriform intraductal cancer and adenocystic areas, it does indicate that the adenocystic pattern is more common than appreciated. Lastly, the intraductal component of such dissimilar-appearing tumors as the NOS variety may often be truly adenocystic. Indeed, this association has been commented upon even by some of the investigators[77] who believe that the distinction between adenocystic and cribriform infiltrating ductal carcinoma is valid.

The several ultrastructural studies performed on lesions regarded as adenocystic carcinoma note the similarity between its secretory elements and those of other ductal carcinomas of the breast.[32,80] Our own material contained two tumors with both adenocystic and tubular elements. The latter were identical to those of the "pure" well-differentiated tubular carcinoma described above (Fig. 14). Histologically, the adenocystic components appeared to be intraductal. Their component cells also resembled the secretory cells of the tubular element, often including paraluminal secretory droplets as well as intracytoplasmic, membrane-bound vacuoles of homogeneous, moderately electron-dense material corresponding to the mucin noted by appropriate tinctorial techniques in these lesions. The secretory cells also exhibited other features noted in tubular carcinoma, including sparse mitochondria, inconspicuous, narrow lacunae of coarse endoplasmic reticulum, cytofilaments, and occasional lipid droplets. Both light and dark secretory cells, as well as rare myoepithelial elements, were present. This is similar to the experiences of Gould[32] and Koss[80] and their associates, who also regarded many of the lumens in the adenocystic variant as "pseudocysts" that were lined by lamina basalis material and effaced by myoepithelial cells or cells possessing myoepithelial features. However, we have been unimpressed with the occurrence of pseudocysts in this type of cancer. Interestingly, only an occasional intracytoplasmic lumen was noted in the material that we studied. The lumens appeared to be lined by secretory elements with microvilli, desmosomal attachment plates, and, frequently, numerous secretory granules. This information indicates, as suggested previously by us[2] on the basis of light microscopic studies, that the adenocystic configuration represents a variation of tubular structure. It is of interest to note that the cellular aggregates of recorded examples of adenocystic carcinoma were all invested by lamina basalis.

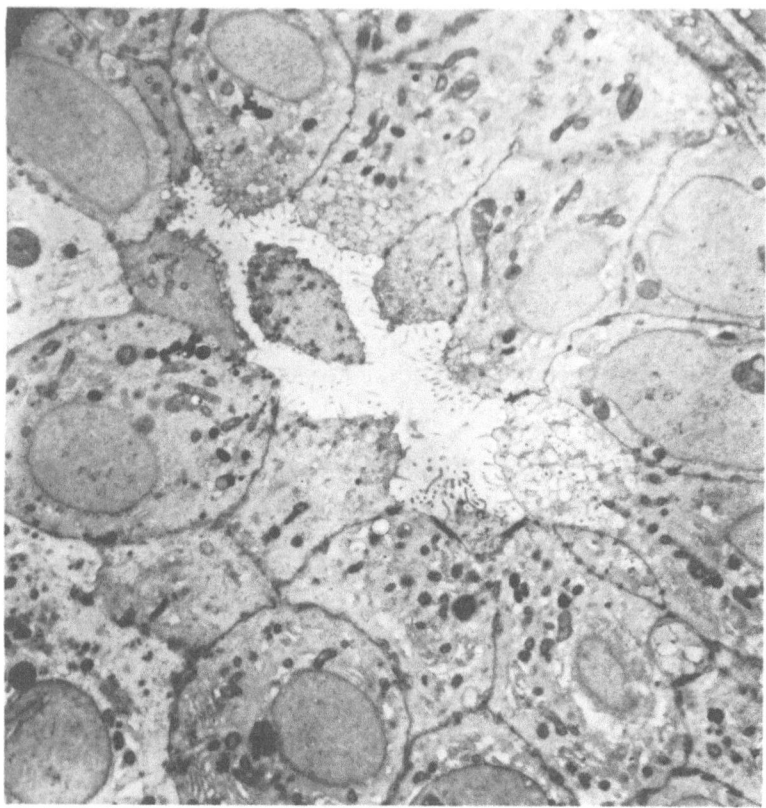

Fig. 14. Electron micrograph of a portion of adenocystic carcinoma revealing well-differentiated tubular structure resembling that found in well-differentiated tubular carcinoma. Noteworthy is the paraluminal honeycombing reflecting mucin secretion. ×5700. (From Fisher.[3]) (Reduced 35% for reproduction.)

We have also noted its presence, but encountered foci in which this structure was lacking. This observation would be in accord with the observations of Ozello[18] concerning the focal interruption of lamina basalis in examples of intraductal carcinoma which he examined and the foci of intraductal carcinoma in infiltrating cancers which we have described above.

2.7. Papillary Carcinoma

Although intraductal papillary growth is not an uncommon component of various histologic types of invasive mammary carcinoma, the truly papillary, invasive carcinoma is a rare neoplasm. Notation of its possible derivation, as well as its distinction from benign intraductal papillomas, is often made.[81-84] We are unaware of any study concerned with a large number of examples of this type of mammary carcinoma. Although some have indicated its favorable prognosis,[9,10,61,81,84] the follow-up observations of Kraus and Neubecker[84] of 21 examples of papillary cancer indicate a disease-free survival rate comparable to that of mammary cancer in general.

Although the frond-like projections characteristic of this pattern may contain fibrous supporting stalks, such structures are lacking in most foci (Fig. 15). Indeed, this delicate or nonexistent fibrovascular core, nuclear hyperchromatism, and absence of double layer of cells and "apocrine" change represent features distinguishing papillary carcinoma from intraductal papillomas.[84] In addition, the invasive nature of the papillary lesions designated as carcinoma in this study was quite apparent in sections stained by the alcian blue–PAS technique, which vividly delineates the ductal basement membrane.

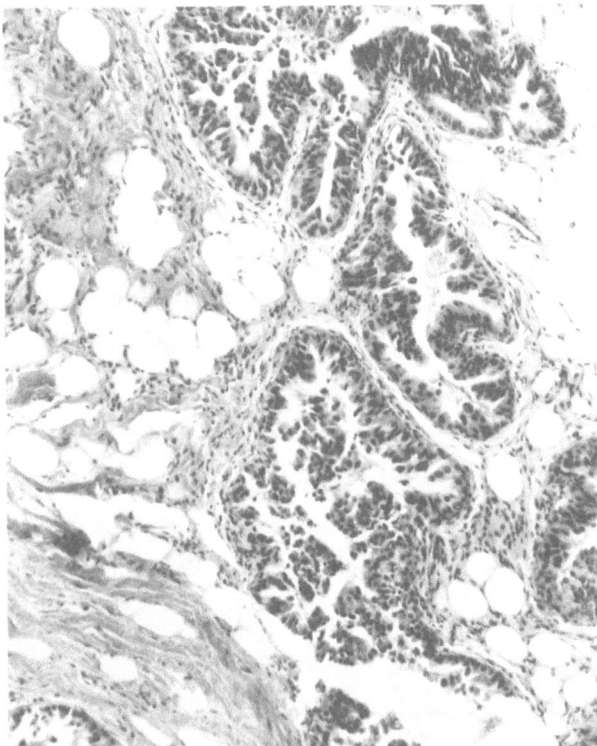

Fig. 15. Papillary carcinoma of the breast characterized by papillary projections without perceptible stromal stalks. ×100.

2.8. Paget's Disease

Epidermal involvement of the nipple by apparently neoplastic cells represents the *sine qua non* of Paget's disease of the breast (Fig. 16). Although there has been controversy concerning the derivation of these cells, most investigators subscribe to the view that they represent extensions of neoplastic elements from subjacent ducts in the nipple[85] and/or metastases from an underlying carcinoma.[10,86–88] Neubecker and Bradshaw[89] have demonstrated the ultrastructural similarities of so-called Paget's cells and those comprising the underlying cancers of the breast, although others[90,91] have been less certain in this regard. Indeed, Sagebiel[91] questioned the neoplastic nature of such cells. The neoplastic involvement of the epidermis of the nipple in this disorder may assume

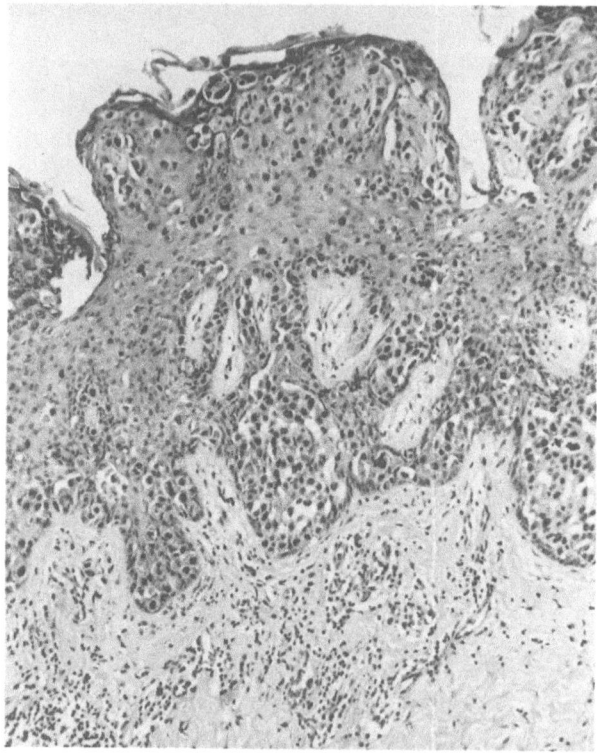

Fig. 16. Portion of nipple from a patient with NOS tumor of the underlying breast. Classical Paget's cells are seen in superficial portions of the epidermis, whereas the tumor cells are more clustered in basal portions, where they resemble the underlying cancer of the breast proper. ×100.

two patterns. The first and most familiar is that characterized by the presence of large neoplastic cells with optically clear cytoplasm—so-called Paget's cells. These may exhibit tinctorial reactions identical to those of cells in the underlying carcinoma,[65] particularly when the latter contain glycoprotein or mucinous substances. In other instances, such cells are unreactive, and differ in this regard from morphologically similar elements in extramammary Paget's disease. They usually lack glycogen, unlike the cells of Bowen's disease, which may morphologically mimic them.[92] The Paget's cells may be further distinguished from those of Bowen's disease by noting their discrete disposition among the epidermal elements, whereas in Bowen's disease, the large neoplastic elements are found in association with other dysplastic or atypical squamous cells. The other form of epidermal involvement in Paget's disease consists of neoplastic cells lacking optically clear cytoplasm but often arranged in a solid, ductal, or acinar configuration. Such intraepidermal collections often morphologically mimic elements of the underlying cancer. The latter appearance would seem to represent strong evidence in support of the view that such epidermal involvement represents an extension of metastasis rather than a de novo epidermal lesion.

As has long been recognized since the original description of the disorder by Paget,[93] there is a greater likelihood for the duration of symptoms to be prolonged in patients with Paget's disease. There is also a greater frequency of multicentric cancer. As might be expected, most of the tumors are in the subareolar area of the breast and exhibit other skin and nipple involvement. Although lymphatic extension is more frequent in the dominant tumor, the axillary nodal status, both clinically and pathologically, does not appear to be distinctively related to this type of mammary lesion.

2.9. Rare Cancers of the Breast

2.9.1. Carcinosarcoma

Carcinosarcoma is a very rare neoplasm of the breast. We encountered only one example in 1667 cases of invasive carcinoma.[2] As noted by Robb and MacFarlane,[94] some purported examples may represent carcinomas with pseudosarcomatous stroma, a possibility that may be raised regarding the identification of carcinosarcoma of other sites as well. Their Case 2 appears comparable to that described by us,[2] except that they could identify some vestiges of fibroadenoma in their lesion. That carcinosarcomas develop from preexisting fibroadenomas remains to be conclusively demonstrated.

2.9.2. Carcinoma in Fibroadenoma

That carcinoma may arise in fibroadenoma has been substantiated by a number of reports,[95-97] although such an event is considerably less common than the occurrence of the sarcomatous change of cystosarcoma phyllodes. Although noninvasive carcinomas, including lobular carcinoma *in situ* and intraductal carcinoma, represent the most common forms of cancer arising in fibroadenoma, examples of infiltrating lobular carcinomas, as well as other forms of infiltrating ductal carcinoma, have been observed.

2.9.3. Sarcomas

Since this presentation is concerned principally with carcinoma of the breast, only brief mention of sarcomatous lesions shall be made. It appears germane to note that stromal sarcomas other than cystosarcoma phyllodes, angiosarcoma, or malignant lymphoma may also be rarely encountered in the breast. Berg and associates[98] discussed 25 examples of such lesions and emphasized their variable fibrous, myxoid, or fatty composition. It appears sufficiently documented to conclude that carcinosarcomas with fibrosarcomatous or osteosarcomatous mesenchymal elements, carcinomas with pseudosarcomatous stroma, carcinomas arising in fibroadenomas, pure stromal sarcomas, and the more familiar cystosarcoma phyllodes (which would appear to represent the malignant mesenchymal analogue of carcinoma arising in fibroadenoma) may all be included in the congerie of rare malignant breast neoplasms. The nosologic polemic of these rare tumor types is further complicated by the recognition of instances of carcinoma with osteoid or cartilaginous stroma—the so-called metaplastic carcinomas.[99]

2.9.4. Metaplastic Carcinoma (Carcinoma with Osseous or Cartilaginous Stroma)

Although cartilage and bone formation is common in mammary tumors of cats and dogs, its occurrence in humans is exceedingly rare. Huvos and associates[99] encountered only 16 examples, an incidence rate of approximately 0.003% of all breast cancers at the Memorial Sloan-Kettering Cancer Center. The osteoid and chondroid foci noted in the cases of their report were apparently well differentiated. They regarded the change as the result of epithelial metaplasia; in this regard, it might be considered as analogous to the derivation of the mesenchymal elements of so-called mixed tumors of salivary glands. Whether the bone-forming sarcomatous elements of the cases of carcinosarcoma recorded by Robb and MacFarlane[94] represent examples of malignant transformation of the benign osteoid component of these so-called metaplastic breast carcinomas is uncertain. Gonzalez-Licea and associates[100] examined such a tumor by electron microscopy and noted that all of the cells, including the stromal components, shared a common feature, notably, the presence of desmosomes which they indicated as support for the epithelial derivation of the cartilage and bone. However, one might note that such intercellular structures may also be found in mesenchymal cells, particularly those of embryonic nature.[101] This tends to limit their significance as an epithelial marker as well as to offer some skepticism concerning the derivation of such mesenchymal elements. In any event, metaplastic breast carcinoma has been regarded as having a less favorable prognosis than the similar-appearing neoplasm occurring in animals.

2.9.5. Pure Squamous-Cell Carcinoma

Although varying degrees of squamous differentiation occur in a modest number of mammary cancers of other histologic types, pure squamous-cell carcinoma is exceedingly rare. Indeed, it is difficult to ascertain accurately the incidence of squamous-cell carcinoma of the breast, since many recorded cases represent examples of other tumor types with squamous metaplasia. Further, the distinction between metaplasia and actual prozoplasia—i.e., squamous elements with malignant characteristics—is not often made. Reported incidences of squamous-cell carcinoma, which vary from 0.5% to 2% of all mammary cancers, reflect these uncertainties. Cornog and associates[102] have recently reviewed the pertinent literature in this regard. They reported on the findings in 24 cases that were designated as "squamous carcinoma of breast." Yet they note that in only three instances was the neoplasm regarded as pure squamous-cell carcinoma. One of these apparently arose in cystosarcoma phyllodes, and in the other two, their anatomic relationships suggested that they may have arisen from the epidermis. The case reported by Jones[103] is of interest in that the lesion was regarded as pure squamous-cell carcinoma with pseudosarcomatous stroma. Whether this lesion represents an example of carcinosarcoma (see Section 2.9.1) or a pure form of squamous-cell carcinoma is uncertain. We have had the opportunity to examine an instance of pure squamous-cell carcinoma of the breast in which none of these other complicating features were present[3] (Fig. 17). Ultrastructurally, the cells contained pronounced tonofilaments and fibrils, as well as large numbers of intracytoplasmic desmosomes as have been noted in cutaneous carcinomas of squamous-cell derivation.

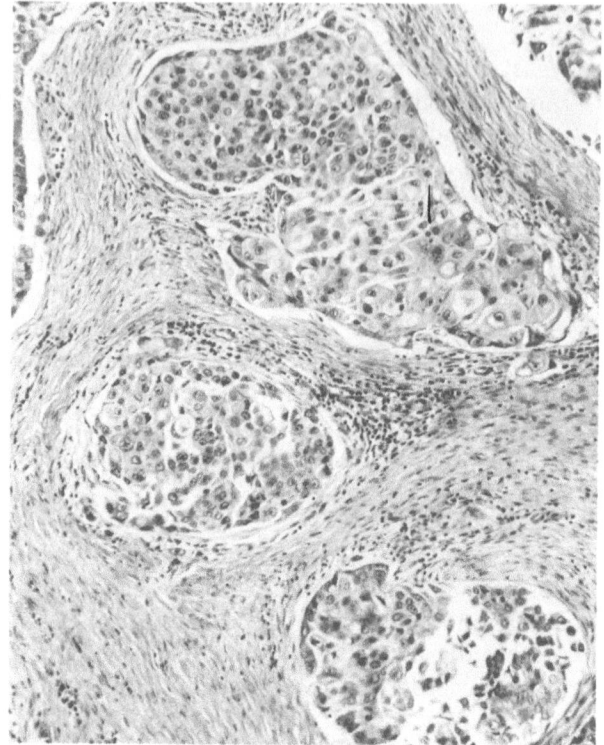

Fig. 17. Portion of squamous-cell carcinoma of the breast. The tumor cells reflect varying degrees of squamous maturation. ×100.

2.9.6. Basal-Cell Carcinoma

Newcombe[104] has reported on the occurrence of a breast tumor whose histopathologic appearance was indistinguishable from that of basal-cell carcinoma of skin. The tumor was characterized by marked ulceration of the skin and extended only for a short distance into the underlying breast tissue. There was involvement of the underlying ducts by basaloid cells as well as elements similar to those of intraductal carcinoma. The author regarded the latter sites as the most likely origin of the tumor. However, the possibility that the involvement of the breast resulted from direct extension of a cutaneous basal-cell carcinoma, or that the lesion represented a collision between the latter and a true intraductal mammary cancer or basaloid form of NOS tumor, cannot be excluded.

2.9.7. Lipid-Rich Carcinoma

Ramos and Taylor[64] have recently called attention to an unusual type of mammary carcinoma which they designated as lipid-rich carcinoma. Although the tumors frequently had areas of intraductal carcinoma and lobular carcinoma *in situ*, the major portions were comprised of large cells with clear, sometimes bubbly, cytoplasm which was positive for neutral lipid when appropriately stained. Electron microscopy of one example revealed intramitochondrial crystals. They indicated that the foamy, "lipophage" appearance of the tumor cells might mimic a malignant reticuloendotheliosis when found in nodal metastases. The prognosis of the 13 patients with this type of mammary carcinoma was regarded as poor. It would appear that the validity of such a tumor type might be strengthened by information concerning the lipid content of cells comprising other histologic types of mammary carcinoma. In this regard, it might be noted that we have observed neutral lipid in cells comprising a variety of mammary cancers, not only in appropriately stained sections examined by light microscopy, but also in electron microscopic preparations. Further, we have noted the intramitochondrial paracrystalline material described by Ramos and Taylor in their example of so-called lipid-rich carcinoma in an example of NOS carcinoma, as well as one of tubular type.[3]

3. Histologic Grading

Von Hansemann (in 1893) is usually credited with first calling attention to the possible relationship between the behavior of malignant neoplasms and their degree of "anaplasia,"[105] although Tough and associates[79] note that a similar correlation was expressed even earlier (in 1891) by Dennis. MacCarty and Sistrunk[106] and White[107] considered not only the degree of differentiation of the neoplastic elements important in grading mammary carcinomas, but also their associated lymphoid infiltration and stromal fibrosis. Greenough,[108] upon whose method most recent investigators have based their technique of grading mammary carcinomas, divided tumors into three grades of malignancy depending upon the degree of tubule formation, size of cells and nuclei, and degree of hyperchromatism and number of mitoses. That survival might be related to the histologic grade of the tumor was confirmed by Scarff and Patey.[109] However, a subsequent study by Scarff and Handley[110] led to the conclusion that staging was perhaps a more important factor in prognosis, but that the best indicator might be found with the use of both staging and histologic grading. Utilization of the method of grading of Greenough was revived in 1950 by Bloom,[111,112] who, at that time as well as subsequently, found a close correlation between survival and grade.[78] The method employed by most investigators is based upon the consideration or actual scoring of the degree of tubule formation and regularity of nuclei and mitoses from 1 to 3. The scores for each of these three features are added together. Marks of 3 to 5 indicate a tumor of low-grade malignancy (Grade 1); 6 and 7, a moderate degree of malignancy (Grade 2); and 8 and 9, a high degree of malignancy (Grade 3). Wolff,[113] as well as Tough and associates,[79] Dabska,[114] and Champion and associates,[115] subsequently confirmed the feasibility as well as prognostic significance of grading as employed by Bloom. However, Wolff[113] has emphasized that grading combined with pathologic staging was more significant than the former alone, whereas Tough and associates added the feature of tumor size to stage and grade as offering a more comprehensive assessment of prognosis.[79] However, they hasten to add that ideally, consideration of the tumor alone should not be utilized, since such an approach is artificial and fails to recognize possible host factors. This view may be amplified by the recognition that the medullary form of mammary carcinoma qualifies by most schemes of grading based upon the properties of the tumor cells *per se* as a highly malignant (Grade 3) lesion, yet its favorable prognosis has been repeatedly emphasized. Eichner and associates[116] compared the results of histologic grading as utilized by Bloom and the assessment of nuclear grade as described by Black and associates[117-119] and found the results comparable insofar as assessing survival rates for five years. This might not be totally unexpected, for as noted above, much of the Greenough–Bloom criteria of grading are based upon nuclear features.

We have utilized a modification of the method employed by Bloom and others. As noted above, degrees of nuclear differentiation are adequately scored by the relatively simple technique of nuclear grading as employed by Black and associates.[117-119] Although these investigators utilized four grades, we have found it practical to combine their Grades 0 and 1 into one grade, Grade 1. Unfortunately, and contrary to conventional methods of grading, this represents the most anaplastic nuclear appearance. Grade 2 nuclei are intermediate in appearance, and those designated as Grade 3, the most well-differentiated forms (for further remarks concerning nuclear grade, see Section 4). A scheme was devised to incorporate the nuclear grade with the presence or absence of tubule formation in deriving the histologic grade, as noted in Table I. As indicated, the so-called adenocystic pattern is also included as a form of tubule formation.

Table I
Criteria for Simplified Histologic Grading of Mammary Cancer

Tubule formation	Nuclear grade (1–3)	Histologic grade (1–3)
Pure, or in part tubular	3	1
Pure, or in part adenocystic	3	1
Pure, or in part tubular	1, 2	2
Pure, or in part adenocystic	1, 2	2
Absent	3	2
Absent	1, 2	3

Approximately two-thirds of all mammary cancers might be designated as histologic Grade 3 according to the scheme utilized.[2] Only a relatively small number (2.3%) are regarded as being well differentiated or Grade 1. The association of Grade 1 tumors in older women, absence of nodal involvement, as well as frequency of histologic types purported

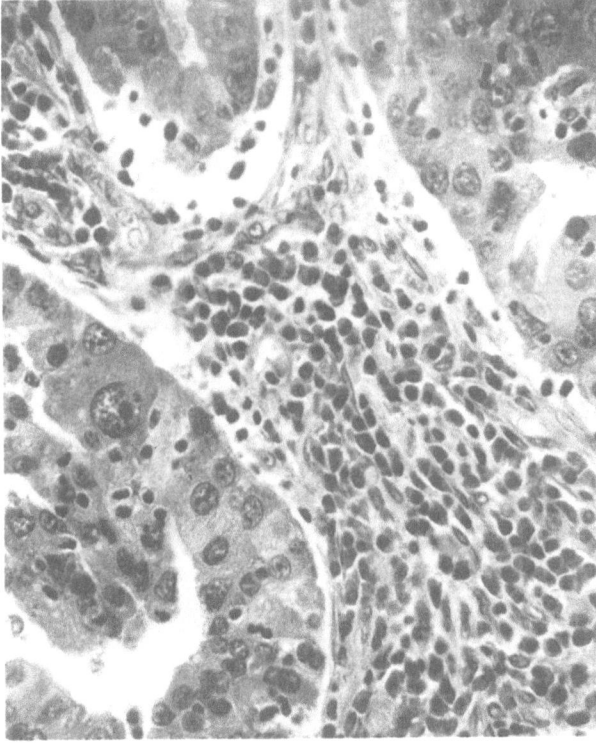

Fig. 18. Nuclei regarded as Grade 1 from the medullary cancer depicted in Fig. 5. ×400.

to exhibit a good prognosis, and the converse with tumors histologically graded as 3 (except for the good prognosis with the medullary type) is consonant with information provided by other investigators. In addition, it was noted that Grade 3 tumors exhibit a greater frequency of lymphatic extension. It is also of interest that Grade 1 tumors exhibit marked elastosis, absent necrosis, and cell reaction, but marked and moderate mucin content, which, when present, is usually of all tinctorial types.

4. Nuclear Grading

In several reports, Black and associates[117-120] have emphasized a clear relationship between nuclear grade of the tumor and sinus histiocytosis of axillary lymph nodes and patient survival. Eichner and associates,[116] as noted previously, regarded estimation of nuclear grade as a simpler and equally efficacious method of grading mammary can-

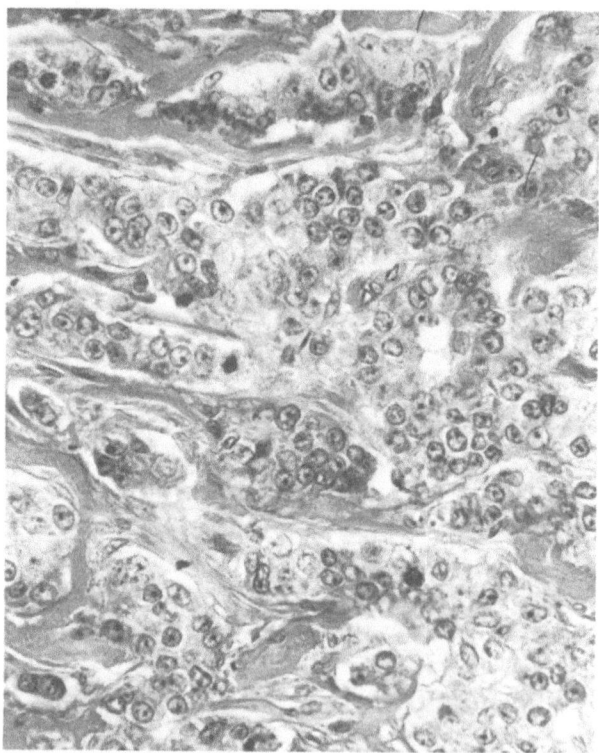

Fig. 19. Nuclei regarded as Grade 2. They are smaller and more uniform than those in Fig. 18. Nucleoli are moderately prominent, however. ×400.

cers as the technique based upon multifactorial features Sommers[121] found more well-differentiated nuclei in intraductal carcinomas as opposed to those in invasive cancers. He related this difference to the enhanced invasion by the less-differentiated mammary carcinoma cells. Tomic and associates[9] considered nuclear grade useful, but not a certain guide to prognosis. They regarded histologic typing, as well as evaluation of other factors, including size, site, infiltrative properties, nodal metastases, and other features, as more significant. Kister and associates[122] were unable to find any statistically significant relationship between nuclear grade and survival in a clinically favorable (Columbia classification) group of cases.

As noted previously, we have utilized a modification of the system of Black and associates for nuclear grading, the major departure being represented by combining their Grades 0 and 1 and 3 and 4, resulting in only three grades (Figs. 18–20). Grade 1 nuclei, the most poorly differentiated, are characterized by pleomorphism, prominent nucleoli,

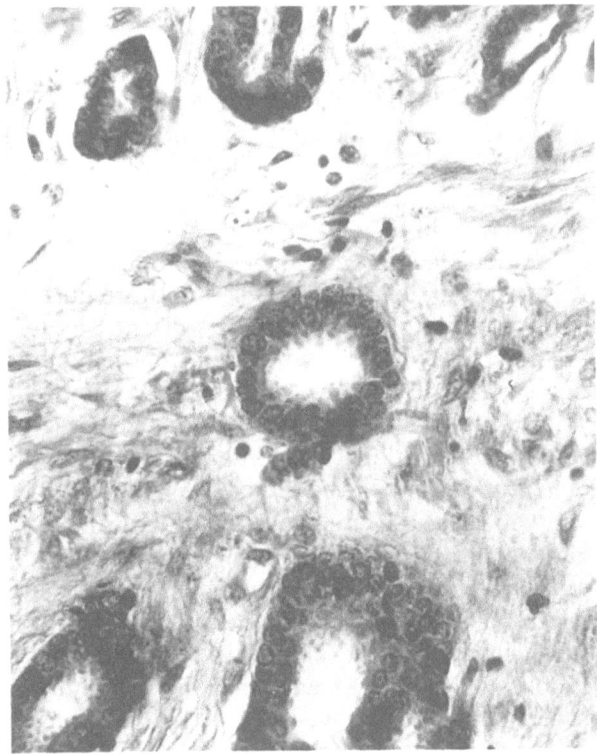

Fig. 20. Nuclei of tubules from the tubular carcinoma depicted in Fig. 11 are regarded as Grade 3. They are small and uniform, without conspicuous nucleoli or mitotic forms. ×400.

large size, and frequent mitoses; Grade 2 nuclei are intermediate; and Grade 3, the well-differentiated nuclei, are small and uniform and exhibit inconspicuous nucleoli and, rarely, mitotic figures. When variations in nuclei are encountered in the same tumor, the less-differentiated forms are regarded as, representative of its grade. It is unfortunate that the scale employed in nuclear grading is the converse of that customarily employed in the grading of differentiation, such as the histologic grade. Nevertheless, to avoid confusion it is considered unwarranted to alter this grading system, despite its unconventionality.

It has been observed that tumors with nuclear Grade 1 are frequently associated with the presence of positive lymph nodes, blood vessel and lymphatic invasion, large tumor size, and young age of the patients—features generally regarded as prognostically ominous.

5. Circumscription

Mammary carcinomas generally assume either a circumscribed or more infiltrative, irregular, or stellate configuration. Dockerty[81] noted that the incidence of axillary nodal involvement was less and the five-year survival rate higher with evidence of encapsulation. Lane and associates[123] grouped 204 examples of mammary cancer into two types according to the appearance of the contour of the tumor, as judged by naked-eye or hand-lens examination of histologic slides. They recognized well-delimited and irregular forms. The former was characterized by a rounded or lobulated border, suggesting an expansile or pushing type of growth, whereas the latter was serrated, irregular, or stellate, with radial projections into the surrounding tissue. The ten-year cure rates were strikingly different: 38% in patients whose tumors were designated as irregular and 80% in those in which they were well delimited. The well-delimited tumors tended to be larger and contained less fibrous stroma but more marked cellular elements. Nuclear atypism was conspicuous in such tumors and was often accompanied by a lymphocytic reaction. Axillary metastases were also less frequent, and when present, were less extensive in the well-delimited group than with tumors regarded as irregular. Unfortunately, apparently about one-third of the cases included in the study were of the medullary type, whose greater cure rate may be related to factors other than their circumscription, e.g., lymphocytic infiltrate. Hamlin,[124] who used three designations (round, serrated, or absent true edge), failed to find any relationship between the configuration of the tumor border and survival. Divergent results were also noted by Silverberg and associates,[125] who found no difference in survival rates of patients whose tumors were or were not circumscribed. However, if medullary and mucinous forms were excluded from the circumscribed group, the prognosis was actually worse. More recently, Gold and associates[126] have assessed the tumor border by mammography and have found a statistically significant increase in axillary metastases in those tumors with highly, rather than slightly, infiltrative borders. As also noted by Lane and associates,[123] a greater proportion of infiltrative tumors were small. However, highly infiltrative tumors of large size metastasized to axillary nodes more often than did smaller infiltrative lesions.

In our own study, it was noteworthy that although 39.8% of mammary cancers studied were grossly regarded as circumscribed, only 16.9% were regarded as such after microscopic evaluation. Microscopically, circumscription was considered only when a fibrous band of variable thickness surrounded the tumor or when its cellular configuration at the periphery was smooth or "pushing" in appearance. This contrasted with the radial projections of tumor cell clusters in surrounding adipose tissue which characterized the stellate lesions. Lack of circumscription or the stellate configuration of breast cancers was found to be more frequently associated with short-term treatment failure (up to 24 months).

6. Tumor Size

Tumor size might be regarded as an obvious discriminant of import for the prognosis of mammary cancer. The efforts devoted to the "early" detection of such lesions certainly impart the impression of an inverse relationship between survival and tumor size. The designation of cancers measuring less than 5 mm as "minimal" cancer also conveys this relationship.[7] Further, support for such a view comes from reports indicating that almost three-fourths of patients with tumors larger than 5 cm already have nodal metastases when first examined.[127] Cady[128] has noted a decrease in the mean size of mammary cancers to 3.0 cm, with a concomitant decrease in the incidence of axillary node involvement during the 20-year period between 1948 and 1968, as compared to earlier decades. Earlier studies, such as that by Eggers and associates,[129] related a 73% five-year survival for patients whose tumors were less than 2 cm, 24% for those with lesions measuring 3–6 cm, and only 15% when tumors measured 7 cm or more. These relationships between size of tumor, nodal metastases, and prognosis have, for the most part, been confirmed by more recent studies.[1,130,131] Yet, it is noteworthy that others[132,133] have failed to recognize such a correlation between tumor size and survival. Although in some instances there are apparent reasons for such a dichotomy (e.g., different types of treatment, different stages of disease, etc.), in others an explanation is less apparent, suggesting that other factors may be operative in relation to survival, in addition to, or regardless of, tumor size. Appreciation of the various histologic types and grades of mammary cancers might be sufficient to suspect that the doubling times or rates of growth of all mammary cancers are not similar. Indeed, Bloom[111] could find no correlation between prognosis and the size of tumors that were designated as being of low or high degree of malignancy. On the other hand, there was a poorer prognosis with tumors larger than 2 cm that were of intermediate histologic grade. Hamlin[124] failed to recognize a correlation between tumor size and mortality in her material, although the majority of patients regarded as Clinical Stage I had small tumors. Fisher and associates[131] observed poorer survival with large tumors when more than three axillary nodes exhibited metastases than if no nodes or only one to three were involved; no striking difference in survival was observed in patients with small or large tumors in whom no nodes or one to three contained metastases. Their data also suggested a greater predilection for axillary metastases with large tumors. Gold et al. [126] have noted more axillary metastases in patients with large tumors (> 6 cm) with an infiltrative border than with tumors measuring < 4.5 cm with a similar type of border as delineated by mammography. Complementary to these findings are the observations of Lane and associates,[123] who found a better prognosis in patients with larger, well-delimited tumors than with those of similar size but an irregular border. However, they also noted that tumors with well-delimited borders in patients exhibiting a long survival period were one-third larger than those that were irregular.

Although it would be highly desirable to obtain information concerning the volume of mammary cancers, it is difficult to obtain measurements of three dimensions of many of these lesions. This is in large part the result of the polymorphous configuration which these cancers often possess. Such shapes are readily apparent from mammographic studies. Because of this, we resorted only to information relative to their maximum diameter as obtained by measurement of the gross specimen.[2] The median size of 3.0 cm coincided with that recorded by Cady[128] for the period 1948–1968, suggesting that there has been little or no greater increase in the detection of small tumors during the past 25 years.

Tumors greater than 4.0 cm in maximum diameter were found in younger women (20–44 years) and were consistently associated with multicentric foci of cancer, blood vessel and lymphatic invasion, marked necrosis in the dominant tumor mass, the presence of four or more axillary lymph nodes containing metastases, and, importantly, the occurrence of short-term treatment failure (up to 24 months). An association, albeit an inconsistent one, was also noted between the occurrence of tumors larger than 4.0 cm and the presence of nipple and skin involvement. As noted previously,[134] no association between tumor size and the involvement of no or one to three axillary lymph nodes was evident. However, in patients with clinically positive axillae, there was a greater likelihood that the nodes contained metastases when their tumors were larger than 4.0 cm. Larger tumors were more frequently found in blacks than in whites or those of other races. Tumors measuring 2.1–4 cm more frequently exhibited a nuclear grade of 1, whereas those less than 2.1 cm were found to be associated with a nuclear grade of 3, absent cell reaction, and clinically and pathologically negative axillae. The duration of symptoms was short (three months or less) in patients with small tumors. Surprisingly, no association with any particular tumor type was found, although the impression has been conveyed that medullary and mucinous types frequently are of large size.

7. Cell Reaction

It has long been recognized that some mammary as well as other cancers may be found to have a lymphoid infiltrate at their periphery or among their cellular elements. As noted previously, MacCarty and Sistrunk[106] in 1922 considered the degree of lymphocyte content of tumors as a criterion for their grading. Moore and Foote[28] described the favorable prognosis associated with medullary cancers, which contain a marked lymphoid infiltrate. They suggested that this cellular reaction might represent a host response to the tumor, an interpretation offered by many early investigators for the presence of inflammatory cells in neoplasms. Subsequently, Black and associates[119,120,135–138] indicated that the lethality of breast cancer may be determined by the interaction of factors relating to the growth potential of the tumor, as reflected by nuclear grade on the one hand, and host inhibitory or resistance factors, such as lymphoid infiltrate of the tumor and sinus histiocytosis of regional nodes, on the other. This conclusion was based upon the study of cases followed either to death or for a minimum of five years after operation. It is of interest, however, that tumors from only 11 of the patients in one study[117] were regarded as having a lymphoid infiltrate greater than 2+. Hamlin,[124] a strong proponent of relating lymphoid infiltrate to host resistence, performed an exhaustive study of the cellular infiltration in 272 tumors, assessing the general pattern and density of infiltrate, including that of plasma cells, lymphocytes, and large pyroninophilic cells or "immunoblasts." Each factor was score 1–3+ and the average utilized to designate the degree of host resistance. This factor was also correlated with other parameters, such as qualitative features of the cellular elements of the axillary nodes, histologic grade according to the method of Bloom, histologic type, age, menopausal status, site and size of tumor, and clinical stage. There was a close correlation between degree or index of "host resistance" and prognosis or survival, a relationship also encountered with the grade of tumor as well. However, the interrelationship of cell reaction to other parameters related to survival was not clear. Berg[139-141] reported that a peripheral plasmacellular infiltrate in poorly differentiated carcinomas was associated with improved survival, and that this was directly proportional to the degree of such reaction. On the other hand, Champion and associates,[115] utilizing a less sophisticated analysis of the lymphoid infiltrate than Hamlin,[124] found this reaction more commonly in tumors of high-grade malignancy which exhibited a poorer prognosis. This cellular reaction had no influence on prognosis when considered in tumors within each grade of malignancy. This view that lymphoid infiltration does not in all instances convey a good prognosis is similar to that expressed previously by Scarff and Torloni.[142] Sommers[121] failed to find any difference in cell reaction in intraductal (incipient) carcinomas, compared to the invasive forms, all of which were regarded as Clinical Stage I. We[143] have recently attempted to correlate the lymphocyte transformation of regional node cells with various histologic parameters in 50 cases of mammary cancer. A significant statistical relationship was noted between lymphocyte transformation and a mild lymphoid infiltrate, which would also minimize the significance of the latter as a measure of host resistance to tumor growth. This impression receives some support from the study of Richters and Sherwin,[144] who observed greater degrees of lymphocyte activity, including cytotoxicity on tumor cells, in explants of mammary carcinomas when regional node cells were added than in their absence, although the explants contained lymphoid infiltrates derived from the primary tumor.

A considerable amount of literature has accumulated regarding a possible role of mast cells in tumor growth and development, most of which is contradictory, as discussed by us in a previous report.[145] Some suggestive evidence that serotonin may affect the growth of established subcutaneous tumors in an experimental animal tumor system was found. Hamlin[124] failed to note any relationship between the mast cell content of the cell reaction in mammary carcinomas and survival trends.

Results of our own studies in regard to cell reaction have prompted the view that this phenomenon appears more closely related to features signifying the degree of malignancy of breast cancer rather than to an immunologic host response *per se*. The failure to encounter any discernible effect of so-called effector cells on tumor cell structure by electron microscopy has been noted in Section 2.2.

8. Stromal Change

As noted previously, early workers attempted to devise prognostic schemes based upon the stromal content of mammary carcinomas. Attention in this regard was directed to their lymphocytic and connective tissue components, the degree of the latter being considered proportional to the degree of host resistance. MacCarty and Sistrunk,[106] as well as Hueper,[146] regarded stromal hyalinization as a favorable prognostic feature. However, Hamlin[124] and Alderson and associates[1] noted a lower mortality in patients with tumor stroma that was fibrovascular rather than dense and collagenous. Okamoto,[147] in a comprehensive histochemical study of the stroma in a vareity of tumors including those of breast, also viewed this response as defensive in nature, although the possibility that it might be promotional could not be excluded. The ratio of tumor-cell to connective-tissue stromal elements in breast cancers has also been used in the past as a basis for the descriptive terminologies employed for mammary cancers, the scirrhous form being relatively acellular, the medullary exhibiting a preponderance of cellular elements, and the simplex variety consisting of roughly equal proportions of both.

Approximately one-half of the cancers have a moderate connective-tissue stromal component. In only rare instances is the stroma absent or negligible, whereas in the remainder of the cases, it is somewhat equally divided as being slight or marked. No significant relationship between degree or type of stromal reaction (i.e., whether or the loose or dense variety) has been observed.[2]

9. Elastica

According to Davies,[148] the presence of elastosis in mammary carcinomas was recognized as early as 1860 by Billroth and subsequently confirmed by a number of investigators, some of whom viewed such change as a premalignant phenomenon,[149-151] since as noted by Orr,[151] such a change was rarely, if ever, encountered in benign mammary disorders. However, Davies[148] has more recently demonstrated from his examination of the uninvolved ducts of 86 breasts harboring cancer, 199 "control" postmortem glands, and 140 examples of mammary dysplasia (fibrocystic disease) obtained by biopsy that the incidence of hyperelastosis, as well as obliteration and fibrous plaques of these structures, was comparable in all. He noted an enhanced prevalence of ductal elastosis to occur with increasing parity. Williams and associates[152] reported massive increases in elastica in all breast cancers examined and a modest amount in apparently benign hyperplastic lesions. Fibroadenomas, on the other hand, failed to exhibit such change. Shivas and Douglas[153] noted a highly significant statistical correlation between the degree of elastosis in mammary cancers which they graded from 0 to 3+ and the survival rate of 103 patients treated by simple mastectomy and irradiation. It is to be noted that their indices or quantitative assessment were based upon focal aggregates of elastosis. The diffuse form was disregarded, since they apparently were more interested in periductal elastosis. Lundmark[154] found 65% of the 414 cancers examined by appropriate technique to exhibit elastosis. There was no apparent correlation between this alteration and the degree of differentiation of the neoplasms and no positive statistically significant relationship to age, although greater degrees of elastosis exhibited a trend to occur in older women. Azzopardi and Laurini[155] recorded an increase in elastica of ducts as well as vessels, particularly that in veins, in 86% of 115 cases of infiltrating cancers examined. Again, the degree of this change was graded on the basis of focal accumulations. Indeed, diffuse disposition of such fibers was regarded as negative or absent elastica. They noted that elastosis was infrequent in medullary and other specialized forms of mammary cancer, and regarded such change as an indicator of early infiltration. They also reemphasized that the yellow streaking often grossly noted in mammary carcinomas was due to elastosis rather than tumor necrosis, as had long been conventionally held.

The biological significance and histogenesis of elastosis in mammary carcinoma are uncertain. As noted above, early investigators regarded it as evidence of a premalignant change, whereas more recently, Azzopardi and Laurini[155] and Bonser and associates[156] considered it to represent a sign of early infiltration of ductal carcinomas. Several authors[154,157] have attempted to relate elastosis to a host defense mechanism, in keeping with the views concerning the nature of the other connective tissue and cellular elements of the stromal response to cancer. It has been quite boldly attributed to factors emanating from the cancer cells which are capable of stimulating its production from fibroblasts and other precursor cells.

The identification of the fibrillary structures referred to above, as well as by previous authors, as elastica has been challenged. Sumegi and Rajka[158] noted that in addition to their affinity for so-called elastic-tissue stains, they were also colored by those methods commonly employed for the identification of amyloid. This led them to designate the material as "elastic amyloid." However, the material was not dichroic after staining with Congo red, which is a significant diagnostic feature of amyloid. Lundmark[154] noted some residual connective tissue elements after digestion with elastase, and was also of the opinion that the structure designated as elastica may indeed have an amyloid moiety. On the other hand, Azzopardi and Laurini[155] have interpreted the results of their enzymatic digestions as signifying its elastic nature, and we[159] have repeatedly noted some residue, even after the digestion of such prototype elastic fibers as ligamentum nuchae with elastase preparations. This controversy is reminiscent of that concerning the identification of the anatomical defect in the systemic disease known as pseudoxanthoma elasticum or the more commonplace cutaneous disorder senile elastosis. Evidence has been presented previously[159-160] to indicate that such material in these conditions does indeed represent elastica. Three basic patterns of elastica occur in breast cancers: a modest deposition of such fibers about the neoplastic ducts only; this same disposition as well as a modest number within the tumor stroma; or a marked abount of elastica which appears diffusely within the stroma with scant or insignificant periductal elastosis. Marked or moderate degrees (Fig. 21) of elastosis have been noted with a marked tumor stromal

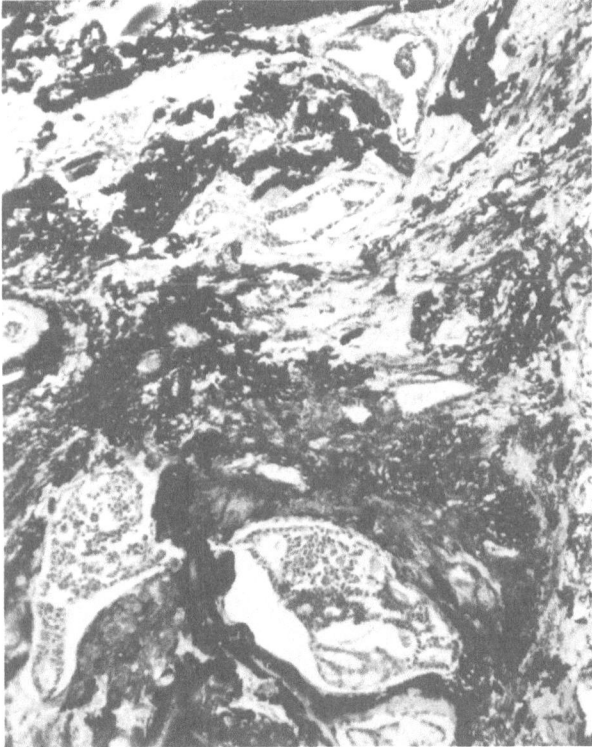

Fig. 21. Marked elastosis in tubular and adenocystic breast cancer. The elastic fibers are periductal as well as in the stroma. Orcein elastica stain, ×100.

component. Also, such special types of carcinoma as the medullary and mucinous types are more frequently associated with absent or slight elastica than with moderate or marked amounts. When the elastica was absent or slight, there was a greater likelihood that the age of the patient was 20–44 years. Although there was a statistically significant association between marked elastica and tumors from patients of older age groups, this was not consistent.[2] This suggests that the breast may reflect changes in elastica comparable to those of other tissues (e.g., the skin).

10. Mucin

Although there have been several studies indicating a relatively favorable prognosis for the mucinous type of mammary carcinoma, little attention has been directed to the possible significance of lesser degrees of mucin which may occur in such tumors. Some early[161,162] as well as more recent[55] investigators considered the mucin content one of the most significant prognostic indicators in breast cancer, although this has been disputed by others.[163] Hamlin[124] has indicated that the presence of mucin was correlated with the degree of differentiation of the breast cancers she studied. However, none apparently contained sufficient amounts of this substance or presented sufficient characteristics to warrant a designation as mucinous carcinoma. Although the presence or absence of mucin does not appear to have any significant association with nuclear or histologic grade, lymphatic extension, or severe cell reaction, these parameters have been found to be significantly frequent when the mucin that was present was only PAS-positive.[2] On the other hand, in the presence of mixed mucin, nuclear grade appeared high (Grade 3) and the combination of both PAS- and alcian-blue-positive material in the same neoplasm was significantly associated with large tumors. Most pure mucinous carcinomas exhibit the mixed mucin reaction as well as alcian-blue-positive material.

11. Calcium

The utilization of mamography has directed attention to the calcium content of mammary cancers, since the appearance of such mineral deposits has been regarded as an important diagnostic feature of those lesions. Yet, the incidence of calcific opacifications in benign breast lesions approximates that noted in cancer. Further, it is to be noted that no consistent qualitative differences between the calcific deposits encountered in malignant and benign breast diseases have been found in specimen mammograms.[164,165] In this regard, it is of interest that the incidence of cancer in blocks of breast tissue selected because of the presence of opacification in areas unrelated to a dominant mass or unusual density is extremely low, being only 0.7% in specimen mammograms.[165] Calcium may be detected by appropriate tinctorial methods such as the von Kossa reaction in approximately 60% of cases, an incidence which approximates that noted by clinical mammography but less than the 86% noted in the specimen mammograms. This obviously reflects a sampling error attendant with the histological method of assessment. Aside from the presence of calcium in instances in which the tumors exhibited necrosis, no other significant relationships between such mineral deposits and other parameters have been noted.[2] It is of interest that a high degree of association between calcium deposition and marked tumor elastosis has been noted and appears to represent another biological instance in which such a phenomenon is associated with calcium deposition.

12. Glycogen

Only a few histochemical studies of mammary carcinomas have been performed. Godlewski[166] considered the disappearance of glycogen and phosphorylases to be related to the immaturity of their cells, since differentiated benign tumors exhibited marked glycogen content and enzyme activity. Foraker[167] performed a battery of histochemical tests on examples of breast cancer and found that although glycogen was stronger and more uniform in normal epithelium, it also occurred in carcinomas, some of which might be classified as poorly differentiated. He failed to detect any histochemical pattern or profile which would allow for the distinction of benign and malignant breast disease. No significant or notable associations between the presence or absence of glycogen within the tumor cells comprising mammary cancers have been noted.

13. Squamous Metaplasia

Squamous metaplasia characterized by large, somewhat polygonal, oxyphilic cells exhibiting intracellular bridges and/or pearl formation occurs in approximately 4% of breast cancers, and has been found to be associated with the presence of glycogen in the tumor cells, a finding which appears to be in accord with the presence of this polysaccharide in squamous epithelium. There is also a greater likelihood that patients whose tumors exhibit such change will be regarded *clinically* as having positive axillary nodal involvement. However, this nodal change appears to be the result of nonneoplastic alteration, since there is also an association between squamous metaplasia and marked sinus histiocytosis, but not nodal metastases. Tumors with squamous metaplasia also exhibit an increased incidence of moderate or marked necrosis, appear to have a prominent cell reaction, involve the overlying skin, and possess poorly differentiated nuclei (nuclear Grade 1).

14. Apocrine Change, Oxyphilia

Some have considered so-called "apocrine" or "sweat gland" carcinoma of the breast as a distinct histologic entity. Proponents[10,29,168–171] of this view invariably indicate that the breast represents a specialized modification of apocrine glands, and note analogies in their structure, development, and responsiveness to hormonal influences such as might occur during menstruation, pregnancy, and lactation. The occurrence of apocrine-like change in fibrocystic disease of the breast is commonplace. Certainly in this light, the designation of mammary tissue as well as tumors arising within the breast as being of "sweat gland" origin would be erroneous, since the structure and function of the latter are eccrine in nature and unrelated to those of the breast. There has been some discussion as to whether the large, swollen oxyphilic cells comprising some carcinomas occur as a result of anomalous development; represent embryonal inclusions of "sweat gland" structures within the breast; or are of normal occurrence, a degenerative phenomenon, or an instance of metaplasia. We have had the opportunity to examine by electron microscopy a mammary cancer comprised of neoplastic cells with relatively large amounts of finely granular, oxyphilic cytoplasm.[3] Ultrastructurally, the cell cytoplasm contained slightly more mitochondria than cells comprising most NOS mammary cancers. Nevertheless, as in the latter, these were irregular in shape and generally vacuolated. In some instances, they contained lamellar cristal stacks and cristal-like matrical particles similar to those noted in so-called lipid-rich carcinomas, although lipid droplets were only occasionally encountered, as were a variety of lysosomes. Some of the latter were lipofuscin bodies, whereas others appeared as multivesicular structures of myelin figures. A few contained a homogeneous electron-dense matrix within their limiting membrane. The coarse endoplasmic reticulum was dilated and vesicles and vacuoles with smooth profiles were numerous. Golgi structures were also prominent. Nuclei were large, with a heterochromatin pattern and large nucleoli. Cell membranes exhibited frequent interdigitations and occasional villi. No lamina basalis was detected, the tumor cells lying apposed to mature collagen and elastic fibers. Thus, these cells possessed some of the features of apocrine cells, notably, an increase in size, as well as a modest increase in number of mitochondria. Although the cells contained membrane-bound bodies similar to those noted in apocrine elements, they were more variable in their structure and less orderly arranged than in the latter, which we feel, contrary to the conclusions of others,[172,173] are indeed morphologically apocrine in structure. It is not inconceivable that these differences may be the result of malignant neoplastic transformation. We are unaware of any ultrastructural studies of apocrine carcinomas of such sites as the skin which might offer some evidence in support or denial of such a possibility.

Nevertheless, most reports of relatively large series of purported examples of "apocrine"[61,169,170] carcinoma indicate that the degree of malignancy and prognosis are similar to those of mammary carcinoma in general. Because of these considerations, as well as those presented previously, we have not attributed special significance to tumors that may exhibit areas containing large, granular oxyphilic cells, except to note their presence.

15. Necrosis

Tumor necrosis of varying degree is not an uncommon feature of mammary carcinoma, occurring in approximately two-thirds of all cases. The presence of marked necrosis is usually associated with tumors of high or most malignant histologic grade. However, this may reflect the greater frequency of necrosis in medullary carcinomas, since such other associated features of this tumor type as squamous metaplasia, severe cell reaction, slight stroma, mucin content, and younger age of occurrence (20–44 years) have also been noted. On the other hand, the NOS type of tumor may also be found to be associated with marked necrosis, as well as features more common to this type such as nipple involvement and a marked intraductal component of the comedo type. In addition, absent or slight necrosis has been found to be consistently associated with the absence of sinus histiocytosis and with a number of tumor types including the mucinous, lobular invasive, and NOS combination varieties. The possible relationship between tumor necrosis and sinus histiocytosis is suggested by this relationship, but has not unequivocally been supported statistically, since the relationship between marked necrosis and the presence of sinus histiocytosis, although noted, is not consistent.

16. Relationship of Fibrocystic Disease to Cancer

The relationship of fibrocystic disease to mammary cancer remains an enigma, despite the voluminous literature devoted to this problem. The pathologic distinction of certain forms of ductal hyperplasia from cancer represents one of the most difficult decisions confronting the surgical pathologist. Unfortunately, in many instances, this judgment is largely subjective, if not capricious. More objective criteria than the customarily stated "severe cellular atypia," "numerous mitoses," and "foci of necrosis" would be highly desirable for this purpose. The management of patients with fibrocystic disease of the breast is also uncertain and disputable. This has resulted from the controversy concerning the premalignant potential of fibrocystic disease, as well as the relatively unreliable pathologic distinction between atypical hyperplasia and cancer. Information concerning the relationship between fibrocystic disease and cancer has generally been derived from three types of studies. Several reports which might be regarded as concurrent in nature indicate the higher incidence of fibrocystic disease in the vicinity of mammary cancers, as well as in areas of the breast remote from the dominant lesion, than in breasts with foci of benign or no disease.[174-187] Estimates of such change accompanying carcinoma have ranged from 20 to 100%, whereas the occurrence of fibrocystic disease in apparently normal breasts recovered from autopsied patients or those removed surgically for benign disease varies between 12 and 29%.[176,184,188] It is of interest that Ryan and Coady[184] noted no difference in the incidence of fibrocystic disease unassociated with mammary cancer in pre- or postmenopausal autopsied patients, which would tend to dispel the notion that such an event should be looked upon with suspicion in the older patient. The findings from these concurrent studies appear to represent more than a fortuitous association between fibrocystic disease and mammary cancer. Yet, a more skeptical view may regard the former evidence as an example of *post hoc ergo propter hoc* reasoning.

Another approach to the investigation of the relationship of fibrocystic disease to cancer has been to determine the incidence of the former in biopsies of patients whose breasts have been subsequently removed for carcinoma. Results of such retrospective studies have generally tended to support such a relationship, although their statistical validity, because of the obvious sampling difficulties, might be challenged. Nevertheless, Foote and Stewart[176] found that 2.5% of 1200 patients with breast cancer had a previous biopsy revealing benign disease, whereas only 1.1% of 120 patients with cancer elsewhere had a previous breast biopsy that revealed benign disease. Black and associates[189] reviewed the breast biopsies obtained years previously from

93 patients with cancer, and found that an appreciable number had *in situ* cancer or "precancerous mastopathy," although the original diagnosis rendered was only that of fibrocystic disease.

Prospective studies, which might be regarded as the most appropriate type of inquiry into this relationship, have yielded the greatest dichotomy of conclusions. On the one hand, some[10,190–193] have failed to note any unusually high incidence of carcinoma developing in breasts that had been the site of previous biopsy for benign fibrocystic disease in patients followed from 5 to as long as 18 years. Indeed, Devitt[190] claims that there is no need for any special vigilance in patients with fibrocystic disease. Others[194–199] note a two to seven times greater frequency of cancer arising in breasts with previous evidence of fibrocystic disease. It does appear noteworthy that many of the investigators subscribing to the view relating fibrocystic disease to cancer of the breast emphasize the significance of the proliferative form in this regard. One suspects that much of the divergent findings may be related to the lack of distinction between the obviously more common cystic type of mammary dysplasia and that characterized by proliferation of ductal and ductular epithelium, variably designated as epitheliosis or papillomatosis. Several studies have been made concerning the association of the various forms of fibrocystic disease with cancer. Foote and Stewart,[176] as well as Humphrey and Swerdlow[177] and Kern and Brooks,[179] found duct papillomatosis, particularly that with atypical features, more common in apparently uninvolved tissue of breasts with cancer than in breast tissue removed for benign fibrocystic disease. Further, sclerosing adenosis, apocrine metaplasia, and lobular hyperplasia were more common in benign fibrocystic disease.

Lobular hyperplasia should also be included as a form of proliferative fibrocystic disease, since it appears to represent the lobular analogue of papillomatosis of larger ducts. The term "papillomatosis" is synonymous with the designation of "epitheliosis" of British investigators, and signifies intraductal collections of epithelial cells arranged in solid cribriform or papillary configurations. The papillary form is distinguished from intraductal papillomas by the location of the latter in the larger ducts, as well as the dense, hyalinized fibrovascular stalk often present in their arborizations. It is to be noted that the premalignant potential of the intraductal papilloma is dubious,[84] yet some investigators do not make any distinction between this lesion and papillomatosis. Utilizing these criteria, we found only a negligible incidence of intraductal papillomas in the vicinity of the dominant mass of 1000 cancers. Although this information might be considered to refute the views of those[61,193,198] who indicate a histogenetic relationship between proliferative fibrocystic disease and intraductal papillomas, it is noteworthy that there are striking ultrastructural similarities between the two,[3] which provides at least some morphological support for their common nature.

The possibility that ultrastructural studies of fibrocystic disease might provide information to resolve this problem is apparent. Yet, there has been a relative paucity of electron microscopic studies in this regard. Our own material contained five examples of proliferative fibrocystic disease in which the intraductal and intraductular aggregates appeared by light microscopy to be unequivocally benign. Ultrastructurally, the cells comprising the lesion were variable, but generally resembled either those of the normal gland or the other nonproliferative forms of fibrocystic disease such as sclerosing and blunt-duct adenosis. It is of interest that in the one example of this banal proliferative fibrocystic disease in which chromosome study was performed, karyotypic abnormalities were encountered which were similar to those found in examples of overt cancer[200] (Figs. 22 and 23).

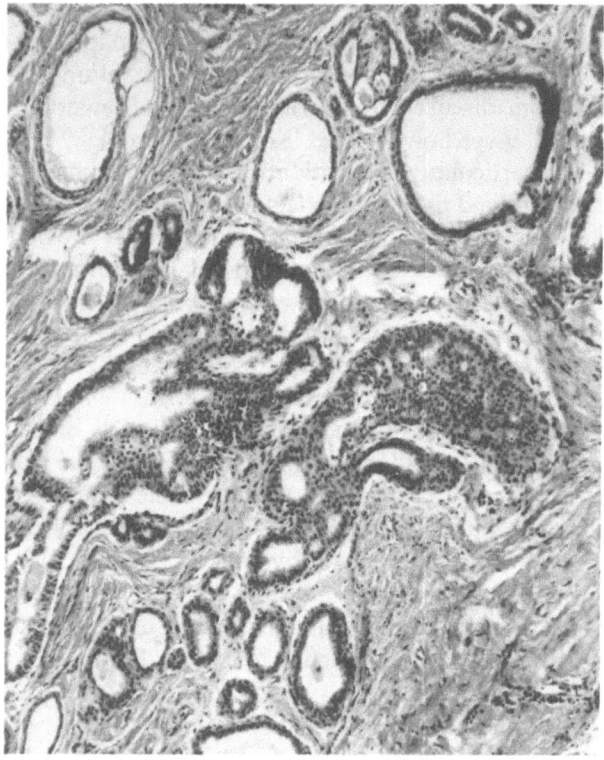

Fig. 22. Focus of relatively banal-appearing proliferative fibrocystic disease. Some non-proliferative foci are also evident. ×100.

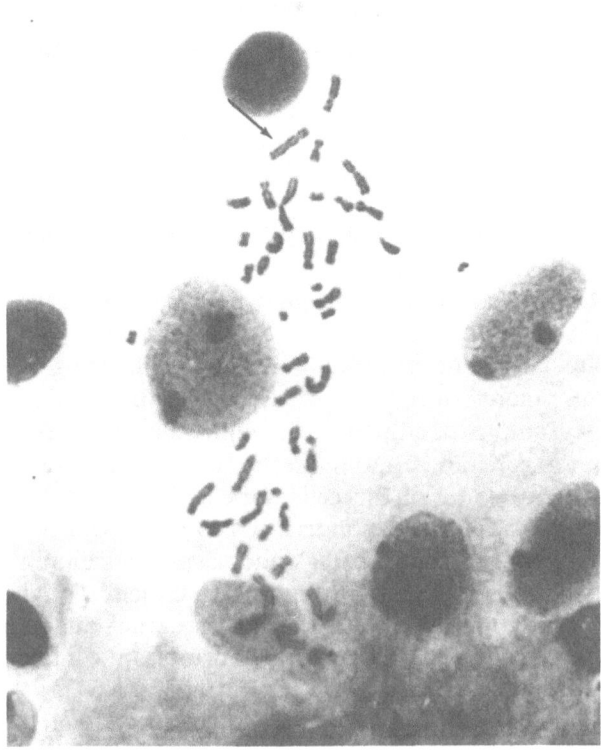

Fig. 23. Chromosomes from a cell of the proliferative fibrocystic disease depicted in Fig. 22. Only 42 chromosomes are present in this instance. A marker form similar to that observed in cultures of cells from overt cancer of the breast is also present (arrow).

There have been a few attempts to ultrastructurally characterize those proliferative intraductal lesions which might be regarded as atypical hyperplasia. Goldenberg and associates,[20] addressing themselves to the distinction between atypical hyperplasia and cancer, reported the presence of giant microvilli on the luminal surface of cells comprising the former. Intracytoplasmic lumens were found only in cells comprising intraductal or invasive cancers. Since such intracytoplasmic lumens were claimed to be found in fibrocystic disease as well as in some normal cells, little diagnostic significance was attributed to this feature, although we have been unimpressed by their presence in such banal situations in our material. The study of Gould and Snyder[16] appears to be most important regarding the diagnostic problem of atypical hyperplasia and intraductal cancer. They compared the features of two examples of subareolar florid papillomatosis, which might be regarded as proliferative fibrocystic disease par excellence, with those of two lesions which by light microscopy also contained foci of carcinoma and with two examples of frank carcinoma of this site. Noteworthy was the presence of myoepithelial cells in all of the tumors. Basal lamina gaps and intracytoplasmic lumens were found in all lesions, but were most frequent in the cancers. Reduplicated basal lamina were more frequent in the papillomatoses.

There were five examples of hyperplastic fibrocystic disease in our material that were regarded by light microscopy as being atypical in that the decision to view the lesion as benign or malignant (i.e., intraductal carcinoma) might be considered somewhat tenuous. In two additional cases, some of the cells—particularly, but not exclusively, those in proximity to the basement membrane—appeared histologically normal, whereas those more centrally disposed were distinctly abnormal. These represented examples of either overt malignant transformation of a duct or extension of carcinoma into it. In the five examples of atypical proliferative change, some of the cells appeared clear with a paucity of organelles. Only a few mitochondria, which were swollen, vacuolated, and irregular, were present. Coarse endoplasmic reticulum was variably dilated, occasionally to cisternal proportions. Other cells exhibited similar changes, but imparted a more dense appearance due to the marked collection of free ribosomal particles. The cytoplasm contained an occasional lipid droplet, centriole, and Golgi structure (Fig. 24). Another cell type was characterized by abundant Golgi vesicles or secretory granules and still another, by the presence of lamellar stacks of narrow lacunae of coarse endoplasmic reticulum. The latter cells appeared to be more frequent near the lumen or central portion of the intraductal aggregates. Plasma membranes were usually interdigitated with desmosomal attachment plates in collections of the normal-appearing cells, whose nuclei were also round or ovoid with a euchromatin pattern. The more atypical cells, for the most part, exhibited simplified cell membranes, although in some, they were frequently thrown into numerous villous folds. Intracytoplasmic lumens per se were uncommon, however. Nuclei of such cells often exhibited many invaginations with coarse clumping of chromatin. In some cells, multinucleated or syncitial forms were noted. Cellular necrosis was recognized and characterized by aggregates of distorted membranes, lipid bodies, and myelin figures. Necrotic foci were noted in individual cells. Surprisingly, cells exhibiting the latter change often exhibited only modest atypia of their nuclei or cytoplasmic organelles.

This same spectrum of ultrastructural change was appreciated in the examples of ducts depicting central cell aggregates that were indisputably recognized as cancer by light microscopy. Again, cells of peripheral portions of these ducts exhibited less profound alteration.

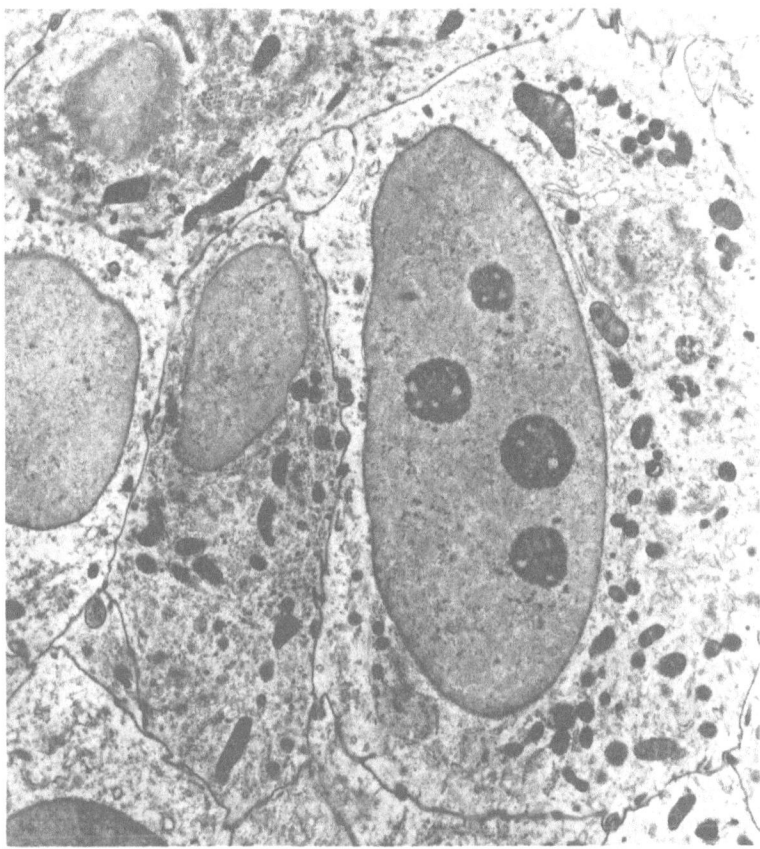

Fig. 24. Electron micrograph of portions of cells comprising atypical proliferative fibrocystic disease. Nuclei are irregular and one contains many large nucleoli. Light and dark forms are present. Mitochondria in some cells are pleomorphic and vary in size. Golgi structures are prominent. These changes approximate those seen in some cancers. ×9000. (Reduced 35% for reproduction.)

Thus, it would appear that the distinction between hyperplasia and cancer is more quantitative than qualitative, a finding analogous to that encountered in the MCA (methylcholanthrene)-induced mammary tumor model in the rat.[201] This information represents strong evidence in support of views indicating the premalignant (malignant?) nature of proliferative fibrocystic disease. It also helps to explain the difficulty in the pathologic distinction between atypical hyperplasia and cancer, and suggests that such delineation may be more pragmatic than real.

17. Noninvasive Cancer in the Vicinity of the Dominant Tumor

Several studies have provided evidence that cancer of the breast may have a relatively wide field of origin.[202-205] Multicentricity in this sense is not to be confused with its use for the designation of those cancers remote from the main mass which appeared to represent independent, *de novo* lesions that do not contribute to its substance. The latter will be discussed under the designation "multicentric cancer" (Section 21). In an attempt to determine if there was any significance to alterations in the breast surrounding the dominant lesion, it was considered worthwhile to note the occurrence of noninvasive cancer. It was obvious that no certain determination could be made as to whether foci of invasive cancer in the vicinity of the main tumor represented evidence of "multicentric" origin or extensions of the tumor proper. On the other hand, the presence of lobular carcinoma *in situ* or intraductal carcinoma in such locations might be more appropriately regarded as representing evidence of the multifocal development of the main tumor mass.

This was found in approximately 40% of cancers examined, and was associated with tumors that were histologically of high grade, stellate, and contained glycogen and calcium, with moderate stroma and necrosis.[2] Noteworthy was the association of noninvasive cancer in the vicinity of the dominant mass with the occurrence of multicentric cancers in remote quadrants. This information tends to support the view noted above that relates such change to the multifocal origin of mammary cancer. Clinically, and pathologically, patients with tumors exhibiting an intraductal component in their vicinity were distinguished as having axillary nodal involvement.

18. Lymphatic Invasion

Although it has long been recognized that mammary cancer exhibits a predilection for lymph nodal metastases, little attention has been directed to the phenomenon of lymphatic invasion within the tumor proper. Such extension may be appreciated in one-third of breast cancers and might be regarded as questionable in an additional 23%. The greater frequency of noncircumscribed, larger tumors (4.1+ cm) of high histologic grade and the NOS type, blood vessel and perineural space invasion, and nipple involvement in the presence of lymphatic extension strongly implicates the latter as an unfavorable pathologic finding in mammary cancer.

19. Blood Vessel Invasion

There have been relatively few reports concerning the incidence and possible significance of blood vessel invasion in mammary carcinoma. Those that are extant appear to originate from one or two groups of investigators, although the material apparently was derived from several sources. Results of such investigations reveal the incidence of such an event to vary from 21 to 46%.[206-209] Some of this divergence appears related to the cases studied. In some, only examples of one clinical stage were selected, whereas in others, no mention of this factor is made. Nevertheless, recognition of such vascular involvement has been claimed to adversely affect survival rates. In this regard, it is interesting to note that in at least one of the studies, blood vessel invasion was prognostically significant only in the presence of nodal metastases, whereas in others, significance was encountered only when such metastases were absent. It is our impression that the incidence of blood vessel invasion cited above is inordinately high. In our own material, this phenomenon was encountered in only 5% of the cases.[2] This appears to be due in large part to the difficulty in distinguishing intravascular extension from intraductal involvement by neoplasm. Recourse to elastic-tissue stains for the assessment of blood vessel invasion, although advisable (if not mandatory) with tumors in other organs, may be misleading in studies of the breast, since the larger ductal structures of this organ also contain a relatively marked mantle of elastic fibers. Blood vessel invasion has been noted to be associated with a significantly greater frequency of a severe cell reaction in the tumor; lymphatic invasion; metastases in four or more axillary nodes; and tumors with marked necrosis, slight elastica and stroma, slight or moderate amounts of mucin, and nuclear grades of 1, but, surprisingly, not with short-term treatment failure.[2]

20. Perineural Space Invasion

Although extension of mammary carcinoma into perineural spaces is well recognized, little information is available concerning its significance or association with other pathologic features. In some organs, such as salivary glands, demonstration of perineural extension is often useful in establishing the malignancy of such well-differentiated carcinomas as the cylindromatous or adenocystic types. In other sites, such as the prostate, this feature may have some diagnostic value, although its significance in this regard, as well as its relationship to prognosis, is not as meaningful as had been once considered.[210]

Perineural extension may occur in as high as 28% of breast cancers, and has been noted to be associated with lymphatic invasion, nipple involvement, and metastases in axillary lymph nodes.

21. Multicentric Cancer and Changes in Quadrants Remote from the Primary Tumor

That many, if not all, breast cancers may be multicentric in origin has been noted previously. Most early studies in this regard appeared to be more concerned with establishing the concept of such multicentricity of the dominant mass, rather than with the occurrence of foci of cancers in quadrants remote from the main lesion. One of the earliest studies addressing itself to this problem was that of Qualheim and Gall,[211] who noted an incidence of cancers in 35% of cases studied pathologically by the total-mount technique in areas that they termed opposite to that of the main mass. Subsequent studies,[164,165,186,203,212,213] with or without specimen mammography, have indicated the incidence of such independent foci of cancer to vary from 0.9 to at least 26.5%. Although Gallager and Martin[203] found areas of atypical hyperplasia and/or cancer in regions near to or remote from the dominant lesion in three-fourths of 34 cases, it is difficult to be certain how many multicentric, independent cancers might have been present, since no clear distinction as to actual site or pathologic type of lesion encountered was provided.

Our own study of this problem revealed a 13.4% incidence of cancer in quadrants remote from the dominant mass. Approximately three-fourths of these were of noninvasive type (i.e., lobular carcinoma *in situ* and intraductal carcinoma). In approximately 12% of the cases of the entire series studied, multiple multicentric cancers were noted. Since these findings were derived from only one random block of the quadrants remote from and excluding that of the dominant mass, it is apparent that such estimates are conservative.

Multicentric cancers were significantly associated with grossly noncircumscribed primary tumors; the presence of nipple involvement; a moderate or marked intraductal component in the primary tumor; noninvasive cancer in the vicinity of the primary tumor; and tumors whose maximum diameters were greater than 4.1 cm. These independent, multicentric cancers were also found to be more frequently associated with proliferative (67.8%), rather than nonproliferative (22.3%), fibrocystic disease in the quadrants harboring them.

Examination of remote quadrants also disclosed the presence of lymphatic tumor emboli in 2% of all cases of breast cancer. This was most prevalent in lesions located beneath the nipple; in 27.8%, it was observed in two quadrants and in 5.6%, it was noted in three. The presence of quadrant lymphatic extension of the primary tumor has received little attention in considerations of the multicentricity of breast cancer. Its detection might be regarded as perhaps even more significant than that of the noninvasive *de novo* cancers insofar as prognosis is concerned, since such emboli may be considered to represent potential metastases. On the other hand, some doubt exists concerning the clinical significance of the foci of noninvasive cancers uncovered in the quadrants remote from the primary lesion.[214] This view appears to be substantiated by noting that in the presence of such tumor emboli, there was a greater likelihood of clinical, as well as pathologic, nodal metastases; the occurrence of blood vessel and lymphatic invasion within the primary tumor; and short-term treatment failure.

It would appear, at least at present, incommodious to consider such procedures as segmental resection for the surgical treatment of large, unencapsulated tumors that exhibit a moderate or marked intraductal component and noninvasive cancer in their vicinity as well as nipple involvement. This opinion has been expressed in a previous report by us[215] concerning multicentric breast cancer.

22. Nipple Involvement

Although retraction and, less frequently, discharge or erosion of the nipple are well-recognized clinical features of mammary cancer, relatively little attention has been directed to the pathologic involvement of this structure, save that which occurs in Paget's disease. As noted previously, the *sine qua non* of the latter is the presence of neoplastic cells within the epidermis of the nipple. Nipple involvement occurs in approximately 12% of all cases of mammary cancer and is manifest as epidermal involvement or Paget's disease in about 2.5%. Epidermal involvement is encountered only when the lymphatics or ducts of this structure are also involved. In the prescence of nipple involvement, there is a greater likelihood that the primary tumor within the breast is not grossly or microscopically circumscribed; it has a moderate or marked intraductal component of papillary or comedo type and a moderate stromal component, and exhibits lymphatic and perineural extension and a slight/moderate cell reaction.[2] The tumors are large, measuring greater than 4.1 cm. As might be expected, the primary tumors are most frequently located beneath the nipple. Nipple involvement is also associated with metastases in four or more lymph nodes and with the presence of multicentric cancer.[2] The most frequent histologic types accompanying nipple extension are the NOS, NOS + tubular, medullary, and mucinous carcinomas. The relationships between the latter two types, whose prognosis is purportedly favorable, and nipple involvement are surprising, particularly in light of the association between nipple involvement and the occurrence of short-term treatment failure.

23. Relationship of Florid Papillomatosis of the Nipple to Cancer

In 1955, Jones[216] called attention to a benign papillary lesion of the nipple ducts which clinically mimicked Paget's disease. Pathologically, the lesion exhibited a florid papillomatous and adenomatous pattern. He regarded the heterogeneity of cell types comprising the lesion, i.e., columnar, polygonal, and cuboidal, to represent its major distinguishing feature from ductal cancers. One of the six cases presented was associated with an apparently independent cancer of the underlying breast tissue. Subsequent reports attested to the benign nature of florid papillomatosis of the nipple ducts.[217-219] Doctor and Sirsat[220] concluded from their study that florid papillomatosis or adenoma of the nipple represented two distinct lesions, the former related to fibrocystic disease and the latter, with its adenomatous pattern, to sweat gland tumors. More recently, Bhagavan and associates,[221] who utilized the designations "papillomatosis" and "adenoma" synonymously, reported two cases which they considered to represent examples of malignant transformation of the benign lesion. In another case, as also noted by Jones[216] and others,[61,217,222] the lesion was associated with an independent cancer of the breast. This, as well as another instance of cancer arising within areas of florid papillomatosis,[223] contradicts the impression of its universally benign nature. Such malignant potential, however, must be exceedingly low, certainly less than its association with independent cancers presenting as dominant masses. In our experience, about 1% of the nipples from breasts with invasive cancer exhibit florid papillomatosis. This relatively high incidence of florid papillomatosis of the nipple indicates that this lesion at least pathologically occurs in association with cancer with greater frequency than has been previously suspected. In this regard, it appears analogous to the frequent association of proliferative fibrocystic disease (which it well may represent) and

cancer of the breast. Its recognition would seem to warrant close evaluation of the underlying breast tissue for carcinomatous change.

24. Involvement of Skin over the Tumor

In the discussion of histologic types of mammary cancer, no mention was made of so-called "inflammatory carcinoma." This appelation
reflects the *clinical* features of an enlarged, tender, warm, and
erythematous breast harboring a cancer that is usually poorly delineated. Contrary to the misconceptions of some, pathologic examination fails to disclose evidence of an inflammatory reaction, but does
reveal extensive lymphatic extension within the neoplasm which is otherwise without distinguishing features. The inflammatory manifestations have been attributed to the blockage of these lymphatic spaces.[10]
Some have regarded this form of mammary cancer as incurable,[10,224-226]
whereas others[227,228] note some patients who have survived their disease for at least five years. Recently, Ellis and Teitelbaum[229] have
clarified this apparent dichotomy. They reviewed material from many of
the patients who appeared free of disease five years following mastectomy and observed that none exhibited infiltration of the dermal lymphatics, whereas this change was encountered in those not surviving
their disease. Because of this, they suggested that the term "inflammatory carcinoma" be discarded in preference to the designation "dermal
lymphatic carcinomatosis" of the breast. Yet, not all patients with dermal lymphatic invasion exhibit the clinical manifestations of inflammatory carcinoma and, as noted above, not all of the latter exhibit such
cutaneous involvement. It would appear from their investigation that
examination of the skin would represent an important feature of the
pathologic examination of the breast with carcinoma, at least from a
prognostic standpoint. Unfortunately, this aspect of the examination is
not too frequently undertaken.

Cutaneous involvement may be encountered in about 4.5% of
cases. This may occur as involvement of lymphatics alone or in combination with the dermis and epidermis. We have not observed the epidermis as the only site of such skin involvement. In the presence of skin
involvement (all types), there is a greater likelihood that the tumor is
beneath the nipple or in the subareolar area, with involvement of this
structure. There is also a statistically significant incidence of squamous
metaplasia and large dominant masses measuring ≥4.1 cm. A significant
association with invasive multicentric cancers and short-term treatment
failure has also been encountered.[2] The latter can be attributed to the

lymphatic involvement of the skin, since only it was associated with short-term treatment failure or recurrence. This finding is in accord with the views expressed above by Ellis and Teitelbaum[229] concerning the significance of this feature in inflammatory cancer.

25. Alterations of Regional Lymph Nodes in Breast Cancer

There is accumulating evidence in experimental systems as well as in humans that indicates that the regional lymph nodes are essential for the initiation as well as maintenance of tumor immunity.[230-233] Lymph nodes draining tumors in syngeneic experimental systems reveal a marked response of pyroninophilic cells (immunoblasts) as early as 3 days following tumor implantation, with a maximal reaction at 7 to 14 days, at which time tumor immunity may be demonstrated.[234] Although lymph follicle formation and sinus histiocytosis are not a conspicuous part of the morphological expression of such immunity in the regional nodes, they are encountered to some degree in those of nonregional sites.[234]

A variety of nodal changes may be encountered in the axillary lymph nodes of women harboring breast cancer. Lymph follicle formation has been observed in association with tumors of low nuclear grade and mild lymphoid infiltrates, and its absence noted in tumors of high nuclear grade with a marked cell reaction.[143] Regional nodes draining mammary cancers exhibit transformation of their lymphoid elements with or without stimulation with phytohemagglutinin.[235] It is of interest that the uptake of tritiated thymidine by nodal cells has been noted to be significantly greater in those cells from the lower levels of the axilla than in those from higher or apical regions.[236] It has been suggested that the high nodes are more closely related functionally to distant or nonregional nodes, and that those of low axillary position more dynamically reflect a response to tumor antigen. Yet, there does not appear to be any significant difference in the presence of lymph follicle formation or sinus histiocytosis in nodes from these various levels. The observations of Berg and associates[237] are of interest in this regard. They found prognosis to be better when there was sinus histiocytosis and/or prominent germinal centers in apical nodes. This was considered important in accounting for the observations relating better survival when apical nodes were enlarged, but not replaced by cancer despite other axillary metastases, than if they were small or undetectable.

Rarer reactions encountered in regional nodes draining mammary cancers are the presence of sarcoid-like granulomas and foci of hyalinization.[238] Hamlin[124] failed to note any relationship between nodal scarring and survival.

25.1. Sinus Histiocytosis

Due to the efforts of Black and associates,[117,119,120,136–138] most attention has been directed to the occurrence and significance of sinus histiocytosis in axillary nodes draining mammary cancers. These investigators, as well as others,[124,238–240] have observed a more or less direct relationship between the intensity of this nodal response and survival. All have considered this reaction to represent a manifestation of the host response, vis-à-vis immunologic reaction, to tumor growth. On the other hand, several investigators[122,241,242] have failed to find any correlation

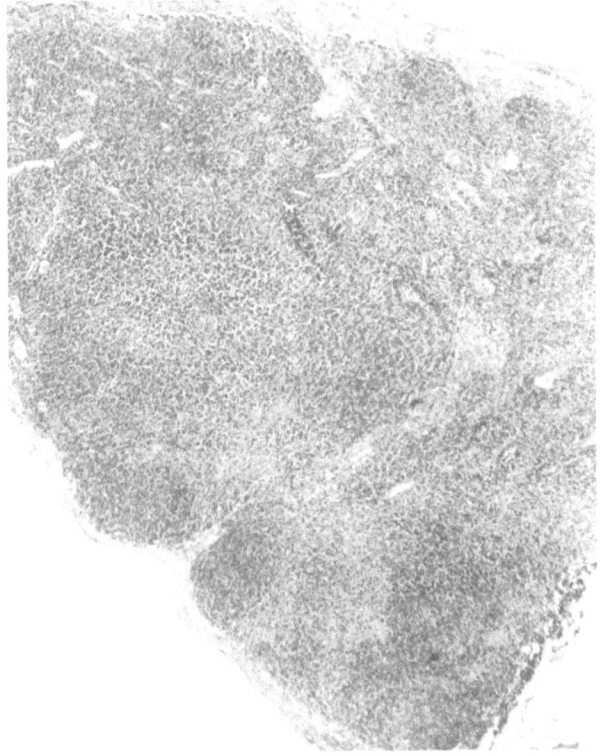

Fig. 25. Axillary lymph node from a patient with breast cancer revealing a dense cortical and paracortical population of lymphoid elements characteristic of the lymphocyte predominance pattern. No sinus histiocytosis is present. ×40.

between sinus histiocytosis and survival in breast cancer. Silverberg and associates[243] concluded that sinus histiocytosis is a valuable prognostic indicator only when other factors that might be considered as significant in this regard are inconclusive. Thus, they found assessment of sinus histiocytosis to be of little prognostic value with well-differentiated tumors or when nodal metastases were absent or many nodes were involved. On the other hand, the presence of sinus histiocytosis suggested an improved survival for those individuals whose tumors exhibited moderate or poor differentiation, or when nodal metastases were only moderate in number. DiRe and Lane[244] found its assessment to be of value only in tumors with irregular borders. It is of interest that the cells comprising sinus histiocytosis ultrastructurally resemble common macrophages, rather than so-called immunoblastic elements.[234] Further, from a functional standpoint, no relationship between this phenomenon and lymphocyte transformation of nodal cells has been recognized.[143]

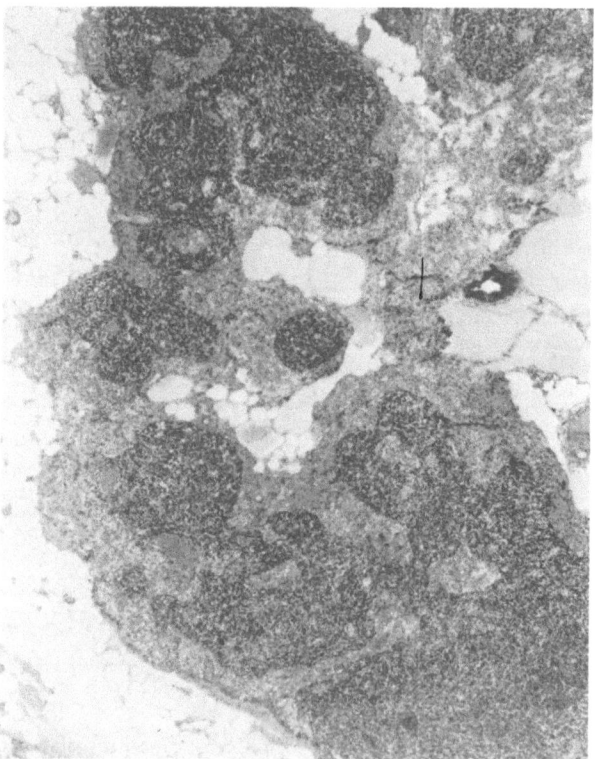

Fig. 26. Axillary lymph node from a patient with breast cancer revealing the so-called unstimulated pattern accompanied by marked sinus histiocytosis. ×40.

Nevertheless, we have noted the presence of marked sinus histiocytosis (Figs. 25 and 26) to be consistently associated with pathologically, but not clinically, negative axillary nodes, as well as with squamous metaplasia and calcium in the tumors that were of intermediate size (2.1–4 cm); necrosis and mucin content of the tumors were slight. When sinus histiocytosis was absent, there was a greater likelihood that four or more nodes contained metastases, necrosis and mucin were absent, and the tumors were large, measuring ≥4.1 cm. The inconsistent relationship of sinus histiocytosis to necrosis tends to minimize this as a causal factor in its pathogenesis. However, there does appear to be a consistently inverse relationship between the degree of sinus histiocytosis and the incidence of nodal metastases. A relationship between the absence of sinus histiocytosis and short-term treatment failure was also noted.[2]

25.2. Significance of Regional Node Histology Other Than Sinus Histiocytosis

Tsakraklides and associates[245] have recently correlated five- and ten-year survival in a group of 227 women with breast cancer with nodal morphological features other than sinus histiocytosis which are considered to reflect immunologic function. Lymph nodes exhibiting lymphocyte predominance (Fig. 25) were associated with high survival, whereas those with lymphocyte depletion, a poor prognosis. Predominance of germinal centers or an unstimulated pattern (Fig. 26) was found in those with intermediate survival. It appears pertinent to note that the retrospective study included patients who received a variety of treatment modalities in addition to radical mastectomy.

The results of our own study of these nodal patterns disclosed differences from those reported previously by Tsakraklides and associates[245] concerning their incidence as well as significance. Our material disclosed a slightly greater (17%) frequency of the lymphocyte predominance pattern and lesser (12%) incidence of the unstimulated appearance than reported by these investigators. Although a few nodes were encountered with features of lymphocyte depletion, in no instance did such nodes represent the majority of change for any particular case. Tsakraklides and associates[245] observed a 4% incidence of lymphocyte depletion. We have no certain explanation for this dichotomy, yet it does appear pertinent to consider the possibility that the variety of treatment modalities in addition to radical mastectomy utilized for the patients in their retrospective study might account for this, as well as the other, differences encountered.

Although Tsakraklides and associates[245] observed a significantly greater overall five- and ten-year survival in patients exhibiting a lymphocyte predominance pattern, our results failed to reveal any relationship between any particular nodal pattern and short-term treatment failure up to and including four years. Whether this lack of association will also be evident with longer periods of observation remains to be demonstrated. Nevertheless, such short-term observations of treatment failure generally reveal discriminants of subsequent significance. In this regard, it is of interest to note that short-term treatment failure for the same group of patients utilized in that study has been noted to be significantly associated with clinically positive axillae, the presence of four or more nodes with metastases, and large ($\geq$4 cm) tumors, all of which, on the basis of past retrospective studies, might be regarded as poor prognostic indices.[2] Analysis of the material failed to reveal any relationship between these parameters and the nodal patterns investigated.[246]

On the other hand, lymphocyte predominance of regional nodes was noted to be significantly associated with tumors comprised of combinations of histologic types, a stellate border, and an absent lymphoid cellular reaction. The latter feature was also shared by tumors associated with nodes that exhibited an unstimulated pattern. This information reaffirms our previous contentions concerning the questionable significance of the cellular infiltrate of the primary tumor as a measure of host immunologic responsiveness,[236] if indeed the lymphocyte predominance pattern signifies activity of a cell-mediated immune response and the unstimulated pattern, a weakly or nonantigenic tumor.[245,247] On the basis of our impressions of the nodes examined, it was not surprising that the lymphocyte and germinal-center predominance patterns were significantly associated with absent sinus histiocytosis, whereas the unstimulated appearance was encountered with the converse or marked sinus histiocytosis. These relationships are paradoxical to the findings of poor prognosis and short-term treatment failure associated with absent sinus histiocytosis, and long-term survival, with a marked degree of such nodal change.[2,117,119,120,136-138] Unlike Tsakraklides and associates,[245] our results also indicated a relationship between the lymphocyte and germinal-center predominance patterns and a patient age of 55 or more years; the unstimulated appearance was encountered in patients between 45 and 54 years of age. This relationship to age cannot be unequivocally construed to represent a possible explanation for the better survival in patients with the lymphocyte predominance pattern noted by Tsakraklides and associates,[245] since no correlations were encountered between these patterns and the younger age group (20–44 years) of patients who purportedly exhibit a poorer prognosis and, in our experience, a greater incidence of short-term treatment failure than individuals aged 55 or more years.[2] The germinal-center pattern was encountered in association with circumscribed tumors with a severe

cellular reaction and not unexpectedly, therefore, of the medullary histologic type. Although this nodal pattern is indicated to be associated
with an intermediate prognosis, a relatively high survival rate for medullary tumors has been repeatedly indicated, and represents another
paradox concerning the relationship of our findings to those recorded by
Tsakraklides and associates.[245]

25.3. Nodal Status

It has been stated that the main route of spread of mammary cancer
is by way of the axilla. Although relatively little is known concerning the
route of vascular dissemination of this neoplasm, certainly this view is
acceptable at least insofar as lymph nodal involvement is concerned. The
significance of the latter as a prognostic discriminant has been repeatedly emphasized. The presence or absence of palpable lymph nodes
within the ipsilateral axilla represents one of the important criteria
utilized for clinical staging. Bloom[111] and Wolf[113] have indicated that
although histologic grading of the malignancy of the cancer and clinical
staging are comparable from the prognostic standpoint, a more accurate
prediction in this regard may be obtained when both are considered.
Bloom also indicated that recognition of the histologic grade might help
to account for some of the unexpected survival periods exhibited by
some patients (i.e., unfavorable clinical stage but a well-differentiated
tumor). On the other hand, others[115] have failed to find any correlation
between nodal status and histologic features of the neoplasm. Cutler
and Myers[248] noted a better prognosis for individuals whose nodes
were clinically regarded as positive but proved to be negative after
pathologic examination, particularly if the contralateral axillary nodes
were also palpable. The uninvolved, large nodes were regarded as a host
response to the tumor. However, Champion and associates[115] found
that a bad prognosis was present in all patients with pathologically
proven nodal metastases, regardless of clinical assessment. They regarded the relatively poor prognosis of patients with clinically palpable
nodes to be due to the higher incidence of nodal metastases in such
enlarged nodes. In this regard, Cutler and Myers[248] have noted that
38% of the axillae regarded clinically as negative exhibit metastases
pathologically; a somewhat smaller estimate has been made of the converse, that is, pathologically negative nodes in 35% of the instances in
which the axillae were regarded clinically as positive.[248] More disagreement between the pathologic and clinical evaluation was observed
with large primary tumors and clinically negative axillae than when the
nodal status was clinically regarded as positive and the tumors were
small. In our study, the incidence of false positive and negative evalua-

tions of the axilla was 24% and 39%, respectively. The overall error in clinical staging was 32%. Perusal of findings by others in regard to five-year survival fails to reveal any great differences in rate between patients with pathologically negative nodes and those in whom clinical estimation of such involvement was also negative. This same relationship also applies to patients with positive clinical and pathologic assessment of the nodal status. This information signifies the prognostic utility of clinical staging in breast cancer.

There has long existed some degree of contention between pathologists and surgeons concerning the number of lymph nodes that should or might be recovered from operative specimens. The pathologist is also confronted by the dilemma of practicality on the one hand and theoretical significance on the other in regard to the necessity to determine whether such nodes contain metastatic foci. However, it has been noted that there is a relationship between prognosis and the number, rather than proportion, of positive axillary nodes. Survival was only

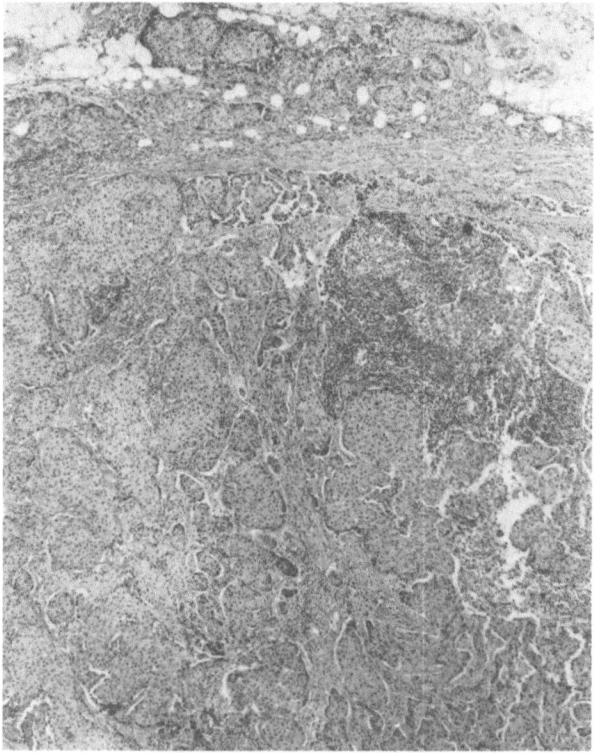

Fig. 27. Extension of metastasis in this axillary lymph node to the perinodal adipose tissue has occurred. ×100.

slightly less when one to three positive nodes were found than if none was present. On the other hand, a marked difference existed when four or more positive nodes were identified.[134]

There are claims relating prognosis to the level of nodal involvement. As generally practiced, Level I is represented by nodes lying below the pectoralis minor muscle, Level II by those within the borders of this structure or beneath it, and Level III by the apical nodes above it. Crude and relative five- and twenty-year survivals have been reported to be inversely proportional to the level of nodal involvement.[66] The prognostic value of involvement of nodes such as those found in the interpectoral region or Rotter's nodes is questionable, at least according to the findings of Kay,[249] who failed to find any relationship between involvement of such structures and survival. A direct relationship between pathologic nodal status and histologic grade has been noted,[118] and indicates that nodal status may be predicted, at least from a statistical standpoint, from the histologic grade of the tumor. No particular

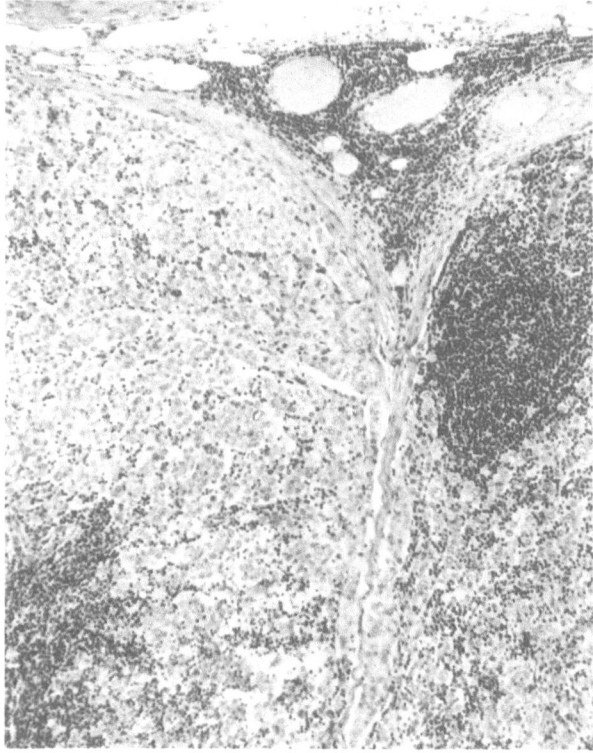

Fig. 28. The metastasis in this axillary lymph node remains within the confines of the node. ×100.

histologic tumor type has been found to be related to the presence or absence of nodal metastases.

25.4. Significance of Extranodal Axillary Metastases

Assessment of axillary nodal metastases according to whether they extend beyond (Fig. 27) or remain within (Fig. 28) the confines of the node appears to represent a useful pathologic discriminant.[250] A statistically significant association ($P < .05$) was revealed between extranodal extension of such metastases and short-term treatment failure, as well as the presence of four or more involved nodes, infiltrating ductal NOS histologic tumor type, stellate tumor border, and nipple involvement. When the metastases were confined to the node, there was a significantly greater likelihood that the cancers were either medullary or tubular histologic types. Associations with severe cell reaction and a nuclear grade of 1 were also noted, but appear to reflect the high frequency of medullary carcinoma in this group.

26. Multiple Cancers (Dominant Masses) in the Same Breast

The occurrence of two distinct carcinomas presenting as dominant masses in the same breast is unusual. Most of the few examples recorded are instances in which one of the tumors represented a cancer arising in a fibroadenoma.[94,251,252] We have observed two patients with two clinically, as well as pathologically, distinct cancers in the same breast in 1667 cases reviewed (0.1%).

27. References

1. M.R. Alderson, I. Hamlin, and M.D. Staunton, The relative significance of prognostic factors in breast carcinoma, *Br. J. Cancer* **25**, 646–656 (1971).
2. E.R. Fisher, R.M. Gregorio, and B. Fisher, The pathology of invasive breast cancer. A syllabus derived from findings of the National Surgical Adjuvant Breast Project (Protocol No. 4), *Cancer* **36**, 1–85 (1975).
3. E.R. Fisher, Ultrastructure of human breast and its disorders, *Am. J. Clin. Pathol.* **66**, 291–375 (1976).
4. J.M. Budinger, A pathologist views diagnosis and prognosis of carcinoma of the breast, *Radiology* **83**, 255–262 (1964).
5. H.R. Butcher, Jr., Effectiveness of radical mastectomy for mammary cancer—An analysis of mortalities by the method of probits, *Ann. Surg.* **154**, 383–396 (1961).
6. W.M. Christopherson, Prognosis of breast cancer based on pathologic type, *Cancer* **24**, 1179–1181 (1969).
7. R.V.P. Hutter, The pathologist's role in minimal breast cancer, *Cancer* **28**, 1527–1536 (1971).

8. C.M. Perez-Mesa, Pathology of mammary carcinoma, *Major Probl. Clin. Surg.* **5**, 70–87 (1967).

9. S. Tomic, S. Vukcevic, and Z. Vidovic, Histoloski i drugi faktori u prognozi raka dojke i histoloski tip raka dojke i prognoza, *Med. Arh.* **26**, 3–13 (1972).

10. C.D. Haagensen, *Diseases of the Breast*, W.B. Saunders, Philadelphia (1956).

11. K.A. Hultborn and B. Tornberg, Mammary carcinoma—The biologic character of mammary carcinoma studies in 517 cases by a new form of malignancy grading, *Acta Radiol. Diag. Suppl. (Stockholm)* **196**, 1–143 (1960).

12. N.T. Kouchoukos, L.V. Ackerman, and H.R. Butcher, Jr., Prediction of axillary nodal metastases from the morphology of primary mammary carcinomas, *Cancer* **20**, 948–960 (1967).

13. B.O. Maehle and F. Hartveit, Prognostic typing in breast cancer—Further investigation of a necropsy series compared with recent surgical specimens, *J. Clin. Pathol.* **26**, 784–791 (1973).

14. F.W. Stewart, Tumors of the breast, in: Atlas of Tumor Pathology, Armed Forces Institute of Pathology, Washington, D.C. (1950).

15. W. Busch and H.J. Merker, Electronenmikroskopische Untersuchungen an menschlichen Mammacarcinomen, *Virchows Arch. (Pathol. Anat.)* **344**, 356–371 (1967).

16. V.E. Gould and R.W. Snyder, Ultrastructural features of papillomatosis and carcinoma of the nipple ducts. The significance of myoepithelial cells and basal lamina in benign, "questionable" and malignant lesions, *Pathol. Annu.* **9**, 441–469 (1974).

17. F. Haguenau, Le cancer du sein chez la femme. Etude comparative au microscope électronique et au microscope optique, *Bull. Cancer (Paris)* **46**, 177–211 (1959).

18. L. Ozzello, Ultrastructure of the human mammary gland, *Pathol. Annu.* **6**, 1–59 (1971).

19. A. Schafer and R. Bassler, Vergleichende elektronen-mikroskopische Untersuchungen am Drusenepithel und am sog. lobularen Carcinom der Mamma, *Virchows Arch. (Pathol. Anat.)* **346**, 269–286 (1969).

20. V.E. Goldenberg, N.S. Goldenberg, and S.C. Sommers, Comparative ultrastructure of atypical ductal hyperplasia, intraductal carcinoma, and infiltrating ductal carcinoma of the breast, *Cancer* **24**, 1152–1169 (1969).

21. S.W. Wellings and P. Roberts, Electron microscopy of sclerosing adenosis and infiltrating duct carcinoma of the human mammary gland, *J. Natl. Cancer Inst.* **30**, 269–287 (1963).

22. T.M. Murad and D.G. Scarpelli, The ultrastructure of medullary and scirrhous mammary duct carcinoma, *Am. J. Pathol.* **50**, 335–360 (1967).

23. A.A. Barton, An electron microscope study of human breast cells in fibroadenosis and carcinoma, *Br. J. Cancer* **18**, 682–685 (1964).

24. T.M. Murad and E. von Haam, Ultrastructure of myoepithelial cells in human mammary gland tumors, *Cancer* **21**, 1137–1149 (1968).

25. A. Ahmed, The myoepithelium in human breast carcinoma, *J. Pathol.* **113**, 129–135 (1974).

26. W. Busch, Elektronenmikroskopische Untersuchungen an der Tumor-Bindegewebs-grenze beim Mammacarcinom der Frau, *Virchows Arch. (Pathol. Anat.)* **346**, 15–28 (1969).

27. A.A. Shivas and A.Mackenzie, The origins of stromal reaction in breast carcinoma, *J. R. Coll. Surg. Edinburgh* **19**, 345–350 (1974).

28. O.S. Moore and F.W. Foote, Jr., The relatively favorable prognosis of medullary carcinoma of the breast, *Cancer* **2**, 635–642 (1949).

29. C.F. Geschickter, *Disease of the Breast—Diagnosis, Pathology, Treatment*, 2nd ed., J.B. Lippincott, Philadelphia (1945).

30. H.J.G. Bloom, W.W. Richardson, and J.R. Field, Host resistance and survival in carcinoma of breast—Study of 104 cases of medullary carcinoma in a series of 1411 cases of breast cancer followed for 20 years, Br. Med. J. **3**, 181–188 (1970).

31. W.W. Richardson, Medullary carcinoma of the breast—A distinctive tumour type with a relatively good prognosis following radical mastectomy, Br. J. Cancer **10**, 415–423 (1956).

32. V.E. Gould, J. Miller, and W. Jao, Ultrastructure of medullary, intraductal, tubular and adenocystic breast carcinomas; comparative patterns of myoepithelial differentiation and basal lamina deposition, Am. J. Pathol. **78**, 401–407 (1975).

33. E.R. Fisher and B. Fisher, Local lymphoid response as an index of tumor immunity, Arch. Pathol. **94**, 136–146 (1972).

34. F.W. Foote, Jr. and F.W. Stewart, Lobular carcinoma in situ—A rare form of mammary cancer, Am. J. Pathol. **17**, 491–496 (1941).

35. R. Muir, The evolution of carcinoma of the mamma, J. Pathol. Bacteriol. **52**, 155–172 (1941).

36. J.R. Benfield, M. Jacobson, and N.E. Warner, In situ lobular carcinoma of the breast, Arch. Surg. **91**, 130–135 (1965).

37. J.T. Godwin, Chronology of lobular carcinoma of the breast—Report of a case, Cancer **5**, 259–266 (1952).

38. R.W. McDivitt, R.V. Hutter, F.W. Foote, Jr., and F.W. Stewart, In situ lobular carcinoma—A prospective follow-up study indicating cumulative patient risks, J. Am. Med. Assoc. **201**, 82–86 (1967).

39. H.W. Miller, Jr. and S. Kay, Infiltrating lobular carcinoma of the female mammary gland, Surg. Gynecol. Obstet. **102**, 661–667 (1956).

40. W. Newman, Lobular carcinoma of the female breast, Ann. Surg. **164**, 305–314 (1966).

41. R.E. Fechner, Infiltrating lobular carcinoma without lobular carcinoma in situ, Cancer **29**, 1539–1545 (1972).

42. R. Ashikari, A.G. Huvos, J.A. Urban, and G.F. Robbins, Infiltrating lobular carcinoma of the breast, Cancer **31**, 110–116 (1973).

43. J.P. Barnes, Bilateral lobular carcinoma in situ of the breast, Tex. Med. **55**, 581–584 (1959).

44. G.F. Robbins and J.W. Berg, Bilateral primary breast cancer—A prospective clinicopathological study, Cancer **17**, 1501–1527 (1964).

45. D. Carter, J.H. Yardley, and W.M. Shelley, Lobular carcinoma of the breast. An ultrastructural comparison with certain duct carcinomas and benign lesions, Johns Hopkins Med. J. **125**, 25–32 (1969).

46. T.M. Murad, Ultrastructure of ductular carcinoma of the breast (in situ and infiltrating lobular carcinoma), Cancer **27**, 18–28 (1971).

47. L. Ozzello, Ultrastructure of intra-epithelial carcinomas of the breast, Cancer **28**, 1508–1515 (1971).

48. H. Tobon and H.M. Price, Lobular carcinoma in situ. Some ultrastructural observations, Cancer **30**, 1082–1091 (1972).

49. J. Kermarec, S. Plouvier, H. Duplay, and R. Daniel, Tumeur mammaire à cellules myo-épitheliales. Etude ultrastructurale, Arch. Anat. Pathol. (Paris) **21**, 225–231 (1973).

50. H.J. Norris and H.B. Taylor, Prognosis of mucinous (gelatinous) carcinoma of the breast, Cancer **18**, 879–885 (1965).

51. S.G. Silverberg, S. Kay, A.R. Chitale, and S.H. Levitt, Colloid carcinoma of the breast, Am. J. Clin. Pathol. **55**, 355–363 (1971).

52. C.F. Geschickter, Gelatinous mammary cancer, Ann. Surg. **108**, 321–⌐⌐6 (1938).

53. M.R. Melamed, G.F. Robbins, and F.W. Foote, Jr. Prognostic significance of gelatinous mammary carcinoma, Cancer **14**, 699–704 (1961).

54. W.C. Johnson and E.B. Helwig, Histochemistry of primary and metastatic mucus-secreting tumors, *Ann. N.Y. Acad. Sci.* **106,** 794–803 (1953).

55. S.S. Spicer, R.D. Neubecker, L. Warren, and J.G. Henson, Epithelial mucins in lesions of the human breast, *J. Natl. Cancer Inst.* **29,** 963–975 (1962).

56. C.M. Gros and J. Girardi, Aspect histochimique et ultrastructure d'un cancer muci-pare mammaire chez la femme, *Bull. Cancer* **54,** 225–246 (1967).

57. J.A. Sykes, L. Recher, P.H. Jernstrom, and J. Whitescarver, Morphological investigation of human breast cancer, *J. Natl. Cancer Inst.* **40,** 195–223 (1968).

58. M. Tellem, A. Nedwich, P.S. Amenta, and J.E. Imbriglia, Mucin-producing carcinoma of the breast. Tissue culture, histochemical and electron microscopic study, *Cancer* **19,** 573–584 (1966).

59. E.R. Fisher and D.A. Sharkey, The ultrastructure of colonic polyps and cancer with special reference to the epithelial inclusion bodies of leuchtenberger, *Cancer* **15,** 160–170 (1962).

60. H.B. Taylor and H.J. Norris, Well-differentiated carcinoma of the breast, *Cancer* **25,** 687–692 (1970).

61. R.W. McDivitt, F.W. Stewart, and J.W. Berg, Tumors of the breast, in: Atlas of Tumor Pathology, Armed Forces Institute of Pathology, Washington, D.C. (1968).

62. P.H.B. Carstens, A.G. Huvos, F.W. Foote, Jr., and R. Ashikari, Tubular carcinoma of the breast—A clinicopathologic study of 35 cases, *Am. J. Clin. Pathol.* **58,** 231–238 (1972).

63. R.A. Erlandson and P.H.B. Carstens, Ultrastructure of tubular carcinoma of the breast, *Cancer* **29,** 987–995 (1972).

64. C.V. Ramos and H.B. Taylor, Lipid-rich carcinoma of the breast. A clinicopathologic analysis of 13 examples, *Cancer* **33,** 812–819 (1974).

65. L.V. Ackerman, *Surgical Pathology,* 4th ed., C.V. Mosby, St. Louis, (1968).

66. H. Cammoun, G. Contesso, and J. Rouesse, Les adénocarcinomes cylindromateaux de sein, *Ann. Anat. Pathol. (Paris)* **17,** 143–154 (1972).

67. B. Friedman and H.A. Oberman, Adenoid cystic carcinoma of the breast, *Am. J. Clin. Pathol.* **54,** 1–14 (1970).

68. J.R. Galloway, L.B. Wooner, and O.T. Clagett, Adenoid cystic carcinoma of the breast, *Surg. Gynecol. Obstet.* **122,** 1289–1294 (1966).

69. L.E. Groshong, Adenocystic carcinoma of the breast, *Arch. Surg.* **92,** 424–427 (1966).

70. J.A. Hayes and V. Brooks, Adenoid cystic carcinoma of the breast, *Arch. Surg.* **94,** 134–145 (1967).

71. C.A. Schulenburg and W.J. Pepler, Adenoid cystic carcinoma of the breast, *Br. J. Surg.* **56,** 395–396 (1969).

72. B. Elsner, Adenoid cystic carcinoma of the breast—Review of the literature and clinico-pathologic study of seven patients, *Pathol. Eur.* **5,** 357–364 (1970).

73. H.R. Nayer, Cylindroma of the breast with pulmonary metastases, *Dis. Chest* **31,** 324–327 (1957).

74. R.T. O'Kell, Adenoid cystic carcinoma of the breast, *Mo. Med.* **61,** 855–858 (1964).

75. W.B. Wilson and J.P. Spell, Adenoid cystic carcinoma of the breast—A case with recurrence and regional metastasis, *Ann. Surg.* **166,** 861–864 (1967).

76. R.R. Verani and J. Van der Bel-Kahn, Mammary adenoid cystic carcinoma with unusual features, *Am. J. Clin. Pathol.* **59,** 653–658 (1973).

77. F.J. Cavanzo and H.B. Taylor, Adenoid cystic carcinoma of the breast—An analysis of 21 cases, *Cancer* **24,** 740–745 (1969).

78. H.J.G. Bloom, The role of histology in the treatment of breast cancer, *Br. J. Radiol.* **29,** 488–497 (1956).

79. I.C. Tough, D.C. Carter, J. Fraser, and J. Bruce, Histological grading in breast cancer, *Br. J. Cancer* **23**, 294–301 (1969).
80. L.G. Koss, C.D. Brannan, and R. Ashikari, Histologic and ultrastructural features of adenoid cystic carcinoma of the breast, *Cancer* **26**, 1271–1279 (1970).
81. M.B. Dockerty, The grading and typing of carcinoma of the breast, *J. Iowa Med. Soc.* **54**, 289–294 (1964).
82. D. Hart, Intracystic papillomatous tumors of the breast, benign and malignant, *Arch. Surg.* **14**, 793–835 (1927).
83. C. Huggins, G. Briziarelli, and H. Sutton, Jr., Rapid induction of mammary carcinoma in the rat and the influence of hormones on the tumors, *J. Exp. Med.* **109**, 25–42 (1959).
84. F.T. Kraus and R.D. Neubecker, The differential diagnosis of papillary tumors of the breast, *Cancer* **15**, 444–455 (1962).
85. K. Inglis, Paget's disease of the nipple with special reference to the changes in ducts, *Am. J. Pathol.* **22**, 1–33 (1946).
86. G.L. Cheatle and M. Cutler, Paget's disease of the nipple, *Arch. Pathol.* **12**, 435–466 (1931).
87. R. Muir, Further observations on Paget's disease of the nipple, *J. Pathol. Bacteriol.* **49**, 299–312 (1939).
88. C. Simard, La maladie de Paget du mamelon; cancer épidermotrope, *Bull. Cancer (Paris)* **19**, 50–81 (1930).
89. R.D. Neubecker and R.P. Bradshaw, Mucin, melanin, and glycogen in Paget's disease of the breast, *Am. J. Clin. Pathol.* **36**, 49–53 (1961).
90. K.H. Hollmann, J.M. Verley, and J. Civatte, La maladie de Paget du mamelon. Etude de deux cas au miscroscope électronique, *Ann. Dermatol. Syphiligr. (Paris)* **96**, 37–44 (1969).
91. R.W. Sagebiel, Ultrastructural observations on epidermal cells in Paget's disease of the breast, *Am. J. Pathol.* **57**, 49–64 (1969).
92. E.R. Fisher and F. Beyer, Jr., Differentiation of neoplastic lesions characterized by large vacuolated intraepidermal (Pagetoid) cells, *Arch. Pathol.* **64**, 140–145 (1959).
93. J. Paget, On disease of the mammary areola preceding cancer of the mammary gland, *St. Bartholomew's Hospital Statistical Reports* **10**, 86 (1974).
94. P.M. Robb and A. MacFarlane, Two rare breast tumours, *J. Pathol. Bacteriol.* **75**, 293–298 (1958).
95. W.P. Doremus, Carcinoma of breast arising in a fibroadenoma, *N. Y. State J. Med.* **65**, 918–920 (1965).
96. R.L. Goldman and M.B. Friedman, Carcinoma of the breast arising in fibroadenomas, with emphasis on lobular carcinoma—A clinicopathologic study, *Cancer* **23**, 544–550 (1969).
97. R.W. McDivitt, F.W. Stewart, and J.H. Farrow, Breast carcinoma arising in solitary fibroadenomas, *Surg. Gynecol. Obstet.* **125**, 572–576 (1967).
98. J.W. Berg, J.J. Decrosse, A.A. Fracchia, and J. Farrow, Stromal sarcomas of the breast—A unified approach to connective tissue sarcomas other than cystosarcoma phyllodes, *Cancer* **15**, 418–424 (1962).
99. A.G. Huvos, J.V. Lucas, Jr., and F.W. Foote, Jr., Metaplastic breast carcinoma—Rare form of mammary cancer, *N. Y. State J. Med.* **73**, 1078–1082 (1973).
100. A. Gonzalez-Licea, J.H. Yardley, and W.H. Hartmann, Malignant tumor of the breast with bone formation. Studies by light and electron microscopy, *Cancer* **20**, 1234–1247 (1967).
101. R. Ross and T.K. Greenlee, Electron microscopy: attachment sites between connective tissue cells, *Science* **153**, 997–999 (1966).

102. J.L. Cornog, J. Mobini, E. Steiger, and H.T. Enterline, Squamous carcinoma of the breast, *Am. J. Clin. Pathol.* **55**, 410–417 (1971).
103. E.L. Jones, Primary squamous-cell carcinoma of breast with pseudosarcomatous stroma, *J. Pathol.* **97**, 383–385 (1969).
104. R. Newcombe, Basal-cell breast carcinoma, *Br. J. Clin. Pract.* **21**, 363–365 (1967).
105. C.D. Haagensen, The bases for the histologic grading of carcinoma of the breast, *Am. J. Cancer* **19**, 285–327 (1933).
106. W.C. MacCarty and W.E. Sistrunk, Life expectancy following radical amputation for carcinoma of the breast—A clinical and pathologic study of 218 cases, *Ann. Surg.* **75**, 61–69 (1922).
107. W.C. White, Late results of operations for ·carcinoma of the breast, *Ann. Surg.* **86**, 695–701 (1927).
108. R.B. Greenough, Varying degrees of malignancy in cancer of the breast, *J. Cancer Res.* **9**, 453–463 (1925).
109. R.W. Scarff and D.H. Patey, The position of histology in the prognosis of carcinoma of the breast, *Lancet* **1**, 801–804 (1928).
110. R.W. Scarff and R.S. Handley, Prognosis in carcinoma of the breast, *Lancet* **2**, 582–583 (1938).
111. H.J.G. Bloom, Prognosis in carcinoma of the breast, *Br. J. Cancer* **4**, 259–288 (1950).
112. H.J.G. Bloom, Further studies on prognosis of breast carcinoma, *Br. J. Cancer* **4**, 347–367 (1950).
113. B. Wolff, Histological grading in carcinoma of the breast, *Br. J. Cancer* **20**, 36–40 (1966).
114. M. Dabska, Prognosis in breast cancer on the basis of histological evaluation of malignancy according to the criteria of Bloom, *Pol. Med. J.* **7**, 908–916 (1968).
115. H.R. Champion, I.W. Wallace, and R.J. Prescott, Histology in breast cancer prognosis, *Br. J. Cancer* **26**, 129–138 (1972).
116. W.J. Eichner, H.M. Lemon, and G. Friedell, Tumor grade in the prognosis of breast cancer, *Nebr. Med. J.* **55**, 405–409 (1970).
117. M.M. Black, S.R. Opler, and F.D. Speer, Survival in breast cancer cases in relation to the structure of the primary tumor and regional lymph nodes, *Surg. Gynecol. Obstet.* **100**, 543–551 (1955).
118. M.M. Black and F.D. Speer, Nuclear structure in cancer tissues, *Surg. Gynecol. Obstet.* **105**, 97–102 (1957).
119. M.M. Black, F.D. Speer, and S.R. Opler, Structural representations of tumor–host relationships in mammary carcinoma—Biologic and prognostic significance, *Am. J. Clin. Pathol.* **26**, 250–265 (1956).
120. M.M. Black and F.D. Speer, Immunology of cancer, *Int. Abstr. Surg.* **109**, 105–116 (1959).
121. S.C. Sommers, Histologic changes in incipient carcinoma of the breast, *Cancer* **23**, 822–825 (1969).
122. S.J. Kister, S.C. Sommers, C.D. Haagensen, G.H. Friedell, E. Cooley, and A. Varma, Nuclear grade and sinus histiocytosis in cancer of the breast, *Cancer* **23**, 570–575 (1969).
123. N. Lane, H. Goksel, R.A. Salerno, and C.D. Haagensen, Clinico-pathologic analysis of the surgical curability of breast cancers—A minimum ten-year study of a personal series, *Ann. Surg.* **153**, 483–498 (1961).
124. I.M.E. Hamlin, Possible host resistance in carcinoma of the breast, a histological study, *Br. J. Cancer* **22**, 383–401 (1968).
125. S.G. Silverberg, A.R. Chitale, and S.H. Levitt, Prognostic significance of tumor margins in mammary carcinoma, *Arch. Surg.* **102**, 450–454 (1971).

126. R.H. Gold, G. Main, C. Zippin, and G.P. Annes, Infiltration of mammary carcinoma as an indicator of axillary node metastasis—A preliminary report, *Cancer* **29**, 35–40 (1972).

127. F.R. Johnstone, Carcinoma of breast—Influence of size of primary lesion and lymph node involvement based on selective biopsy, *Am. J. Surg.* **124**, 158–164 (1972).

128. B. Cady, Changing patterns of breast cancer—A point of view, *Arch. Surg.* **104**, 266–269 (1972).

129. C. Eggers, I. deCholnoky, and D.S. Jessup, Cancer of the breast, *Ann. Surg.* **113**, 321–340 (1941).

130. T.G. Brightmore, W.P. Greening, and I. Hamlin, An analysis of clinical and histopathological features in 101 cases of carcinoma of breast in women under 35 years of age, *Br. J. Cancer* **24**, 644–669 (1970).

131. B. Fisher, N.H. Slack, and I.D.J. Bross, Cancer of the breast—Size of neoplasm and prognosis, *Cancer* **24**, 1071–1080 (1969).

132. B.F. Hoopes and A.B. McGraw, The Halsted radical mastectomy—Five-year results in 246 consecutive operations at the same clinic, *Surgery* **12**, 892–905 (1942).

133. C.A. Kunath, Problem of cancer of the breast—Radical mastectomy in 90 cases, *Arch. Surg.* **41**, 66–78 (1940).

134. B. Fisher and N.H. Slack, Number of lymph nodes examined and the prognosis of breast carcinoma, *Surg. Gynecol. Obstet.* **131**, 79–88 (1970).

135. S.J. Cutler, M.M. Black, and I.S. Goldenberg, Prognostic factors in cancer of the female breast, *Cancer* **16**, 1589–1597 (1963).

136. M.M. Black, S. Kerpe, and F.D. Speer, Lymph nodes structure in patients with cancer of breast, *Am. J. Pathol.* **29**, 505–521 (1953).

137. M.M. Black and F.D. Speer, Sinus histiocytosis of lymph nodes in cancer, *Surg. Gynecol. Obstet.* **106**, 163–175 (1958).

138. M.M. Black and F.D. Speer, Lymph node reactivity in cancer patients, *Surg. Gynecol. Obstet.* **110**, 477–487 (1960).

139. J.W. Berg, Inflammation and prognosis in breast cancer—A search for host resistance, *Cancer* **12**, 714–720 (1959).

140. J.W. Berg, Active host resistance to breast cancer, *Int. J. Cancer* **18**, 854–861 (1962).

141. J.W. Berg, Morphological evidence for immune response to cancer—An historical review, *Cancer* **28**, 1453–1456 (1971).

142. R.W. Scarff and H. Torloni, *Histological Typing of Breast Tumours*, World Health Organization, Geneva (1968).

143. E.R. Fisher, E. Saffer, and B. Fisher, Studies concerning the regional lymph node in cancer—VI. Correlation of lymphocyte transformation of regional node cells and some histopathologic discriminants, *Cancer* **32**, 104–111 (1973).

144. A. Richters and R.P. Sherwin, The significance of autochthonous lymphocyte interactions with human breast cancer cells in primary tissue cultures, *Cancer* **27**, 274–277 (1971).

145. E.R. Fisher and B. Fisher, Role of mast cells in tumor growth, *Arch. Pathol.* **79**, 185–191 (1965).

146. W.C. Hueper, The clinical significance and application of histologic grading of cancers, *Ann. Surg.* **95**, 321–326 (1932).

147. Y. Okamoto, Stromal response in relation to invading forms of tumors: A histochemical and histopathological study, *Gann* **57**, 563–576 (1966).

148. J.D. Davies, Hyperelastosis, obliteration and fibrous plaques in major ducts of the human breast, *J. Pathol.* **110**, 13–26 (1973).

149. M. Askanazy, Die Beziehungen der gutaritigen Erkrankungen der Brustduse zum Mammakarcinom, *Beitr. Pathol.* **87**, 396–424 (1931).

150. J.G. Jackson and J.W. Orr, The ducts of carcinomatous breasts, with particular reference to connective-tissue changes, *J. Pathol. Bacteriol.* **74**, 265–273 (1957).

151. J.W. Orr, The significance of connective tissue changes within the ducts in the relation to mammary carcinoma, in: *International Symposium on Mammary Cancer* (L. Severi, ed.), Perugia (1958).

152. G. Williams, F.H. Green, and A. Ahmed, Studies of elastic tissue in human breast lesions, *J. Pathol.* **107**, xv (1972) (abstract).

153. A.A. Shivas and J.G. Douglas, The prognostic significance of elastosis in breast carcinoma, *J. R. Coll. Surg. Edinburgh* **17**, 315–320 (1972).

154. C. Lundmark, Breast cancer and elastosis, *Cancer* **30**, 1195–1201 (1972).

155. J.G. Azzopardi and R.N. Laurini, Elastosis in breast cancer, *Cancer* **33**, 174–183 (1974).

156. G.M. Bosner, J.A. Dossett, and J.W. Jull, *Human and Experimental Breast Cancer*, Pitman Medical, London (1961).

157. R. Muir and A.C. Aitkenhead, The healing of intra-duct carcinoma of the mamma, *J. Pathol. Bacteriol.* **38**, 117–127 (1934).

158. I. Sumegi and G. Rajka, Amyloid-like substance surrounding mammary cancer and basal cell carcinoma, *Acta Pathol. Microbiol. Scand. Sect. A* **80**, 185–192 (1972).

159. E.R. Fisher, G.P. Rodnan, and A.I. Lansing, I. Identification of the anatomic defect in pseudoxanthoma elasticum, *Am. J. Pathol.* **34**, 977–991 (1958).

160. E.R. Fisher and H.L. Wechsler, The so-called collagen diseases and elastoses of skin, in: *The Skin* (E.B. Helwig and F.K. Mostofi, eds.), pp. 366–410, Williams and Wilkins, Baltimore (1971).

161. P. Delbet and L. Mendaro, *Les Cancers du Sein*, Masson, Paris (1927).

162. R. Leroux and M. Perrot, A propos de la classification prognostique des cancers du sein, *Bull. Cancer (Paris)* **17**, 180–212 (1928).

163. I. Bertrand and A. deNagy, Recherches sur quelques tests concernant le prognostic histologique des cancers du sein, *Nouv. Presse Med.* **39**, 991–995 (1931).

164. E.R. Fisher, W.A. Dow, and H. Posada, Correlations between specimen roentgenograms (mammograms) and pathologic findings in breast disease, *Pathobiol. Annu.* **8**, 453–472 (1973).

165. E.R. Fisher, H. Posada, and H. Ramos, Evaluation of mammography based upon correlation of specimen mammograms and histopathologic findings, *Am. J. Clin. Pathol.* **62**, 60–72 (1974).

166. H.G. Godlewski, Histochemical studies of phosphorylases in cancerous and precancerous lesions in the uterine cervix and mammary gland, *Int. J. Cancer* **20**, 706–709 (1964).

167. A.G. Foraker, A histochemical study of breast carcinoma. *Surg. Gynecol. Obstet.* **102**, 1–8 (1956).

168. J. Ewing, *Neoplastic Disease—A Treatise on Tumors*, 3rd ed., W.B. Saunders, Philadelphia (1928).

169. J.F. Higginson and J.R. McDonald, Apocrine tissue, chronic cystic mastitis and sweat gland carcinoma of the breast, *Surg. Gynecol. Obstet.* **88**, 1–10 (1949).

170. B.J. Lee, G.T. Pack, and I. Scharnagel, Sweat gland cancer of the breast, *Surg. Gynecol. Obstet.* **56**, 975–996 (1933).

171. M. Wald and B.A. Kakulas, Apocrine gland carcinoma (sweat gland carcinoma) of the breast, *Aust. N. Z. J. Surg.* **33**, 200–204 (1964).

172. F. Archer and M. Omar, Pink cell (oncocytic) metaplasia in a fibroadenoma of the human breast: electron-microscope observations, *J. Pathol.* **99**, 119–124 (1969).

173. W.J. Pier, Jr., J.C. Garancis, and J.F. Kuzma, The ultrastructure of apocrine cells in intracystic papilloma and fibrocystic disease of the breast, *Arch. Pathol.* **89**, 446–462 (1970).

174. A. Behrend, Cystic disease of the breast—Its relation to the development of carcinoma, *Int. Surg.* **40**, 549–553 (1963).
175. O.T. Clagett, N.C. Plimpton, and G.T. Root, Lesions of the breast—The relationship of benign lesions to carcinoma, *Surgery* **15**, 413–419 (1944).
176. F.W. Foote, Jr. and F.W. Stewart, Comparative studies of cancerous versus noncancerous breasts—II. Role of so-called chronic mastitis in mammary carcinogenesis, influence of certain hormones on human breast structure, *Ann. Surg.* **121**, 197–222 (1945).
177. L.J. Humphrey and M. Swerdlow, Relationship of benign breast disease to carcinoma of the breast, *Surgery* **52**, 841–846 (1962).
178. C.M. Karpas, H.P. Leis, A. Oppenheim, and W.L. Mersheimer, Relationship of fibrocystic disease to carcinoma of the breast, *Ann. Surg.* **162**, 1–8 (1965).
179. W.H. Kern and R.N. Brooks, Atypical epithelial hyperplasia associated with breast cancer and fibrocystic disease, *Cancer* **24**, 668–675 (1969).
180. J.W. Logie, Mastopathia cystica and mammary carcinoma, *Cancer Res.* **2**, 394–397 (1942).
181. W.C. MacCarty and E.H. Mensing, The relationship between chronic mastitis and carcinoma of the breast, in: *Collected Papers of the Mayo Clinic* (W.B. Mellish, ed.), p. 7, W.B. Saunders, Philadelphia (1915).
182. C.W. McLaughlin, Jr., J.R. Schenken, and J.K. Tamisiea, A study of precancerous epithelial hyperplasia and noninvasive papillary carcinoma of the breast, *Ann. Surg.* **153**, 735–744 (1961).
183. H. Nizze Von, Zum morphologischen Verhalten des erhaltenen Brustdrusengewebes bei Fibroadenomen, fibrosierende Adenosen, Epithel-proliferationen und Mammakarzinomen, *Arch. Geschwulstforsch.* **41**, 34–42 (1973).
184. J.A. Ryan and C.J. Coady, Intraductal epithelial proliferation in the human breast—A comparative study, *Can. J. Surg.* **5**, 12–19 (1962).
185. S.G. Silverberg, A.R. Chitale, and S.H. Levitt, Prognostic implications of fibrocystic dysplasia in breast removed for mammary carcinoma, *Cancer* **29**, 574–580 (1972).
186. M. Tellem, L. Prive, and D.R. Meranze, Four-quadrant study of breasts removed for carcinoma, *Cancer* **15**, 10–17 (1962).
187. S. Warren, The relation of "chronic mastitis" to carcinoma of the breast, *Surg. Gynecol. Obstet.* **71**, 257–273 (1940).
188. V.K. Frantz, J.W. Pickren, G.W. Melcher, and H. Auchincloss, Jr., Incidence of chronic cystic disease in so-called "normal breasts"—A Study based on 225 post mortem examinations, *Cancer* **4**, 762–783 (1951).
189. M.M. Black, T.H.C. Barclay, S.J. Cutler, B.F. Hawkey, and A.J. Asere, Association of atypical characteristics of benign breast lesions with subsequent risk of breast cancer, *Cancer* **29**, 338–343 (1972).
190. J.E. Devitt, Fibrocystic disease of the breast is not premalignant, *Surg. Gynecol. Obstet.* **134** 803–806 (1972).
191. A.C. Estes and C. Phillips, Papilloma of lacteal duct, *Surg. Gynecol. Obstet.* **89**, 345–348 (1949).
192. J.W. Hendrick, Intraductal papilloma of breast, *Surg. Gynecol. Obstet.* **105**, 215–223 (1957).
193. J.B. MacGillivray, The problem of "chronic mastitis" with epitheliosis, *J. Clin. Pathol.* **22**, 340–347 (1969).
194. S.E. Buhl-Jorsensen, K. Fischermann, H. Johansen, and B. Petersen, Cancer risk in intraductal papilloma and papillomatosis, *Surg. Gynecol. Obstet.* **127**, 1307–1312 (1968).

195. H.H. Davis, M. Simons, and J.B. Davis, Cystic disease of the breast—Relationship to carcinoma, *Cancer* **17**, 957–978 (1964).
196. W. Kiaer, *Relation of Fibroadenomatosis (Chronic Mastitis) to Cancer of the Breast*, Munksgaard, Copenhagen (1954).
197. E.F. Lewison, The relationship between breast cancer and benign breast disease, *Am. Surg.* **25**, 71–74 (1959).
198. E.V. Pellettiere, II, The clinical and pathologic aspects of papillomatous disease of breast—A study of 97 patients treated by local excision, *Am. J. Clin. Pathol.* **55**, 740–748 (1971).
199. M. Swerdlow and L.J. Humphrey, Fibrocystic disease and carcinoma of the breast, *Arch. Surg.* **87**, 457–460 (1963).
200. E.R. Fisher and J. Paulson, Unpublished observations.
201. E.R. Fisher, R.H. Shoemaker, and A. Sabnis, Relationship of hyperplasia to cancer in MCA-induced mammary tumorogenesis, *Lab. Invest.* **33**, 33–42 (1975).
202. G.L. Cheatle and M. Cutler, *Tumours of the Breast—Their Pathology, Symptoms, Diagnosis and Treatment*, J.B. Lippincott, Philadelphia (1931).
203. H.S. Gallager and J.E. Martin, The study of mammary carcinoma by mammography and a whole organ sectioning—Early observations, *Cancer* **23**, 855–873 (1969).
204. G.W. Nicholson, Carcinoma of the breast, *Br. J. Surg.* **8**, 527–528 (1921).
205. R.A. Willis, *Pathology of Tumours*, 2nd ed., Butterworths, London (1953).
206. J.R. Bell, G.H. Friedell, and I.S. Goldenberg, Prognostic significance of pathologic findings in human breast carcinoma, *Surg. Gynecol. Obstet.* **129**, 258–262 (1969).
207. G.H. Friedell, A. Betts, and S.C. Sommers, The prognostic value of blood vessel invasion and lymphocyte infiltrates in breast carcinoma, *Cancer* **18**, 164–166 (1965).
208. S.J. Kister, S.C. Sommers, C.D. Haagensen, and E. Cooley, Re-evaluation of blood vessel invasion as a prognostic factor in carcinoma of the breast, *Cancer* **19**, 1213–1216 (1966).
209. U. Ruiz, S. Babeau, M.S. Schwartz, E. Soto, R.A. McAuley, and G.H. Friedell, Blood vessel invasion and lymph node metastasis—Two factors affecting survival in breast cancer, *Surgery* **73**, 185–190 (1973).
210. D.P. Byar and F.K. Mostofi, Carcinoma of the prostate—Prognostic evaluation of certain pathologic features in 208 radical prostatectomies, *Cancer* **30**, 5–13 (1972).
211. R.W. Qualheim and E.A. Gall, Breast carcinoma with multiple sites of origin, *Cancer* **10**, 460–468 (1957).
212. R.H. Koehl, R.E. Snyder, R.V. Hutter, and F.W. Foote, Jr., The incidence and significance of calcifications within operative breast specimens, *Am. J. Clin. Pathol.* **53**, 3–14 (1970).
213. R.L. Stratton, Multicentricity in cancer of the breast, *J. Kans. Med. Soc.* **74**, 48–52 (1973).
214. W.M. Kramer and B.F. Rush, Mammary duct proliferation in the elderly—A histopathologic study, *Cancer* **31** 130–137 (1973).
215. E.R. Fisher, R. Gregorio, C. Redmond, F. Vellios, S.C. Sommers, and B. Fisher, Pathologic findings from the National Surgical Adjuvant Breast Project (Protocol No. 4)—I. Observations concerning the multicentricity of mammary cancer, *Cancer* **35**, 247–254 (1975).
216. D.B. Jones, Florid papillomatosis of the nipple ducts, *Cancer* **8**, 315–319 (1955).
217. F.C. Nichols, M.B. Dockerty, and E.S. Judd, Florid papillomatosis of nipple, *Surg. Gynecol. Obstet.* **107**, 474–480 (1958).
218. K.H. Perzin and R. Lattes, Papillary adenoma of the nipple (florid papillomatosis, adenoma, adenomatosis)—A clinicopathologic study, *Cancer* **29**, 996–1009 (1972).

219. H.B. Taylor and A.G. Robertson, Adenomas of the nipple, *Cancer* **18**, 995–1002 (1965).
220. V.M. Doctor and M.V. Sirsat, Florid papillomatosis (adenoma) and other benign tumours of the nipple and areola, *Br. J. Cancer* **25**, 1–9 (1971).
221. B.S. Bhagavan, A. Patchefsky, and L.G. Koss, Florid subareolar duct papillomatosis (nipple adenoma) and mammary carcinoma—Report of three cases, *Hum. Pathol.* **4**, 289–295 (1973).
222. R.S. Handley and A.G. Thackray, Adenomas of nipple, *Br. J. Cancer* **16**, 187–194 (1962).
223. A. Gudjonsdottir, I. Hagerstrand, and G. Ostberg, Adenoma of the nipple with carcinomatous development, *Acta Pathol. Microbiol. Scand. Sect. A* **79**, 676–680 (1971).
224. A. Porritt, Early carcinoma of the breast, *Br. J. Surg.* **51**, 214–216 (1964).
225. N. Treves, The inoperability of inflammatory carcinoma of the breast, *Surg. Gynecol. Obstet.* **109**, 240–242 (1959).
226. C. Wang, Management of inflammatory carcinoma of the breast, *J. Am. Med. Assoc.* **201**, 533–535 (1967).
227. K.W. Barber, Jr., M.B. Dockerty, and O.T. Clagett, Inflammatory carcinoma of the breast, *Surg. Gynecol. Obstet.* **112**, 406–410 (1961).
228. W.T. Fitts, Jr., Inflammatory carcinoma of the breast, *Surg. Gynecol. Obstet.* **107**, 95–96 (1958).
229. D. Ellis and S.L. Teitelbaum, Inflammatory carcinoma of the breast—A pathologic definition, *Cancer* **33**, 1045–1047 (1974).
230. S.D. Deodhar, G. Crile, Jr., and C.G. Esselystyn, Jr., Study of the tumor cell–lymphocyte interaction in patients with breast cancer, *Cancer* **29**, 1321–1325 (1972).
231. B. Fisher and E.R. Fisher, Studies concerning the regional lymph node in cancer—I. Initiation of immunity, *Cancer* **27**, 1001–1004 (1971).
232. B. Fisher and E.R. Fisher, Studies concerning the regional lymph node in cancer—II. Maintenance of immunity, *Cancer* **29**, 1496–1501 (1972).
233. B. Fisher, E.A. Saffer, and E.R. Fisher, Studies concerning the regional lymph node in cancer—IV. Tumor inhibition by regional lymph node cells, *Cancer* **33**, 631–636 (1974).
234. E.R. Fisher, H. Reidbord, and B. Fisher, Studies concerning the regional lymph node in cancer—V. Histologic and ultrastructural findings in regional and non-regional nodes, *Lab. Invest.* **38**, 126–133 (1973).
235. B. Fisher, E.A. Saffer, and E.R. Fisher, Studies concerning the regional lymph node in cancer—VII. Response of regional lymph node cells from breast and colon cancer patients to PHA stimulation, *Cancer* **30**, 1202–1215 (1972).
236. B. Fisher, E.A. Saffer, and E.R. Fisher, Studies concerning the regional lymph node in cancer—VII. Thymidine uptake by cells from nodes of breast cancer patients relative to axillary location and histopathologic discriminants, *Cancer* **33**, 271–279 (1974).
237. J.W. Berg, A.G. Huvos, L.M. Axtell, and G.F. Robbins, A new sign of favorable prognosis in mammary cancer—Hyperplastic reactive lymph nodes in the apex of the axilla, *Ann. Surg.* **177**, 8–12 (1973).
238. W.B. Wartman, Sinus cell hyperplasia of lymph nodes regional to adenocarcinoma of the breast and colon, *Br. J. Cancer* **13**, 389–397 (1959).
239. O.T. Anastassiades and D.M. Pryce, Immunological significance of the morphological changes in lymph nodes draining breast cancer, *Br. J. Cancer* **20**, 239–249 (1966).
240. L. Masse, C. Masse, and J.P. Chassiagne, Le prognostic de cancers du sein en fonction de la surcharge en histiocytes des sinus des ganglions axillaires, *Chirurgie* **86**, 940–952 (1960).

241. J.W. Berg, Sinus histiocytosis—A fallacious measure of host resistance to cancer, *Cancer* **9**, 935–939 (1956).

242. R.D. Moore, R. Chapnick, and M.D. Schoenberg, Lymph nodes associated with carcinoma of the breast, *Cancer* **13**, 545–549 (1960).

243. S.G. Silverberg, A.R. Chitale, A.D. Hind, A.B. Frazier, and S.H. Levitt, Sinus histiocytosis and mammary carcinoma—Study of 366 radical mastectomies and an historical review, *Cancer* **26**, 1177–1185 (1970).

244. J.J. DiRe and N. Lane, The relation of sinus histiocytosis in axillary lymph nodes to surgical curability of carcinoma of the breast, *Am. J. Clin. Pathol.* **40**, 508–515 (1963).

245. V. Tsakraklides, P. Olson, J.H. Kersey, and R.A. Good, Prognostic significance of the regional lymph node histology in cancer of the breast, *Cancer* **34**, 1259–1266 (1974).

246. E.R. Fisher, R.M. Gregorio, C. Redmond, A. Dekker, and B. Fisher, Pathologic findings from the National Surgical Adjuvant Breast Project (Protocol No. 4). II. The significance of regional node histology other than sinus histiocytosis in invasive mammary cancer, *Am. J. Clin. Pathol.* **65**, 21–30 (1976).

247. H. Cottier, J. Turk, and L. Sobin, A proposal for a standardized system of reporting human lymph node morphology in relation to immunological function, *Bull. W.H.O.* **47**, 375–417 (1972).

248. S.J. Cutler and M.H. Myers, Clinical classification of extent of disease in cancer of the breast, *J. Natl. Cancer Inst.* **39**, 193–207 (1967).

249. S. Kay, Evaluation of Rotter's lymph nodes in radical mastectomy specimens as a guide to prognosis, *Cancer* **18**, 1441–1444 (1965).

250. E.R. Fisher, R.M. Gregorio, C. Redmond, W.S. Kim, and B. Fisher, Pathologic findings from the National Surgical Adjuvant Breast Project (Protocol No. 4). III. The significance of extranodal extension of axillary metastases, *Am. J. Clin. Pathol.* **65**, 439–444 (1976).

251. A.D. Govan, Two cases of mixed malignant tumour of the breast, *J. Pathol. Bacteriol.* **57**, 397–404 (1945).

252. I.A. More and A.T. Sandison, Triple carcinoma of the breast, one arising within a fibro-adenoma, *J. Pathol.* **109**, 263–265 (1973).

Systemic Adjuvant (Combined Modality) Therapy in the Treatment of Primary Breast Cancer

BERNARD FISHER AND NORMAN WOLMARK

1. Introduction

Despite the use of expansive surgical procedures on women with primary breast cancers, noteworthy gains relative to survival and freedom
from disease have not occurred during the past three or four decades.
Elsewhere in this volume, it has been documented that operation alone
is all too frequently inadequate to effect a cure. There is increasing acceptance of the consideration that most, if not all, such patients have
disseminated disease at the time of diagnosis. Consequently, improvement in survival is only apt to result from the employment of effective
systemic therapy in conjunction with those modalities used to control
locoregional disease, i.e., operation and radiation. The use of chemo-,
immuno-, or hormonal therapy in conjunction with operation has been
inappropriately designated as "adjuvant" therapy. Recent advances in
knowledge support the contention that operation and/or radiation, by
reducing tumor burden, may actually serve as the "adjuvant" to systemic therapy. Consequently, the term "combined modality" therapy
seems more appropriate to describe the various conglomerate treatment
regimens. Nonetheless, because of its common usage and the general
familiarity with its connotation, the term "adjuvant therapy" will be
employed in this review.

BERNARD FISHER AND NORMAN WOLMARK · Department of Surgery, University
of Pittsburgh, Pittsburgh, Pennsylvania.

This report serves as a companion piece to Chapter 1, which has presented an appraisal of the role of operation in the treatment of primary breast cancer. It provides information regarding what has been and is being accomplished by the use of systemic therapy and considers what the prospects for the future might be. Moreover, an overview of basic considerations relative to the use of such therapy is presented.

2. Tumor Cell Kinetics and Adjuvant Chemotherapy

The effectiveness of adjuvant chemotherapy is determined by the response of micrometastases to cytotoxic agents. An important consideration is the relationship of the primary tumor to such metastatic foci. Do they respond differently to chemotherapy? What is the effect of ablation of a primary tumor on the sensitivity of residual metastatic cells to cytotoxic agents? Answers to these and other questions, as well as support for the concept of the use of adjuvant chemotherapy, are provided by data obtained from studies regarding tumor cell kinetics. Mendelsohn,[1] and subsequently, Skipper and Schabel,[2,3] have defined the concept of a growth fraction in tumor cell populations. In that

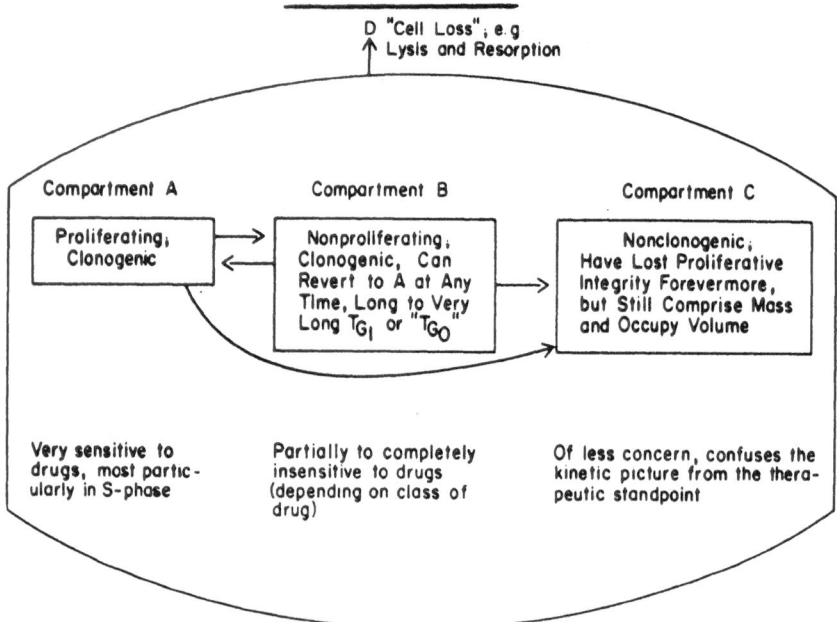

Fig. 1. The proliferative behavior of subpopulations of tumor cells influences both growth rate and sensitivity to therapy. (From Skipper.[3])

hypothesis (Fig. 1), tumors are regarded as consisting of three cell compartments: *Compartment A* consists of proliferating clonogenic cells undergoing active anabolism. Cells in that compartment contribute to the increase in total cell number of a tumor population. Tumor growth occurs when proliferating cells in the compartment exceed cell loss. Cell-cycle-specific chemotherapeutic agents destroy cells in the compartment. *Compartment B* is comprised of a population of nonproliferative cells not engaged in active anabolism. Those cells do not contribute to population growth, but are in equilibrium with cells in compartment A and retain their potential for proliferation. While sensitive to cell-cycle-nonspecific agents to some extent, they are more resistant to cytostatic manipulation. For cell-cycle-specific agents to effectively control tumor growth, cells in compartment A must be depleted with resultant transformation of noncycling cells in compartment B to proliferating cells in compartment A. Those cells then become vulnerable to chemotherapeutic agents. *Compartment C* is composed of permanently nonproliferating, nonclonogenic cells which do not contribute to tumor growth but only to tumor volume, and consequently, are of seemingly lesser clinical significance.

The growth fraction of a tumor has been defined as the ratio of proliferating to nonproliferating cells: A/(B+C). The greater the growth fraction, the more sensitive is a cell population to chemotherapy. The growth fraction of a given population of cells in a growing solid tumor is not constant and is related to total tumor volume. The changing growth rate of tumor cells fits the Gompertz equation, which describes exponential tumor growth that is exponentially inhibited. With increasing volume of a tumor, the growth fraction of a tumor progressively decreases and the tumor doubling time increases (Fig. 2). There results a loss of sensitivity to chemotherapy. Of significance is the demonstration that micrometastases (with a population of $\leq 10^6$ cells) approach exponential log-phase (non-Gompertzian) growth and that their cells are more sensitive to chemotherapy than are their more crowded counterparts in large primary tumors.

Cell-kill by chemotherapeutic agents follows first-order kinetics. A constant proportion of the total tumor cell population is killed by a constant dose of drug, regardless of the size of the total population. First-order kinetics apply only to those populations which grow in exponential fashion with constant growth fractions and tumor doubling times, i.e., micrometastases as opposed to large-volume primary tumors.

Another factor which determines the responsiveness of a tumor population to chemotherapy is the variation of cell-cycle time or the degree of synchronization of cell cycles. Cells that cycle at similar vel-

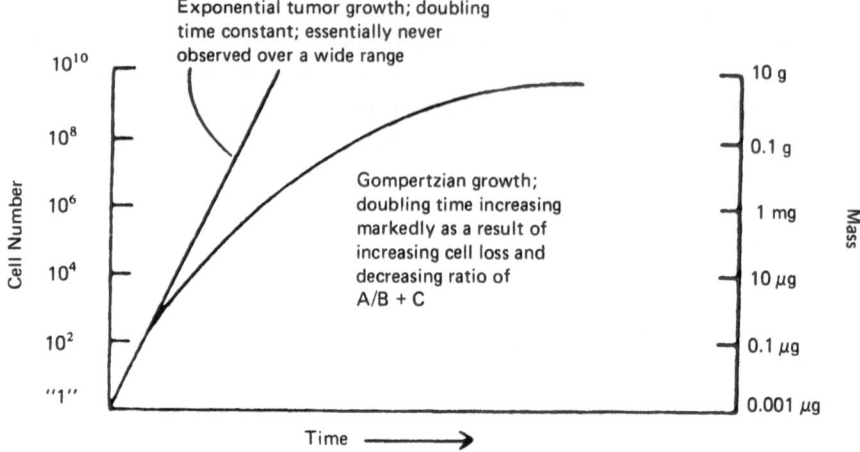

Fig. 2. Growth rates of tumors and their implications. (From Skipper.[3])

ocities (synchronized) have the greatest sensitivity to chemotherapy and, conversely, the more heterogeneous the population in that regard, the less likely it is that there will be an effective response. The reduction of tumor cell burden by surgical removal and/or radiation of a primary tumor may profoundly affect the growth fraction and synchronization of cells in micrometastases so that they become more sensitive to chemotherapy.

Endpoints utilized in clinical trials to test the effectiveness of chemotherapy against either late or early disease may fail to reflect striking events occurring at the cellular level. A 50% regression of a measurable tumor mass resulting from administration of a chemotherapeutic agent may be associated with a 99.99% reduction in clonogenic cells. In early disease, while administration of drugs as adjuvants may be associated with overall results (disease-free interval and/or survival) that are not dramatic, they may be of great import from a biological standpoint. This is best exemplified by findings from the National Surgical Adjuvant Breast Project (NSABP) clinical trial employing short-course triethylenethiophosphoramide (thio-TEPA) (described in detail elsewhere). Premenopausal women with four or more positive nodes demonstrated a prolongation of their disease-free interval and at ten years, had a better survival than did nontreated controls. Since similar doses of thio-TEPA were effective in curing only animals with less than ten viable leukemia cells and had no effect on solid tumors,[3] the clinical findings seem to have biological significance.

Recently adjuvant chemotherapy protocols have been initiated in which there is prolonged administration of cytostatic agents. It has been shown experimentally that tumor cell populations between 10^6 and 10^7 cells may be considered amenable to single-agent chemotherapy. Moreover, it has been estimated that about 75% of women having Stage II breast cancers harbor between 10^6 and 10^7 residual cells following primary tumor removal and could thus be benefited by single-agent therapy (Fig. 3). Based on kinetic studies and data derived from animal tumor models, it would seem that the logical starting point for evaluating the worth of adjuvant chemotherapy in breast cancer would be to implement clinical trials utilizing single agents. After having determined their effectiveness, it would seem proper to proceed with the evaluation of multiple agents in a logical stepwise fashion so that each new effort is based on sound biological hypotheses. Such an orderly approach should permit definition of subsets of patients who may be as responsive to single agents as to combinations of drugs.

The following summarizes information regarding tumor cell kinetics which lends support to the concept of adjuvant chemotherapy and provides a rational basis for the planning meaningful protocols.

1. Growth fractions and doubling times of primary tumors may differ from those in micrometastases. Consequently, responsiveness to chemotherapy may differ.

2. The magnitude of response of a primary tumor in the plateau of Gompertzian growth need not reflect the response of micrometastases in exponential growth.

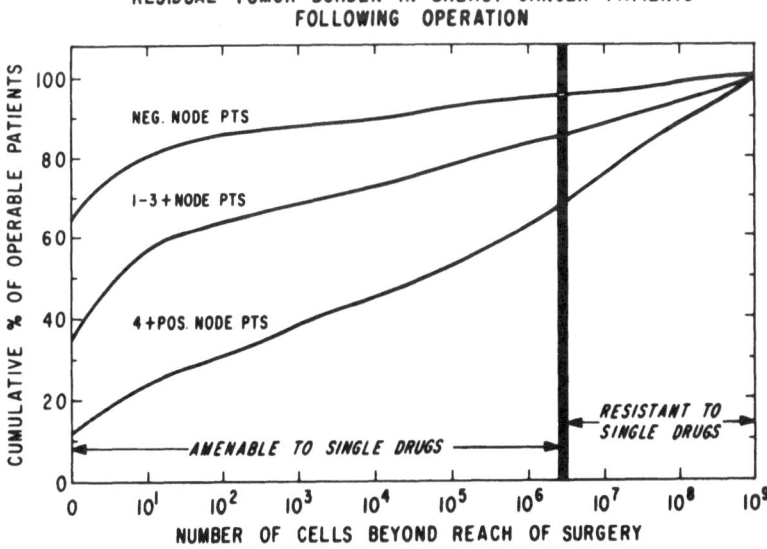

Fig. 3. Number of cells beyond reach of surgery (based on H.E. Skipper's data).

3. First-order kinetics relative to cell-kill by cytocidal agents apply to those cells with constant growth fractions in exponential growth, i.e., micrometastases of $\leq 10^6$ cells.

4. The degree of synchronization of cell-cycle times of a primary tumor and its micrometastases may differ. On this basis, they may respond to cyclical chemotherapy differently.

5. Ablation of a primary tumor with a resultant decrease in total tumor cell burden may alter the growth characteristics of residual micrometastases. A decrease in tumor doubling time, an increase in growth fraction, and an improved synchronization of cell-cycle times may result. Such changes may enhance the sensitivity of micrometastases to chemotherapy.

6. Micrometastases approaching exponential growth kinetics could be sensitive to single-agent chemotherapy. Consequently, there exists the rationale for first evaluating the effect of single agents as adjuvants.

3. Surgical Adjuvant Therapy in Animal Model Systems

Results obtained from investigations in a variety of experimental animal systems employing different species of tumors and chemotherapeutic agents have provided evidence to substantiate the worth of chemotherapy used following operation to eradicate residual neoplastic cells. They have helped formulate principles which supply a basis for the use of systemic agents in conjunction with surgery in the human. The following reviews those accomplishments.

In 1957, Shapiro and Fugmann,[4] employing mammary adenocarcinoma 755 implanted into C57Bl mice, noted that whereas surgical removal of tumors alone or the use of 6-mercaptopurine (6-MP) alone failed to produce "cures" of 15-day-old tumors, the combination of the two resulted in a 57% "cure" rate. Employing the same model, Chirigos et al.[5] confirmed the findings of Shapiro and Fugmann and provided evidence to indicate that the results were better than what might have been expected simply on the additive effect of surgery and chemotherapy. Others have obtained similar results employing single agents as adjuvants to surgery in their models.[6-14] Karrer, Humphreys, and Goldin, for example, have observed that operation followed by cyclophosphamide increased the cure rate of BDF_1 mice with metastases from a primary Lewis lung carcinoma.[9-11] Chemotherapy alone or delayed surgery failed to similarly increase survival.[9] Mayo and associates, utilizing the same tumor system, found that operation plus methyl-CCNU [1-(2-chloroethyl)-3-(4-methylcyclohexyl)-1-nitrosourea] was more effective in increasing survival than either modality alone.[12]

Using a model system which is unusually refractory to chemotherapy alone (B-16 melanoma in BDF_1 mice), Griswold demonstrated that the combination of surgery plus Me-CCNU was extremely effective in prolonging survival of mice, whereas neither modality alone produced an effect of consequence.[13] Recently, Straus et al. studied the effects of operation, operation and cyclophosphamide (Cytoxan; CTX), and CTX alone as functions of time and dose on survival time, cure rate, toxicity, surgical mortality, and other parameters in C57Bl mice with Ca-755 tumors.[14] Again it was observed that post-operative chemotherapy increased survival longer than the additive increase of chemotherapy alone and surgery alone. Moreover, it was shown that the effectiveness of adjuvant therapy was dependent on time administered relative to operation, schedule of employment, and dose utilized.

Results have also accumulated from animal models to indicate that multiple-agent chemotherapy is more effective when given following surgery than is the use of a single agent. Mayo et al.[12] found that in the Lewis lung model, the addition of CTX to Me-CCNU was a more effective surgical adjuvant than was either agent alone, and Martin and associates[15] observed that STEM (streptonigrin, thioguanine, endoxan or cyclophosphamide, and mytomycin C) produced more cures of CD_8F mice with spontaneous adenocarcinomas when given after surgery than did combinations of fewer drugs in conjunction with surgery. Subsequently, the same investigators found that the addition of a fifth agent, actinomycin D, to the therapeutic regimen—i.e., surgery plus STEAM—was even more effective.[16]

4. Early Trials of Systemic Adjuvant Therapy

The historic background that set the stage for the first generation of clinical trials of adjuvant therapy is worthy of consideration. The earliest demonstration of blood-borne tumor cells was in 1869 by Ashworth, who found them in a patient with malignant skin tumors.[17] Aside from a few sporadic case reports of abnormal cells in the blood of patients with tumors[18-20] and the finding by Pool and Dunlop in 1934 of abnormal cells in the blood of 17 of 40 cancer patients,[21] the true nature of which was uncertain, little interest in tumor cells in the blood was entertained. Not until 1955, when Fisher and Turnbull[22] and Engell[23] reported the presence of tumor cells in the blood of patients with cancer did a surge of interest in that subject take place.

In the next few years following those findings, innumerable investigators demonstrated tumor cells in the peripheral blood of patients with operable and advanced lesions,[24-26] in hepatic vein blood,[27] in the blood of patients with all types of neoplasms,[28-32] and in that of children with cancers.[33] Of special interest was the demonstration that showers of the cancer cells were found in the blood during pelvic[34] and rectal[35] examinations, uterine curettage,[36] transurethral resection,[37] rigorous cleansing of the skin over a tumor prior to operation,[35] and operation itself.[38]

It was thus believed that tumor cells dislodged during operation were a prime factor in the failure of cure despite meticulous surgical skill, and if those hematogenously circulating tumor cells could be destroyed, improvement in results would follow. With reports of the favorable effects of chemotherapeutic agents on the destruction of disseminated tumor cells in experimental animals,[39-41] a rationale for embarking upon clinical trials of adjuvant therapy was established.

Consequently, in 1957, under the auspices of the National Institutes of Health, Cancer Chemotherapy National Service Center, representatives of 23 institutions in the United States adopted a common protocol to determine the efficacy of administering chemotherapy in conjunction with "curative" cancer surgery to decrease recurrence and extend survival of patients with cancer of the breast. It was anticipated that such a therapeutic regimen could destroy tumor cells dislodged into the blood and lymph during surgical manipulation. That effort became known as the National Surgical Adjuvant Breast Project (NSABP), a title which has since been used to identify the cooperative group in the United States which has, for almost 20 years, carried out clinical trials to evaluate the worth of a variety of treatment modalities utilized in the management of patients with primary breast cancer. The group has expanded over the years so that at present, it consists of almost 400 surgeons, radiation and medical oncologists, as well as pathologists from 70 institutions in the United States, Canada, and other countries.

Patients were considered eligible for inclusion into the initial protocol only if the tumor was confined to the breast or breast and axilla; the tumor was movable in relation to the chest wall without extensive skin involvement or ulceration; axillary nodes, if present, were movable in relation to the chest wall and blood vessels, and there was no evidence of edema of the arm; there was histologic evidence of a malignant lesion; and a Halsted radical mastectomy, removing breast, pectoral muscles, and axillary contents *en bloc*, had been performed and the age of the patient was between 30 and 70 years.

Patients were excluded from the study because of (a) a previous or concomitant malignant lesion, regardless of site, except squamous-cell and basal-cell carcinomas of the skin; (b) previous treatment of carcinoma of the breast other than performance of a biopsy to confirm diagnosis no more than seven days prior to definitive operation; (c) preoperative white blood cell count of ≥5000 or platelet count of ≥150,000/mm³, or both; (d) being considered a poor surgical risk; and (e) tumors of the breast other than carcinoma or the presence of extensive subepidermal skin involvement and pregnancy or lactation. Thio-TEPA (TSPA), because of its effectiveness in palliation of advanced mammary cancer, was at that time deemed the drug most likely to be beneficial and was chosen for evaluation. The first patient was entered on study April 4, 1958, and patient entry was terminated October 7, 1961. Women were randomized in double-blind fashion between two treatment groups: (1) conventional Halsted radical mastectomy and TSPA, and (2) radical mastectomy with or without placebo (control). Patients received TSPA intravenously (i.v.) in a dose of either 0.8 or 0.6 mg/kg of body weight— 0.2 or 0.4 mg/kg at the time of operation and 0.2 mg/kg on each of the first two postoperative days. Since analysis of data revealed no difference in those receiving one or the other dose, results were combined. Direct recurrence- and survival-rate calculations were obtained from 826 acceptable study patients grouped according to nodal and menopausal status, and the results have been reported in detail.[42] Positive-node patients were further subdivided into those having one to three or four or more such nodes. At the end of five years, there was no significant difference in recurrence rate between patients receiving TSPA or placebo in any of these six principal categories. If, however, recurrence rates for TSPA and placebo groups were plotted against time following surgery (similar to a plot of life-table values), significant information was revealed which was not obtained by examination of data only at the end of five years. Whereas there was no significant difference between the two treatment groups at any time in five of the six menopausal and nodal categories, a difference was discernible between the TSPA and placebo groups of premenopausal patients who had four or more positive nodes. TSPA-treated patients in that category (Fig. 4) demonstrated a recurrence rate between the eighteenth and thirty-sixth postoperative months which was approximately 40% less than that in the placebo group. After that time, the number of recurrences in the TSPA-treated patients gradually increased so that by 48 months, the groups were no longer significantly different. The effect of TSPA in this category was best demonstrated by the observation that 50% of patients in the placebo series had recurrences by the thirteenth month after surgery, whereas recurrences did not occur in half of the TSPA patients until the forty-fifth month of follow-up. While the difference between the treated and control groups relative to treatment failure was no longer statistically significant after five years, it was 20%. A 33% difference in the survival rate that was significant ($P < 0.05$) was observed at that time between the TSPA-treated and control groups: 56.5% for the former versus 24.3% for the

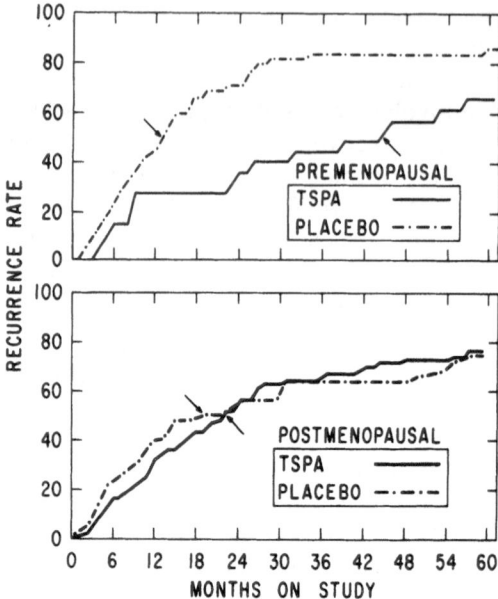

Fig. 4. Recurrence rates up to 60 months of follow-up for patients with four or more positive nodes who received thio-TEPA (TSPA).

latter. At that time, it was anticipated that subsequent years of follow-up study probably would reveal a diminution of the beneficial effects of TSPA to the point where no difference between the two groups would be evident. Recently, results obtained from a ten-year follow-up of patients entered into the TSPA study were reported and did not entirely substantiate that prediction. Only 0.7% of the initial 826 patients evaluated were lost to follow-up at five years, and only 4.7% of patients had no ten-year follow-up information. Contrary to expectations, the ten-year findings revealed a persistence of the difference in treatment failure and survival rates. After ten years, 21% fewer patients in the TSPA groups had treatment failures and 21% more of them survived. Thus, it would seem that the initial suppression of treatment failures had a lasting effect that was reflected in patient survival. The data also suggested that the limited chemotherapy employed was more effective in patients having smaller tumors. Such a finding is in keeping with experimental observations and with modern concepts of chemotherapy which suggest that a therapeutic regimen should be more effective in a host with a minimal tumor burden.

With completion of patient entry into the TSPA study in 1961, a new protocol was begun. It evaluated the worth of 5-fluorouracil (5-FU) compared to TSPA as an adjunct to operation. Again, only a short course of chemotherapy was employed. TSPA-treated patients received a total dose of 0.8 mg/kg of body weight—0.4 mg/kg on the day of operation and 0.2 mg/kg on each of the next two days. Those who were administered 5-FU received 15 mg/kg i.v. on each of four consecutive days, beginning seven days postoperatively, for a total of 60 mg/kg.

Fifty-two percent of patients who received 5-FU suffered local complications and significantly more patients receiving that drug demonstrated systemic complications. Moreover, 42% of patients administered 5-FU became leukopenic and almost half of those had counts of <2500. Of 16 deaths occurring within 60 days following operation in the 1725 patients, eight were recipients of 5-FU and all demonstrated drug toxicity.

As in the first study, only TSPA-treated premenopausal patients with four or more positive nodes had less recurrences than did untreated patients. Results with 5-FU were not impressive, and recurrence rates were the same as in patients receiving placebo.

In retrospect, the findings with TSPA must be considered remarkable in view of the small amount of drug employed for only a brief interval. Skipper had commented[44] that if such an amount of TSPA given in split doses over three days "can significantly delay recurrence and death after surgery in premenopausal patients with ≥4 positive nodes, the odds are good that we might do much better in this patient category (and others) with surgery followed by an optimal regimen of this drug or better yet, a more effective alkylating agent or combination of drugs."

At the time, however, the results were considered by many to be disappointing. Consequently, efforts directed toward design and implementation of a protocol employing prolonged chemotherapy were met with frustration, in spite of our emphasis that the earlier findings did not repudiate the concept of systemic adjuvant chemotherapy. During the next few years, despite a concerted attempt, it was impossible for oncologists to reach an agreement as to what drug(s) should be employed, let alone to decide what regimen with a particular drug would be acceptable. Partly because of that lack of unanimity, and partly because of the fear that since the first adjuvant study had not resulted in a positive contribution and "we could ill afford another failure," little interest could be mounted to carry out such a study. Notwithstanding that climate, in 1968 the NSABP began a feasibility study with methotrexate (MTX) in patients having positive axillary nodes. That drug was administered orally (0.2 mg/kg of body weight) twice a week, no less than three and no more than five days apart, beginning one month after mastectomy. Because of the high incidence of severe toxic manifestations encountered early, a lack of enthusiasm for use of that drug resulted and the effort was aborted.

Until recently, only a few other adjuvant chemotherapy trials had been carried out and the findings had not been consistent. A report by Nissen-Meyer *et al.* of a study by the Scandinavian Adjuvant Chemotherapy Study Group was of interest.[45] Eleven hospitals in Finland, Norway, and Sweden began a cooperative clinical trial in 1965 to evaluate the effect of a short course of chemotherapy after mastectomy for breast cancer. Patients were randomized between a group that received chemotherapy and a non-chemotherapy-treated control group. Each hospital was permitted to employ its own standard method of surgical, radiologic, and endocrinologic treatment of such tumors. Thus, variations in management were allowed between hospitals, but within each hospital, the initially established treatment schedule was to be followed. Operations varied from radical mastectomy to simple mastectomy, with combinations thereof. Postoperative radiation therapy varied between conventional and cobalt-60 treatment. In most, but not all, of the hospitals, surgical or radiologic castration was performed in Stage II cases. The authors were of the opinion that those variations were of minor importance, since each hospital was providing an equal number of patients to the chemotherapy and control groups. Originally, the plan was to permit each hospital to choose the drug considered most effective and most familiar. Ten of the hospitals decided to use CTX, 30 mg/kg of body weight, given by one daily i.v. injection for six days. Another hospital utilized another drug, but abandoned it in favor of the CTX because of toxicity after the first 15 patients were treated. In ten of the hospitals, patients were randomized immediately after surgical treatment and the patients received injections on the day of operation and on each of the next five days. This "surgical subseries" consisted of 621 patients at time of reporting. In the eleventh institution, patients were admitted for postoperative radiotherapy after surgical treatment in other hospitals. In that institution, the randomization and administration of chemotherapy took place two to four weeks after surgical treatment. That group became known as the "radiologic subseries" and was composed of 108 patients. According to the authors, results from this heterogeneous patient population indicated a trend in favor of those patients in the surgical subseries who received chemotherapy (i.e., a higher percent free of disease). No such trend was noted in the "radiologic" subseries. The data presented for the surgical subseries showed that the control group of 323 patients had 71 recurrences and 45 deaths and the chemotherapy group, 298 patients with 50 recurrences and 40 deaths, indicating a 5% difference in recurrence rates between the groups and no difference in survival rates. A more recent report of the results of that study[46] has demonstrated a decreased relapse rate in the group of 534 patients receiving chemotherapy compared with 554 control patients. There was no difference in the survival of the groups.

In 1971, Finney reported results of a trial in England in which all patients (Stages I and II) were treated by surgery and postoperative irradiation, but half of them also received pre- and postoperative chemotherapy.[47] CTX was administered (2–3 mg/kg i.v.) daily for four days preoperatively, on the day of operation, and for five days postoperatively. After three years, results of the group receiving chemotherapy were worse than those of the control group. It is only fair to state that the number of patients was few (83 in both groups), and information concerning comparability of patient groups was lacking.

Other trials of short-course adjuvant chemotherapy are those of Garin et al. of the U.S.S.R.,[48] Rieche et al. of Germany,[49] and Yoshida et al. of Japan.[50] The Japanese investigators employed mitomycin C following radical mastectomy and the other two groups administered CTX. Garin et al.[48] also treated a group of patients with TSPA. Overall, it may be stated that for a variety of reasons—e.g., lack of data and statistical analysis and inconsistencies in treatment regimens and patient selection—these studies make little, if any, substantive contribution to our knowledge regarding adjuvant chemotherapy.

At least five of the earlier trials have utilized more prolonged chemotherapy following surgery. Mrazek and McDonald,[51] between 1956 and 1964, divided 156 patients into treated and control groups. Mechlorethamine hydrochloride (nitrogen mustard) was given to the treated patients—one-half the "usual" dose at operation and the remainder on the first and second postoperative days. Every three months after operation, treated patients received courses of nitrogen mustard to bone marrow tolerance for a mean of 2.9 courses/patient. All patients were followed for eight to thirteen years. No patient who received chemotherapy had a recurrence, and all deaths in that group were unrelated to cancer. There was a recurrence of cancer in 36% of the control group, and only 57% survived.

Donegan[52] instituted a prospective trial in 1962 to determine the value of prolonged treatment with TSPA as an adjuvant to radical mastectomy. After an initial course of therapy begun on the day of surgery (0.4 mg/kg) and for two successive days (0.2 mg/kg per day), patients received 0.2 mg/kg per week for a minimum of one year. Forty-one control and 55 treated patients comprised the study. The author found that the overall recurrence rate was higher among treated patients than among controls, prompting him to suggest that prolonged systemic adjuvant chemotherapy may interfere with host resistance. In 1974, he updated his findings[53] and reported results from 75 controls and 90 treated patients observed from one to ten years. It was not possible to establish that TSPA was of value as a surgical adjuvant. Local recurrence was reduced, but overall recurrence was not altered, either in its frequency or time of appearance. A notable trend associated with treatment was improved disease-free survival among treated patients without axillary metastases. This led him to suggest that the adjuvant may be most effective when residual cancer is minimal.

In a trial whose results are difficult to evaluate, Kholdin et al.[54] reported that the use of postoperative chemotherapy nearly doubled the survival of patients with either negative or positive regional lymph node involvement. They presented results from 392 patients treated between 1964 and 1970 following radical mastectomy and radiation with thio-TEPA, 20–40 mg i.v. at operation and 0.3 mg/kg every day until a total dose of 240–280 mg was reached. This course of therapy was repeated for three or four times every six to eight weeks. Some patients were additionally treated by oophorectomy and long-term androgen and corticosteroid therapy. Cyclophosphamide was also administered to others. The findings were compared with 504 patients who received irradiation between 1949 and 1956. Since this study was not carried out in a randomized fashion and there are many aspects which require clarification, its importance defies assessment.

Ansfield[55] treated 60 patients with positive axillary nodes (number not stated) with six courses of 5-FU, beginning two to four weeks following mastectomy. Each course consisted of 12 mg/kg per day for five consecutive days, followed by half doses every other day to the point of slight toxicity or until 11 such half doses were given with 30-day intervals between courses. He compared the findings from 31 patients at risk after 55 years (56% with no recurrence) with previously reported NSABP data (33%) and concluded that 5-FU, so given, was highly beneficial as an adjuvant. The findings are suggestive that such adjuvant therapy is of value, but cannot be interpreted as being conclusive, since information is lacking to justify such a consideration.

A similar comment may be made concerning the brief report of Ramirez,[56] who treated patients with positive axillary nodes with a "loading course" of 5-FU, 12 mg/kg per day for five days, followed by 6 mg/kg every other day to slight toxicity starting 18 to 22 days after surgery, and maintained on weekly 5-FU, 15 mg/kg per week for one year. Patients received postoperative radiation one week after completion of the "loading course." At the time of reporting, there was an incidence of recurrence of 8.5%. Since there were no controls and the mean or median times following surgery are not provided, little can be said concerning this study.

5. Recent and Present Trials of Systemic Adjuvant Therapy

This was the state of affairs in late 1971, when it was deemed urgent by the NSABP that a trial be begun at once utilizing prolonged chemotherapy following surgery in women with clinically "curable" breast cancers; for, while results from trials conducted prior to that time were less than exciting, the concept of using prolonged chemotherapy continued to have experimental and clinical justification. It was increasingly more apparent that it was not so much the cells that were disseminated at the time of surgery which were of significance, but that it was the nondiscernible micrometastases present at operation which needed to be destroyed and that prolonged administration of chemotherapy provided the best opportunity for this. While there was, at that time, general agreement relative to the need for the beginning of trials of prolonged combined modality therapy, there existed no unanimity of opinion relative to the best agent, combination of agents, or schedule of administration to employ. Consequently, intense deliberation occurred before a protocol was adopted. We have emphasized that the choice of a regimen to be employed in a clinical trial of adjuvant therapy is a great responsibility which requires broad consultation, since by the very nature of such trials, there is a vast commitment of patient resources to many years of observation which could be considered to have been wasted should no positive findings occur.

Several considerations were deemed paramount in the selection of a modality to be employed in a surgical adjuvant trial. First, it was considered essential that such a therapy should have been demonstrated to have had a beneficial effect in advanced breast cancer. A comparison of modalities meeting that criterion (Table I) provided a number of choices.

Table I
Therapeutic Modalities Effective in Advanced
Breast Cancer

Modality	Percent response
1. Androgens	20
2. Single-agent chemotherapy	30
3. Estrogens	35
4. Hormonal ablative surgery	30–40
5. Oophorectomy	40–50
6. Combination chemotherapy	75

Because it could be employed regardless of menopausal status, and also for other reasons, it was considered that for a first trial, chemotherapy be employed in preference to hormonal manipulation.

Having made the initial decision, consideration was then given to what drug(s) might be employed in patients with advanced disease. The choices and their relative effectiveness are many (Table II).

In deciding upon a suitable agent for adjuvant therapy, it was felt that toxicity was of prime importance as a consideration. Rightly or wrongly, it was deemed at that time that surgeons and their patients were unlikely to accept a drug or drugs which produced the kind of toxicity observed and accepted in patients with advanced disease, since women receiving adjuvant therapy were well and were leading essentially normal lives. The toxicity patterns of those drugs receiving consideration were documented (Table III).

Next, the pharmacologic characteristics of these agents were re-

Table II
Effectiveness of Single Agents against Advanced Breast Cancer[a]

Drug	Number of patients evaluated	Number of objective responses	Percent responses
Alkylating agents			
Cyclophosphamide	327	97	30
Thio-TEPA	162	48	30
Nitrogen mustard	92	32	35
Phenylalanine mustard	86	20	23
Chlorambucil	54	11	20
Antimetabolites			
Methotrexate	259	87	34
5-Fluorouracil	1052	310	29
6-Mercaptopurine	45	6	13
Arabinosyl cytosine	64	6	9
Antibiotics			
Mitomycin C	60	23	38
Mithramycin	32	5	16
Actinomycin D	44	5	11
Adriamycin	150	55	37
Vinca alkaloids			
Vincristine	164	32	20
Vinblastine	95	19	20

[a]Data from Carter.[62]

Table III
Toxicity Patterns of Active Drugs against Breast Cancer

Adriamycin	Marrow Alopecia Stomatitis Cardiac Gastrointestinal
Cyclophosphamide	Marrow Gastrointestinal Alopecia Cystitis
5-Fluorouracil	Marrow Gastrointestinal Stomatitis
Methotrexate	Marrow Gastrointestinal Stomatitis
Vincristine	Neurotoxicity
Prednisone	Cushingoid appearances Hypertension Diabetes Peptic ulceration
Phenylalanine mustard	Marrow Gastrointestinal
Vinblastine	Marrow
Thio-TEPA	Marrow Gastrointestinal
CCNU	Delayed marrow Gastrointestinal
Dibromodulcitol	Marrow

viewed (Table IV). Certainly, the ideal adjuvant would be one which could be taken orally (p.o.).

Lastly, there was general agreement that if a single agent were to be employed, one which was cell-cycle-stage nonspecific offered the best chance for success. Consequently, that characteristic of the drugs was examined (Table V).

Table IV
Pharmacologic Characteristics of Drugs
Potentially Useful in Surgical Adjuvant Studies

Oral	Parenteral
Cytoxan	Cytoxan
5-Fluorouracil	5-Fluorouracil
Methotrexate	Methotrexate
Phenylalanine mustard	Phenylalanine mustard
Predinisone	Prednisolone
CCNU	Adriamycin
Dibromodulcitol	Vincristine
	Vinblastine
	Thio-TEPA

Having examined these parameters regarding the various drugs in a more or less systematic way (Table VI), it was concluded that of the several alkylating agents which demonstrated effectiveness in patients with advanced disease—CTX, nitrogen mustard, L-phenylalanine mustard (L-PAM), chlorambucil, or TSPA—there was little to choose from in terms of their accomplishments. A survey of available clinical information concerning those agents revealed that each produced a 20–30% objective response rate. In the extensive quantitative studies of Schmidt et al.,[57] in which 59 alkylating agents were evaluated against 20 animal neoplasms, CTX and L-PAM demonstrated the highest therapeutic indices. Because L-PAM could be administered orally at high intermittent doses for a prolonged period without causing alopecia or undue gastrointestinal toxicity, and because it had been noted by Sears et al.[58] to

Table V
Cell-Cycle Specificity of Drugs Potentially Useful
in Surgical Adjuvant Studies

Cell-cycle-stage specific	Cell-cycle-stage nonspecific
Methotrexate	Adriamycin
Vincristine	Cytoxan
Vinblastine	Phenylalanine mustard
5-Fluorouracil	Thio-TEPA
	Prednisone
	CCNU
	Dibromodulcitol
	5-Fluorouracil

Table VI
Summary of Factors Influencing Drug Selection for Adjuvant Therapy[a]

	Activity	Cell-cycle specificity	Unfavorable toxicity pattern	Positive pharmacologic characteristics
Adriamycin	++	0	++	+
Cytoxan	++	0	+	0—p.o.
5-Fluorouracil	++	+ −0	0	0—p.o.
Methotrexate	++	+	0	0—p.o.
Vincristine	+	+	+	0
Prednisone	+	0	++	0—p.o.
Phenylalanine mustard	+	0	0	0—p.o.
Vinblastine	+	+	0	0
Thio-TEPA	++	0	0	0
CCNU	+ −0	0	0	++—p.o.
Dibromodulcitol	+	0	0	+—p.o.

[a]From Carter.[62]

produce tumor regressions in breast cancer patients of all ages with soft tissue, osseous, and visceral metastatic disease, it was the drug selected for use. It was not anticipated that this drug and the regimen in which it was to be employed would prove to be *the ultimate* in surgical adjuvant therapy. As Skipper cogently pointed out[44]: "It would be foolhardy to expect to hit upon the best drug(s) and best regimen in the first, second or third clinical trial carried out. Hopefully, such trials could be planned in a manner so that we learn and improve design and end-results in stepwise fashion." Those responsible for preparation of the L-PAM protocol believed, however, that the agent to be used was one which might demonstrate a positive result and, at the same time, would be acceptable to enough investigators so that a group capable of conducting this and other trials could be formed.

At the same time, a great deal of consideration was given to the use of combination chemotherapy instead of a single agent, since there was convincing evidence to indicate that the use of multiple agents produced a significantly greater remission rate in patients with advanced disease than did single agents. The original studies by Greenspan and associates[59,60] and the subsequent confirmatory report by Cooper in 1969[61] established that simultaneous two-, three-, or four-drug therapy results in objective regressions in 60–85% of unselected metastatic cases with or without previous hormonal ablative responses. A variety of other reports (reviewed by Carter[62]), mainly from the Clinical Cooperative Groups in the United States, have, for the most part, failed to observe quite as great a remission rate. The Eastern Cooperative Group (ECOG) under the leadership of Carbone reported a 50% response rate when CTX, 5-FU, and MTX were simultaneously employed, and the Acute Leukemia Group B (Leone) observed a 52% remission rate with 5-FU, vincristine (VCR), and prednisone. The Mayo Clinic reported a 50% remission rate when CTX, VCR, and prednisone were used.

As has been pointed out by Schabel,[63] the advantages of combination chemotherapy are that their use results in (a) less than additive toxicity to vital normal cells, (b) potentiation of biochemical activity against tumor cells, and (c) destruction of tumor cells resistant to one or more of the drugs in the combination.

On the face of it, there would be every reason to anticipate that combination chemotherapy, which produces such a high rate of regression in advanced disease, would be exceedingly more effective in the presence of a minimal tumor burden (micrometastases), and, consequently, should be employed as adjuvant therapy. For the reasons elaborated above (toxicity, patient and physician acceptance) and because there remained the possibility that drugs moderately or only marginally effective when employed as single agents in advanced disease might be effective as combinations in the adjuvant setting, a "game plan" was devised which started with the use of a single agent. The plan was to progress in stepwise fashion, first comparing a single agent with no treatment, then two agents versus a single one, and eventually, three versus two. Hopefully, it could thus be ascertained what is required to attain a maximal therapeutic effect with acceptable toxicity.

5.1. L-PAM Protocol

Because of the interest which the L-PAM trial has generated as a result of a preliminary report of findings, a detailed accounting of it is presented. Data were obtained from women undergoing treatment at 37 institutions in the United States and Canada. All women having a radical mastectomy (conventional or modified) for potentially curable breast cancer and having one or more axillary nodes proved histologically to contain tumor were considered eligible for inclusion in the evaluation, provided they fulfilled specific criteria described in the protocol. These included tumors confined to the breast or breast and axilla; tumors movable in relation to the underlying muscle and chest wall; axillary nodes movable in relation to the chest wall and neurovascular bundle; no arm edema; white cell count ≥ 4000; platelet count of $\geq 100,000$; blood urea nitrogen ≤ 25 mg/100 ml; geographic accessibility for follow-up observation; absence of psychiatric or addictive disorders prohibiting the attainment of informed consent; and patient's consent to participate.

Women were considered to be ineligible for inclusion in the study because of the following: if they were over 75 years of age; were pregnant or lactating, had previously been treated for their current neoplasm or had a prior or concomitant cancer other than an effectively managed basal or squamous-cell skin tumor, had a bilateral breast cancer or a tumor other than a carcinoma, the tumor was inflammatory, there was skin ulceration >2 cm, or there was *peau d'orange* involving more than one-third of the skin of the breast, they were excluded. They were also ineligible for participation if satellite or parasternal nodules were present, there was fixation of axillary lymph nodes (over 2 cm), or there were lymph nodes elsewhere suspected of containing tumor unproved by biopsy to be negative. Moreover, if they were poor surgical risks, precluding their being subjected to any of the treatment options, or if nonmalignant systemic disease made prolonged follow-up study unlikely, they were unacceptable.

The experimental design of the study was such that after stratification according to age ($\leq$49 and $\geq$50 years), patients in each age group within each participating institution were randomized so that one-half received L-PAM and the other, placebo (Fig. 5). Neither the physician nor the patient was aware of the treatment administered, so as to ensure lack of bias in subsequent observations. Initially, only patients having four or more tumor-positive axillary nodes were placed on protocol. After the study had progressed for three months, those having one to three positive nodes were also included. Consequently, patients were also stratified according to their nodal status (one to three or four or more positive nodes). The first patient was entered into the evaluation on September 22, 1972.

Patients assigned to L-PAM therapy received 0.15 mg/kg per day for five consecutive days every six weeks. Dosage was determined accord-

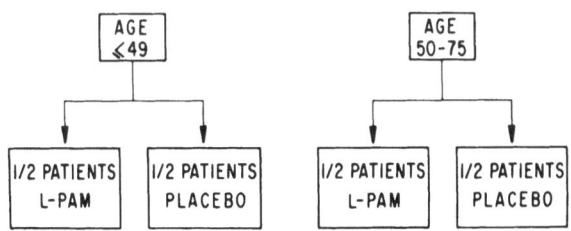

DOSE = 0.15mg/kg/DAY, P.O., X 5 q 6 WEEKS

Fig. 5. Clinical trial of prolonged therapy with L-phenylalanine mustard (L-PAM) as adjuvant to surgery.

ing to the patient's actual or ideal body weight, whichever was less. The entire daily dose was taken by mouth at bedtime. Treatment was begun no sooner than two weeks and not later than four weeks after operation and was to be continued until there was documented evidence of treatment failure, or for two years, whichever occurred first. Placebo was similarly administered.

The drug dose was modified according to the presence and degree of toxicity. The latter was categorized according to a drop in white cell or platelet count (or both) obtained before the onset of each new course of therapy. If no toxicity occurred, the patient received 100% of her calculated dose. If Grade 1 toxicity occurred, as evidenced by a decrease either in white cell count to between 2500 and 3999 or in platelet count to between 75,000 and 99,999, 50% of the calculated dose was given. After Grade 2 toxicity, when the white cell count was <2500 or the platelet count was <75,000, drug was discontinued and resumed only upon evidence of increase in those counts. If after three consecutive courses of therapy no toxicity was observed, the drug dosage was increased to 0.2 mg/kg of actual or ideal body weight per day, whichever was less.

Since a specific aim of that study was to ascertain whether the administration of L-PAM could prolong the disease-free interval of patients, when evidence indicating that achievement had occurred (September, 1974), a progress report of findings was presented.[64] At that time, it was observed (Table VII) that treatment failures had occurred in 22% of 108 patients receiving placebo and 9.7% of 103 women given L-PAM $(P = 0.01)$. A statistically significant difference $(P = 0.02)$ existed in favor of L-PAM relative to disease-free interval.

In premenopausal women (Table VIII), the difference with respect to disease-free interval of treated and control groups was highly significant $(P = 0.008)$. Treatment failures occurred in 30% of premenopausal patients receiving placebo and 3% of those treated with L-PAM $(P =$

Table VII
Proportion of Treatment Failures, Average Follow-Up Time, and Failure Rates for All Patients According to Treatment Groups[a]

Group	Proportion failing	Average follow-up period/patient (mo)	Failure rate $(\times 10^3)$
Placebo	24 of 108 = 0.22	8.4	0.22/8.4 = 2.6
L-PAM	10 of 103 = 0.097	9.1	0.097/9.1 = 1.1
P value	0.01		0.02

[a]From Fisher et al.[64]

Table VIII
Proportion of Failures, Average Follow-Up Time, and Failure Rates According
to Menopausal Status[a]

Status	Proportion of failures	Average follow-up period/patient (mo)	Failure rate ($\times 10^3$)
Premenopausal			
Placebo	11 of 37 = 0.30	8.6	0.30/8.6 = 3.5
L-PAM	1 of 30 = 0.03	9.3	0.03/9.3 = 0.4
P value	0.008		0.008
Postmenopausal			
Placebo	13 of 63 = 0.21	8.3	0.21/8.3 = 2.5
L-PAM	7 of 66 = 0.11	8.8	0.11/8.8 = 1.2
P value	0.15		0.17
Intramenopausal			
Placebo	0 of 8 = 0	9.2	—
L-PAM	2 of 6 = 0.33	11.0	0.33/11.0 = 3.0
P value	0.16		—
P value for all menopausal groups	0.02		

[a]From Fisher et al.[64]

0.008). Whereas a similar trend was observed in postmenopausal patients, the difference was not statistically significant.

Of interest was the finding that results were achieved with minimal alteration of the well-being of patients, despite the fact that 60% of women demonstrated myelosuppression (Grades 1 and 2 toxicity). Nausea and vomiting was reported in 30% of the patients treated with L-PAM. Ten percent of all courses of therapy were associated with that discomfort.

The question has frequently been asked as to the location of the treatment failures in patients who received L-PAM. At the time of the report, there were too few to make any correlation between the relationship of treatment and the location of such treatment failures. They approximated the distribution of those in the untreated group.

5.2. CMF Protocol

In 1973, Bonadonna and his associates at the National Cancer Institute in Milan, Italy embarked upon a clinical trial to evaluate the effectiveness of CTX, MTX, and 5-FU—CMF—as an adjuvant. The patient selection and experimental design were essentially similar to those out-

lined for NSABP Protocol #5 (above). Patients were randomized following radical mastectomy so as to receive either 12 cycles of CMF or no
treatment. Each cycle of drug therapy consisted of CTX (100 mg/M^2 p.o.
from day 1 to 14), MTX (40 mg/M^2 i.v. on days 1 and 8), and 5-FU (600
mg/M^2 i.v. on days 1 and 8). There was a two-week rest period between
cycles. A recent report of data from that trial[65] indicated (Table IX) that
whereas 24% of control patients had treatment failures by 14 months
following operation, only 5.3% of CMF-treated patients demonstrated a
recurrence. In contrast to the toxicity obtained when only the single
agent L-PAM was employed, as might be expected, greater side effects
were noted. Alopecia occurred in more than 50% of patients, cystitis in

Table IX
Characteristics of 179 Control Patients and 207 Patients Treated with CMF (Cyclophosphamide, Methotrexate, and Fluorouracil), with Observed Failure Proportions[a]

| | Evaluable patients | | | | |
| | Control | | CMF | | |
Characteristic	no.	%	no.	%	P value
Total with recurrence	43/179	24.0	11/207	5.3	$<10^{-6}$
Nodes					
1–3	21/125	16.8[b]	5/139	3.6	$<10^{-3}$
≥4	22/54	40.7[b]	6/68	8.8	$<10^{-4}$
Age					
≤49 years	17/74	22.9	6/95	6.3	$<10^{-2}$
≥50 years	26/105	24.7	5/112	4.4	$<10^{-4}$
Menopause					
Pre	20/82	24.3	5/95	5.2	$<10^{-3}$
Post	23/97	23.7	6/112	5.3	10^{-4}
Mastectomy					
Radical	26/132	19.6[c]	9/148	6.1	$<10^{-3}$
Extended	17/47	36.1[c]	2/59	3.3	$<10^{-4}$
Stage					
T$_1$	4/22	18.1	1/18	5.5	0.23
T$_2$	31/136	22.7	7/153	4.5	10^{-5}
T$_3$	8/21	38.1	3/36	8.3	$<10^{-2}$
Histology					
Ductal	39/158	24.6	9/180	5.0	$<10^{-6}$
Lobular	4/15	26.6	2/21	9.5	0.18
Other	0/6	—	0/6	—	
Mean follow-up period (mo)	14.0		13.7		

[a] From Bonadonna et al.[65]
[b] 1–3 nodes versus 4 or more: $P = 10^{-3}$.
[c] Radical versus extended: $P = 0.03$.

30%, and nausea and vomiting in almost all. About one-third of patients showed a repeated tendency to discontinue treatment or diminish the dose because of prolonged nausea and loss of appetite. Whereas 68% demonstrated leukopenia, only 4% had white blood cell counts below 2500. Similarly, 66% had thrombocytopenia but in only 12% was this below 75,000.

At the time of the publication of the L-PAM information, it was pointed out by the authors that many questions were raised by the findings (Table X) which only time could resolve. The findings of Bonadonna *et al.* reiterate the importance of those questions.

Inevitably, following the publication of the findings of the two studies, there was a comparison of the results. It must be emphasized that the two studies are not competitive, but are compatible in that they both have demonstrated, at least for the time of follow-up of each, an advantage in the use of adjuvant chemotherapy following operation. A careful review of material presented in the two reports indicates that the patient populations employed were not entirely comparable in that in the NSABP data, 32% were premenopausal, 7% were intramenopausal, and 61% were postmenopausal. In the Milan data, 46% were pre-menopausal and 54% were categorized as postmenopausal. Moreover, the percentage of patients with one to three positive nodes was 47% in the NSABP study and 68% in the Milan study. Thus, caution must be exercised in comparing the overall results of the two studies.

Table X
Questions Raised by the Preliminary Results of Adjuvant Therapy Trials

1. Will differences in disease-free rates be sustained?
2. Will they be manifested in survival rates?
3. Will undesirable sequelae such as an increase in second neoplasms occur?
4. Will there be a predilection for recurrences to occur at certain sites?
5. Will recurrences be more difficult to treat effectively?
6. Does such therapy prolong the disease-free state following operation but shorten survival following recurrence so that there is little or no total survival benefit?
7. How long should such therapy be given?
8. Is the sequencing of drugs more meritorious than the repetitive use of the same agent(s)?
9. Will immunostimulating agents permit greater tolerance to chemotherapy by the host?
10. Will such agents enhance host immune response and, when employed with chemo-therapy, result in an additive or synergistic effect as in animal models?
11. How relevant is information from patients with advanced disease to those with minimal disease after operation?
    a. Is the response of an overt mass predictive of the sensitivity of cells in micro-metastases?
    b. Might drugs marginally or not effective in advanced cancers be so following removal of a primary tumor?

While there seems to be little difference in the results insofar as premenopausal patients are concerned, the Milan data do demonstrate an advantage for those who are postmenopausal. A recent update of the NSABP data, so that mean follow-up times are comparable, continues to confirm the initial observations.

5.3. Additional NSABP Protocols

With completion of patient entry into NSABP Protocol #5 (placebo versus L-PAM), NSABP Protocol #7 was implemented, as part of our original plan to systematically proceed in stepwise fashion so as to determine maximum chemotherapeutic effectiveness with acceptable toxicity. Utilizing the same criteria of patient acceptability and keeping all other aspects of the protocol compatible with Protocol #5, patient entry began in February, 1975. By March, 1976, over 600 patients had been randomized between L-PAM and L-PAM plus 5-FU, and patient entry was terminated. The L-PAM was administered as the only agent at a dose of 6 mg/M^2 p.o. When combined with 5-FU, 4 mg/M^2 was given orally. The 5-FU dosage was 300 mg/M^2 i.v. Drugs were given on five consecutive days every six weeks for two years. To date, the toxicity of the two-drug combination is only a little greater than that of L-PAM alone and is entirely acceptable. Because patients have been entered into this protocol for only a year, no definitive data have as yet been forthcoming.

Shortly, the NSABP will implement three new protocols testing different adjuvant therapy regimens. Again, in keeping with our original plan for an orderly stepwise increase in the chemotherapy given, and to test the hypothesis that a three-drug combination is better than two or one, L-PAM (4 mg/M^2 p.o.) plus 5-FU (300 mg/M^2 i.v.) will be compared with L-PAM (4 mg/M^2 p.o.) plus 5-FU (300 mg/M^2 i.v.) plus MTX (25 mg/M^2 i.v.). As in previous protocols, the L-PAM and 5-FU will be given on five consecutive days every six weeks and the MTX, on days one and five of each cycle.

Since increasing evidence implicates the role of immunity in a variety of aspects of tumor biology, another NSABP clinical trial will compare chemotherapy with and without *Corynebacterium parvum* in the management of patients with surgically "curable" breast cancer who have one or more positive axillary nodes. The rationale for this employment of immunotherapy alone or in combination with chemotherapy is sound. There are several reasons for utilizing nonspecific immune stimulation in combination with surgery in the treatment of primary breast cancer at this time. A correlation has been established between immunodepression and cancer. It has been shown both experimentally and clinically that nonspecific immune stimulants may increase or restore the general immune status in cancer patients. While manipulation of "specific" immune mechanisms may be more appropriate, such is unlikely to take place in a state of nonspecific immune deficiency. Thus, it may be necessary to restore or improve nonspecific immunocompetence to attain the greatest host immune response.

The reasons for employment of *C. parvum* are related to its reputed relatively high degree of effectiveness and its reputed relatively low toxicity as compared to BCG. *C. parvum* has been demonstrated repeatedly to stimulate reticuloendothelial system function in various experimental tumor systems.[66-68] It has also been demonstrated to enhance resistance of mice to infection,[69] and to augment both delayed hypersensitivity and antibody production.[70] *C. parvum* can inhibit tumor growth in animal tumor systems[71-73] and has been shown to augment the effectiveness of cytostatic chemotherapeutic agents.[74,75]

Experience is accumulating with the use of *C. parvum* in humans. It has been demonstrated to prolong survival in metastatic disease when administered together with combined chemotherapy to a greater degree than chemotherapy alone.[76] Mean survival of 39 cases of disseminated epidermoid bronchogenic carcinoma treated by chemotherapy alone was compared to 43 cases receiving in addition to the same combination chemotherapy (five-drug), a weekly injection of *C. parvum*. In the *C. parvum* group, there was a survival rate of 85% at one year and 41% at two years. The chemotherapy control group had a 41% and 16% survival, respectively. It has been similarly employed against a variety of other solid tumors with significant results. Recently, objective tumor regressions have been noted when *C. parvum* was used i.v., even in the absence of chemotherapy.[77]

Side effects with the use of *C. parvum* administered subcutaneously have been uncommon. Significant local inflammation has occurred in only 3 of more than 400 cases treated by Israel and Edelstein.[76] No allergic reactions were encountered. An increase in the conversion of skin-test-negative to -positive has been reported with the use of *C. parvum*.[78] Accelerated tumor growth has not been observed in patients given *C. parvum*.

Due to the paucity of specific information available relative to *C. parvum* toxicity, a Phase I study was recently carried out by us in patients with advanced disease.[79] From 273 injections of *C. parvum* (5 mg/M^2) in 40 patients, it was observed that following i.v. infusion of *C. parvum*, (a) a febrile response and chills occurred in almost all patients and did not appreciably diminish in intensity following repetitive administrations; (b) nausea, vomiting, and headache were experienced; (c) a "flu-like" syndrome lasting 24 to 48 hours occurred following almost all courses of

C. *parvum;* (d) blood pressure elevations occurred on occasion and were related to the severity of other side effects; hyper- or hypotension was not a problem; and (e) no anaphylactic reactions or other untoward side effects were observed.

Pretreatment with a single administration of 100 mg of hydrocortisone prior to C. *parvum* infusion markedly, and in some instances dramatically, diminished the toxicity, reduced the duration of temperature elevation (Fig. 6), and made acceptable the use of i.v. C. *parvum* on an outpatient basis. The use of C. *parvum* in patients with cerebral metastases may be hazardous. Subcutaneously administered C. *parvum* resulted in a significant number of undesirable local reactions. Evaluation of delayed cutaneous hypersensitivity response, immunoglobulins, complement, E, and EAC rosette-forming cells during C. *parvum* administration failed to demonstrate significant change from preinjection values. Results were similar whether hydrocortisone pretreatment was or was not employed. It must be pointed out, however, that those measurements were made on patients having advanced disease who had received a variety of therapeutic regimens which could depress host immune responses. More recently, it has been observed by us in further Phase I trials that 50 mg of hydrocortisone (Solu-Cortef) also obtunds the side effects. There seems to be no evidence from accumulating data[80] to be concerned that such a dose of cortisone would interfere with C. *parvum* effectiveness. A baseline of information has been gathered from animal models[81,82] to provide guidelines for the timing, frequency, and dose of C. *parvum* to be employed.

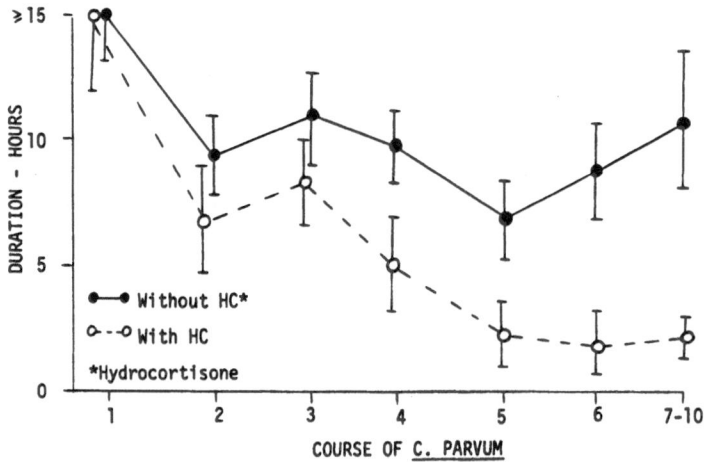

Fig. 6. Relation of duration of temperature elevation following i.v. C. *parvum* to course of therapy.

Patients will be randomized so that they receive L-PAM plus 5-FU in doses and schedules as described in the other NSABP protocols. One-half the patients receiving L-PAM plus 5-FU will also receive C. *parvum* (2.5 mg/M² i.v. every three weeks for one year and every six weeks the second year).

Another protocol which will hopefully be implemented in the next few months is one which evaluates the worth of tamoxifen when employed with chemotherapy. Tamoxifen (ICI 46474, Novaldex) is the *trans*-isomer of 1-(p-β-dimethylaminoethoryphenyl)-1,2-diphenylbut-1-ene. It is a synthetic nonsteroidal compound with potent antiestrogen activity demonstrated in several mammalian species.[83] Its mode of action is by blockade of estrogen receptors. In animal systems, it has been shown to inhibit binding of estradiol to uterine cytosol receptors[84] and has inhibited the growth of dimethylbenzanthracene (DMBA)-induced mammary tumors in rats.[85]

In 1971, Cole *et al.*[86] first reported an effect of tamoxifen when employed in patients with metastatic breast cancer. Of 46 patients so treated, 10 showed a good response, and of equal importance was the low incidence of troublesome side effects. Ward[87] reported that at a dosage of 10 mg twice daily, 60% of patients with metastatic breast cancers had "an arrest or reversal of tumor growth." With 20 mg twice daily, 77% of patients were so affected. As noted by Cole *et al.*, side effects were trivial and no patient showed virilization or fluid retention. Recently, Band and associates[88] have obtained results confirmatory of those obtained by others, and, in addition, noted that responses seemed to be correlated with the presence of estrogen receptors. A dose of 10 mg twice daily was highly effective.

In all reports, the most common toxic effects noted were hot flashes, mild nausea and fluid retention, and in some instances, thrombocytopenia or leukopenia which reverted to normal despite continuous drug administration. Others who have extensively employed this agent have likewise observed no significant toxicity with its use.[89,90] Consequently, as a result of reports of tamoxifen's demonstrated effectiveness in advanced disease, a trial of its use in early disease seems warranted.

Patients with surgically "curable" breast cancer who have one or more positive axillary nodes will be randomized between L-PAM plus 5-FU and L-PAM plus 5-FU plus tamoxifen. The dosage of L-PAM and of 5-FU is identical to that in other protocols; 10 mg of tamoxifen will be administered by mouth twice a day.

Due to increasing awareness of the rationale for combined modality therapy, additional studies to those of the NSABP have been begun around the world and particularly in the United States. The Clinical

Cooperative Groups are especially active in that regard. Frequency of implementation and alterations in protocol design make it impossible to insure complete documentation and accuracy. The following summarizes information that has come to our attention. Only a few studies have as yet produced data concerning the efficacy of the regimens being tested. They are not presented to supply the reader with a complete "registry" of all trials, but are for the purpose of indicating the spectrum of investigations that are under way.

5.4. Other Adjuvant Chemotherapy Trials (Table XI)

The Southwest Oncology Group (SWOG), under the leadership of Dr. Barth Hoogstraten, has begun a protocol to compare combination chemotherapy with a single agent in patients with operable breast cancer who have one or more positive axillary nodes. Patients are stratified according to the number of nodes involved, whether or not they receive postoperative radiation, and menopausal status. They are randomized so that they receive either L-PAM (5 mg/M^2 p.o. daily for five days every six weeks) or the combination of 5-FU (300 mg/M^2 i.v. weekly), MTX (15 mg/M^2 i.v. weekly), vincristine (VCR) (0.625 mg/M^2 i.v. weekly), CTX (60 mg/M^2 p.o. daily), and prednisone (30 mg/M^2 from day 1–14, 20 mg/M^2 from day 15–28, 10 mg/M^2 from day 29–42, and then discontinued). Following ten weeks of the five-drug therapy, the VCR

Table XI
Clinical Trials of Adjuvant Therapy for Stage II Breast Cancer
in Progress

Group (Investigator)	Treatment arms
1. SWOG (B. Hoogstraten)	a. L-PAM b. CMF + VCR + prednisone
2. COG (R. Johnson)	a. L-PAM b. CMF + VCR
3. Mayo Clinic (D. Ahmann)	a. L-PAM b. CTX, 5-FU, prednisone c. CTX, 5-FU, prednisone + postoperative radiation
4. Case-Western Reserve (C. Hubay)	a. No treatment b. CMF + tamoxifen (1/2 get BCG after first year)
5. ALGB (J. Holland)	a. CMF + VCR + prednisone b. CMF c. CMF + MER

and prednisone are discontinued and the CMF combination is given weekly. All therapy is discontinued after one year. No results are as yet available.

The Central Oncology Cooperative Group (COG), under the chairmanship of Dr. Robert Johnson, has initiated a protocol in which breast cancer patients with any number of positive axillary nodes are randomized into two groups. They receive either (a) L-PAM (0.15 mg/kg p.o. daily for five days every six weeks for one year) or (b) 5-FU (10 mg/kg i.v. weekly for seven weeks on days 1, 7, 14, 21, 28, 35, and 42), MTX (0.5 mg/kg i.v. weekly for seven weeks on the same days as the 5-FU), VCR (0.025 mg/kg i.v. weekly for four weeks on days 1, 7, 14, and 21), and CTX (2 mg/kg p.o. on days 1–42). The drugs are given in six-week cycles, followed by four-week rest periods, for one year.

Under the direction of Dr. David Ahmann, patients with positive axillary nodes are randomized into a three-armed protocol at the Mayo Clinic, Rochester, Minnesota. They receive either (a) L-PAM (6 mg/M^2 p.o. daily for five days), (b) CTX (150 mg/M^2 p.o. daily for five days), 5-FU (300 mg/M^2 i.v. daily for five days), and prednisone (300 mg daily for seven days, or (c) CTX, 5-FU, and prednisone as in (b) plus postoperative radiation.

Dr. Charles Hubay and associates at Case-Western Reserve in Cleveland, Ohio are carrying out a trial in which patients with any number of positive axillary nodes are stratified according to whether or not their tumors display estrogen receptor sites. They are randomized to either a "no treatment" control group or to a treatment group. The patients in the latter group receive 5-FU (400 mg/M^2 i.v. on days 1 and 8 of each month), MTX (25 mg/M^2 i.v. on days 1 and 8 of each month), CTX (60 mg/M^2 p.o. on days 1–14 of each month), and tamoxifen (20 mg twice daily every day of the month). A cycle of treatment consists of two weeks of therapy and two weeks of rest (except for tamoxifen). After one year of therapy, half of the patients in the treatment arm continue treatment for an additional year with BCG (Tice strain). They receive one ampule (2–8 × 10^8 organisms), via the tine technique, weekly for four consecutive weeks and subsequently, once a month.

The Acute Leukemia Cooperative Group B (ALGB), under the chairmanship of Dr. James Holland, has begun a trial to evaluate long-term systemic adjuvant chemotherapy with or without MER (methanol-extractable residue of tubercle bacilli). Patients with any number of positive axillary nodes are stratified according to age, tumor size, and nodal status. They are randomized following operation into one of three treatment arms. They receive either (a) CTX (80 or 10 mg/M^2 p.o. daily), 5-FU (500 mg/M^2 i.v. weekly), MTX (40 mg/M^2 i.v. weekly; 30 mg if over age 60), VCR (1 mg/M^2 i.v. weekly), and prednisone (40 mg/M^2 p.o. daily), (b) CMF as in (a) above, or CMF as in (a) or (b) plus MER (200 mg daily in each of five sites every second week). An induction phase of therapy from the first through the sixth week is followed by a three-week rest period. The therapy is resumed utilizing a four-week cycle. The drug is given for two weeks and the patient is rested for two weeks. After the first year of therapy, patients in all groups receive CMF for an additional year. No information concerning results has been reported.

5.5. Trials of Immunotherapy

In addition to the trials described above, there are others (Table XII) which employ immunotherapy as adjuvants following operation for primary breast cancer. These are listed in the International Registry of Tumor Immunotherapy of the National Cancer Institute compiled by Dr. Dorothy Windhorst of the Immunology Branch of that institution.

As yet, there is no information reported from them and there is little knowledge as to how many patients have been accrued, how many

Table XII
Trials of Immunotherapy as Adjuvants to Operation

Group (Investigator)	Treatment arms	Stage of breast cancer
1. UCLA Medical Center (Sparks)	a. CMF + BCG (tine) b. CMF + BCG + tumor cell vaccine	III
2. Duke University (Wells)	a. CMF + prednisone b. CMF + prednisone + C. parvum + allogeneic tumor cells	"Early"
3. M.D. Anderson Hospital (Gutterman)	a. Adriamycin b. Adriamycin + BCG (scarify) c. BCG	II
4. The London Hospital (Hermon-Taylor)	a. No treatment b. BCG (Glaxo, percutaneous, p.o.)	I and II
5. Evanston Hospital (Scanlon)	a. L-PAM b. CTX + FU + prednisone c. CTX + FU + prednisone + BCG (daily)	II and III
6. Sloan-Kettering (Oettgen)	a. L-PAM b. CTX + FU + adriamycin c. Levamisole (p.o.)	II
7. Institute Gustave Roussy (Lacour)	a. No treatment b. Radiation c. Radiation + poly(A)·poly(U)(i.v.) d. Poly(A)·poly(U)	T_2, T_3 N_0, N_1

more are necessary for completion of the study, or special problems encountered. Hopefully, all of this will, in due time, become available.

6. Comments and Speculations

The next decade may well represent the most critical and significant period in the history of breast (as well as other) cancer therapy. The present spectrum of combined modality trials, added to those which are proliferating at an ever more rapid pace throughout the world, is setting the stage for that crisis situation. Should many or most of those trials started with the most noble of intentions fail to be continued to a point where meaningful data are obtained—or, even worse, because of their improper design or implementation produce information of questionable credibility—valuable time will have been lost, patient resources will have been squandered, and, above all, therapeutic confusion and disenchantment will prevail. On the other hand, should a sufficient number of the protocols be impeccably carried to completion and meaningful data obtained, the next ten years could be even more crucial. For there will result verification or repudiation of not only the concepts and principles upon which the use of adjuvant therapy is based, but of the very worth of those modalities which, at present, represent our total therapeutic resources and hopes for cure of the diseases.

If, for example, as unlikely as it may seem, despite the multiplicity of trials evaluating different chemotherapeutic combinations in a variety of ways, should a significant prolongation of freedom from disease which is reflected in a major improvement in survival fail to be observed, the entire chemotherapeutic approach to the treatment of breast cancer will be subject to challenge. The present regression of metastases for 6 to 18 months following combination chemotherapy in up to 85% of patients with advanced disease should not obscure the dismal fact that long-term control for three or more years after the onset of chemotherapy is achieved in less than 15% of those treated for recurrence. The five-year survivorship after the onset of chemotherapy for recurrent metastases is less than 5%, despite best efforts. Consequently, if adjuvant chemotherapy fails to make a dramatic impact on the disease-free survival of patients with "minimal" disease, the outlook is indeed bleak for those with advanced tumors—unless, of course, new agents become available.

Similar considerations relate to the use of immunotherapeutic and hormonal agents. Obviously, unless they can aid in the "cure" of more "curable" lesions, their worth in advanced disease will be nil.

More optimistically, it is likely that from the multiplicity of trials there will come information regarding which regimens are most effective against a particular subset of breast cancer patients with a minimum of toxicity. It is not unreasonable to predict that the same magnitude of chemotherapy employed in patients with four or more positive nodes having a highly unfavorable prognosis will not be required for the patient with one node positive. Most urgently needed for the proper synchronization of available therapeutic modalities so as to make such a concept a reality is the availability of a biological assay that can indicate with precision the amount and the location of residual tumor following operation. It may be predicted that as information becomes available from more of the trials currently in progress, the physician caring for such patients will be faced with a disturbing situation worse than the surgical dilemma of the last decade or two. A debate, for example, that CMF is categorically better than L-PAM or that CAMP (CTX, adriamycin, MTX, prednisone) is better than CMF could well rival the simple versus radical mastectomy polemic. Hopefully, since results are being obtained from carefully controlled studies, in contrast to the method by which the surgical data were generated, such controversies will be avoided.

We have pointed out that to date, the most important aspect of the findings achieved with L-PAM and more recently with CMF is not the statistical magnitude of the differences, or even that the results could be obtained with acceptable toxicity, but that it has been demonstrated that the rationale for using prolonged chemotherapy as an adjunct to operation is a sound one. Different agents in various combinations, refinements of administration, sequencing of drugs, etc., will undoubtedly produce increasingly better results. This will follow as a corollary to the observations obtained, but the initial step forward has been achieved.

One of the pressing decisions to be made is whether or not systemic therapy should be employed at the present time in patients with negative axillary nodes. Since, as has been pointed out, 25% of these patients have treatment failures by ten years, it is our opinion that a trial of such therapy be begun at once. Obviously, such a trial will require significantly greater numbers of patients followed for much longer times than those utilizing women with a more unfavorable prognosis. It will also require the greatest of circumspection in preparation of a protocol.

As systemic therapy becomes more effective, the more likely it becomes that lesser operative procedures could be comparable. As a consequence, increased disease control could be accomplished together with better cosmesis and quality of life. It is not unreasonable to anticipate that the use of systemic therapy will make more remote the chance that at some time in the not too distant future, when diagnostic methodology has improved so that earlier cancers are detected and when there is better understanding regarding the proper use of anti-cancer agents in concert so as to maintain maximum effectiveness, surgery may play a subsidiary role in the management of solid tumors and may be entirely supplanted by other modalities.

It may be stated that at present, there would seem to be justifiable reason for optimism concerning the future of women who develop breast cancer. Paradoxically, however, there will be no permanent prescription or recipe for the management of this disease in the foreseeable future, simply because it is likely that as a result of this initial move forward, as well as activity from other sources, progress will proceed in various directions with increasing momentum and it is impossible to predict the ultimate nature of the next plateau.

In conclusion, the answer to the universal question, "Should *all* women with primary breast cancer receive systemic therapy in addition to surgery?", must be a qualified one. The answer can, for the present?, be "yes" only if this is carried out in a clinical trial situation. Since it has not yet been shown that any therapeutic regimen cures *more*, let alone *all*, patients, a multiplicity of additional trials carried out in a *coordinated* fashion are necessary to make further gains. Where will patients for those trials come from if each is treated by her physician without making a contribution to our knowledge? How will it be possible to resolve the plethora of new questions raised by each additional bit of information? In our opinion, adjuvant therapy for breast cancer as of the spring of 1976 is still a component of clinical research in oncology.

7. References

1. M.L. Mendelsohn, The growth fraction: A new concept applied to tumors, *Science* **132**, 1496 (1960).
2. H.E. Skipper and F.M. Schabel, Jr., Quantitative and cytokinetic studies in experimental tumor models, in: *Cancer Medicine* (J.F. Holland and E. Frei, III, eds.), pp. 629–650, Lea and Febiger, New York (1973).
3. H.E. Skipper, Kinetics of mammary tumor cell growth and implications for therapy, *Cancer* **28**, 1479–1499 (1971).
4. D.M. Shapiro and R.A. Fugmann, A role for chemotherapy as an adjunct to surgery, *Cancer Res.* **17**, 1098–1101 (1957).
5. M.A. Chirigos, J. Colsky, S.R. Humphreys, J.P. Glynn, and A. Goldin, Evaluation of surgery and chemotherapy in the treatment of mouse mammary adenocarinoma 755, *Cancer Chemother. Rep.* **22**, 49–53 (1962).
6. H. Druckrey, B.T. Kirk, D. Schmahl, and D. Steinhoff, Kombination von operation und chemotherapie biem krebs: Modeliver suche an einem resistenten tumor der ratte, *Muench. Med. Wochenschr.* **100**, 1913–1918 (1958).
7. N. Brock, Neue experimentelle ergebnisse mit N-Lost-Phosphamidestern, *Stahlentherapie* **41**, 347–350 (1959).

8. Y.N. Molkov, Prevention by aurantin of recurrence and metastases after surgical removal of transplantable tumors, *Vopr. Onkol.* **6**, 19–25 (1960).

9. K. Karrer, S.R. Humphreys, and A. Goldin, An experimental model for studying factors which influence metastasis of malignant tumors, *Int. J. Cancer* **2**, 213–223 (1967).

10. K. Karrer and S.R. Humphreys, Continuous and limited courses of cyclophosphamide (NSC-26271) in mice with pulmonary metastasis after surgery, *Cancer Chemother. Rep.* **51**, 439–449 (1967).

11. S.R. Humphreys and K. Karrer, Relationship of dose schedules to the effectiveness of adjuvant chemotherapy, *Cancer Chemother. Rep.* **54**, 379–392 (1970).

12. J.G. Mayo, W.R. Laster, Jr., C.M. Andrews, and F.M. Schabel, Jr., Success and failure in the treatment of solid tumors. III. "Cure" of metastatic Lewis lung carcinoma with methyl-CCNU (NSC-95441) and surgery–chemotherapy, *Cancer Chemother. Rep.* **56**, 183–195 (1972).

13. H.E. Skipper, Combination therapy: Some concepts and results, *Cancer Chemother. Rep. Part 2* **4**, 137–145 (1974), as mentioned by D.P. Griswold, Jr.

14. M.J. Straus, V. Sege, and S.C. Choi, The effect of surgery and pretreatment or posttreatment adjuvant chemotherapy on primary tumor growth in an animal model, *J. Surg. Oncol.* **7**, 497–512 (1975).

15. D.S. Martin, P.W. Hayworth, and R.A. Fugmann, Enhanced cures of spontaneous murine mammary tumors with surgery, combination chemotherapy, and immunotherapy, *Cancer Res.* **30**, 709–716 (1970).

16. R.A. Fugmann, D.S. Martin, P.E. Hayworth, and R.L. Stolfi, Enhanced cures of spontaneous murine mammary carcinomas with surgery and five-compound combination chemotherapy, and their immunotherapeutic interrelationships, *Cancer Res.* **30**, 1931–1936 (1970).

17. T.R. Ashworth, A case of cancer in which cells similar to those in the tumours were seen in the blood after death, *Aust. Med. J.* **14**, 146 (1869).

18. H. Marcus, Krebzellen im stromenden blut, *Z. Krebsforsch.* **16**, 217–230 (1917).

19. K. Schleip, Zur diagnose von knochenmarkstumoren aus dem blut-befunde, *Z. Klin. Med.* **59**, 261–282 (1906).

20. G.R. Ward, The blood in cancer with bone metastases, *Lancet* **1**, 676 (1913).

21. E.H. Pool and G.R. Dunlop, Cancer cells in bloodstream, *Am. J. Cancer* **21**, 99–102 (1934).

22. E.R. Fisher and R.B. Turnbull, Jr., Cytologic demonstration and significance of tumor cells in the mesenteric venous blood in patients with colorectal carcinoma, *Surg. Gynecol. Obstet.* **100**, 102–108 (1955).

23. H.C. Engell, Cancer cells in the circulating blood, *Acta Chir. Scand. Suppl.* **201**, 1–70 (1955).

24. G.E. Moore, A.A. Sanberg, and J.R. Schubarg, Clinical and experimental observations of the occurrence and fate of tumor cells in the bloodstream, *Ann. Surg.* **146**, 580–587 (1957).

25. J.C. Pruitt, A.W. Hilberg, and R.F. Kaiser, Malignant cells in peripheral blood, *N. Engl. J. Med.* **259**, 1161–1164 (1958).

26. R. Reiss, Demonstration of carcinoma cells in the bloodstream, *J. Mt. Sinai Hosp. N.Y.* **26**, 171–176 (1959).

27. W.S. Fletcher and J.W. Stewart, Tumor cells in the blood with special reference to pre- and post-hepatic blood, *Br. J. Cancer* **13**, 33–37 (1959).

28. H.T. Langston, J.F. Laws, E.A. McGrew, C. Heidenreich, and M. Slominski, The incidence of blood vessel invasion in bronchogenic carcinoma, *Surg. Gynecol. Obstet.* **107**, 704–708 (1958).

29. T.P. Morley, The recovery of tumor cells from venous blood draining cerebral gliomas, *Can. J. Surg.* **2**, 363–365 (1959).

30. A.W. Diddle, D.M. Sholes, Jr., J. Hollingsworth, and S. Kinlaw, Cervical carcinoma; cancer cells in the circulating blood, *Am. J. Obstet. Gynecol.* **78**, 582–585 (1959).

31. W. Coutts, E. Silva-Inzunza, R. Bulnes, and D. Rosenberg, Cytologic investigation of malignant cells in peripheral blood and testicular substance from patients orchiectomized for prostatic carcinoma, *J. Urol.* **82**, 607–609 (1959).

32. M. Romsdahl, S. Potter, R. Malmgren, E. Chu, C. Brindley, and R. Smith, A clinical study of circulating tumor cells in malignant melanoma, *Surg. Gynecol. Obstet.* **111**, 675–681 (1960).

33. W. Grove, A. Watne, O. Jonasson, and S. Roberts, The vascular dissemination of cancer in children, *Am. Med. Assoc. Arch. Surg.* **78**, 698–702 (1959).

34. S. Roberts, A. Watne, R. McGrath, E. McGrew, and W.H. Cole, Technique and results of isolation of cancer cells from the circulating blood, *Am. Med. Assoc. Arch. Surg.* **76**, 334–346 (1958).

35. L. Long, O. Jonasson, S. Roberts, R. McGrath, E. McGrew, and W.H. Cole, Cancer cells in the blood; results of simplified isolation technique, *Am. Med. Assoc. Arch. Surg.* **80**, 910–919 (1960).

36. S. Roberts, L. Long, O. Jonasson, R. McGrath, E. McGrew, and W.H. Cole, The isolation of cancer cells from the bloodstream during uterine curettage, *Surg. Gynecol. Obstet.* **111**, 3–11 (1960).

37. O. Jonasson, L. Long, S. Roberts, E. McGrew, and J. McDonald, Cancer cells in the circulating blood during operative management of genitourinary tumors, *J. Urol.* **85**, 1–12 (1961).

38. N.C. Delarue, The free cancer cell, *Can. Med. Assoc. J.* **82**, 1175–1182 (1960).

39. E.P. Cruz, G.O. McDonald, and W.H. Cole, Prophylactic treatment of cancer; the use of chemotherapeutic agents to prevent tumor metastasis, *Surgery* **40**, 291–296 (1956).

40. G.O. McDonald, E.P. Cruz, and W.H. Cole, The effect of cancer inhibitor drugs on the "take" of Walker carcinosarcoma 256 in rats, *Surg. Forum* **7**, 486–489 (1956).

41. G.O. McDonald, C. Livingston, C.F. Boyles, and W.H. Cole, The prophylactic treatment of malignant disease, with nitrogen mustard and triethylenethiophosphoramide (Thio-TEPA), *Ann. Surg.* **145**, 624–629 (1957).

42. B. Fisher, R.G. Ravdin, R.K. Ausman, N.H. Slack, G.E. Moore, and R.J. Noer, Surgical adjuvant chemotherapy in cancer of the breast: Results of a decade of cooperative investigation. *Ann. Surg.* **168**, 337–356 (1968).

43. B. Fisher, N. Slack, D. Katrych, and N. Wolmark, Ten year follow-up of breast cancer patients in a cooperative clinical trial evaluating surgical adjuvant chemotherapy, *Surg. Gynecol. Obstet.* **140**, 528–534 (1975).

44. H.E. Skipper, Some thoughts on surgery–chemotherapy trials against breast cancer, in: Monograph, Southern Research Institute, Birmingham, Alabama (1971), p. 1.

45. R. Nissen-Meyer, K. Kjellgren, and B. Mansson, Preliminary report from the Scandinavian Adjuvant Chemotherapy Study Group, *Cancer Chemother. Rep.* **55**, 561–566 (1971).

46. B. Mansson, K. Kjellgren, and R. Nissen-Meyer, Cyclophosphamide as adjuvant to primary surgery for breast cancer, a cooperative controlled clinical study, in: Proceedings of the 11th International Cancer Congress, Florence, Italy, Vol. 3 (1974), p. 531.

47. R. Finney, Adjuvant chemotherapy in the radical treatment of carcinoma of the breast—a clinical trial, *Am. J. Roentgenol.* **111**, 137–141 (1971).

48. A.M. Garin, N.I. Darev, and A.P. Bashenovoc, A summary of the comparative studies of the efficacy of different techniques in treatment of early forms of the mammary gland cancer, *Vopr. Onkol.* **3**(19), 87–93 (1973).

49. K. Rieche, H. Berndt, and B. Prahl, Continuous postoperative treatment with cyclophosphamide in breast carcinoma. A randomized clinical study, *Arch. Geschwulstforsch.* **40**, 349–354 (1972).

50. Y. Yoshida, S. Mivra, and H. Muroi, Late results in combined chemotherapy for cure of breat cancer (axillary lymph node metastases and therapeutic effect), in: 10th Annual Meeting of the Japanese Society for Cancer Therapy (1973) (abstract 177).
51. R.G. Mrazek and G.O. McDonald, Surgery and adjuvant chemotherapy in treatment for breast carcinoma, in: Abstracts of the Tenth International Cancer Congress, Houston, Texas (1970), p. 501.
52. W.L. Donegan, Prolonged surgical adjuvant chemotherapy with Thio-TEPA for mammary carcinoma: A progress report, in: Abstracts of the Tenth International Cancer Congress, Houston, Texas (1970), p. 500.
53. W.L. Donegan, Extended surgical adjuvant Thio-TEPA for mammary carcinoma, Arch. Surg. 109, 187–192 (1974).
54. S.A. Kholdin, L.Y. Deemarsky, and J.L. Bavly, Adjuvant long-term chemotherapy in complex treatment of operable breast cancer, Cancer 33, 903–906 (1974).
55. F.J. Ansfield, 5-FU as an adjuvant to mastectomy in high-risk patients, Proc. Am. Assoc. Cancer Res. and Am. Soc. Clin. Oncol. 15, 177 (1974) (abstract).
56. G. Ramirez, Combined chemotherapy–radiotherapy as an adjuvant to mastectomy in patients with positive nodes, Proc. Am. Assoc. Cancer Res. and Am. Soc. Clin. Oncol. 16, 224 (1975) (abstract).
57. L.H. Schmidt, R. Fradkin, R. Sullivan, and A. Flowers, Comparative pharmacology of alkylating agents, Cancer Chemother. Rep. Suppl. 2, 1–1528 (1965).
58. M.E. Sears, A. Haut, and N. Eckles, Melphalan (NSC-8806) in advanced breast cancer, Cancer Chemother. Rep. 50, 271–297 (1966).
59. E.M. Greenspan, M. Fieber, G. Lesnick, and S. Edelman, Response of advanced breast carcinoma to the combination of the antimetabolite methotrexate and the alkylating agent Thio-TEPA, Mt. Sinai J. Med. N.Y. 30, 246–267 (1963).
60. E.M. Greenspan, Combination cytotoxic chemotherapy in advanced disseminated breast carcinoma, Mt. Sinai J. Med. N.Y. 33, 1–26 (1966).
61. R.G. Cooper, Combination chemotherapy in hormone resistant breast cancer, Proc. Am. Assoc. Cancer Res. abstract 57 (1969).
62. S.K. Carter, Reported at National Surgical Adjuvant Group Meeting, Bethesda, Maryland (October 10–11, 1973).
63. F.M. Schabel, Jr., Synergism and antagonism among antitumor agents, in: Pharmacological Basis of Cancer Chemotherapy (27th Annual Symposium on Fundamental Cancer Research at M.D. Anderson Hospital, Houston, Texas), pp. 595–621, Williams and Wilkins, Baltimore (1975).
64. B. Fisher, P. Carbone, S.G. Economou, R. Frelick, A. Glass, H. Lerner, C. Redmond, M. Zelen, D.L. Katrych, N. Wolmark, P. Band, E.R. Fisher, and Other Cooperating Investigators, L-Phenylalanine mustard (L-PAM) in the management of primary breast cancer; a report of early findings, N. Engl. J. Med. 292, 117–122 (1975).
65. G. Bonadonna, E. Brusamalino, P. Valagussa, A. Rossi, L. Brugnatelli, C. Brambilla, M. DeLena, G. Tancini, E. Baietta, R. Musumeci, and U. Veronesi, Combination chemotherapy as an adjuvant treatment in operable breast cancer, N. Engl. J. Med. 294, 406–410 (1976).
66. B.N. Halpern, A.R. Prevot, G. Biozzi, C. Stiffel, D. Mouton, J.C. Morard, Y. Bouthillier, and C. Decreusefond, Stimulation of the phagocytic activity of the RES provoked by C. parvum, J. Reticuloendothel. Soc. 1, 77–96 (1963).
67. M.T. Scott, Biological effects of adjuvant C. parvum. I. Inhibition of PHA, mixed lymphocytes and GVH reactivity, Cell. Immunol. 5, 459–468 (1972).
68. L.H. Smith and M.F.A. Woodruff, Comparative effect of 2 strains of C. parvum on the phagocytic activity and tumor growth, Nature 219, 197–198 (1968).
69. C. Adlam, E.S. Broughton, and M.T. Scott, Enhanced resistance of mice to infection

with bacteria following pretreatment with *C. parvum, Nature (London) New Biol.* **235,** 219–220 (1972).

70. T. Neveu, A. Branellec, and G. Biozzi, Adjuvant effect of *C. parvum* on antibody production and delayed hypersensitivity conjugated proteins, *Ann. Inst. Pasteur (Paris)* **106,** 771–777 (1964).

71. B. Halpern, G. Biozzi, C. Stiffel, and D. Mouton, Inhibition of tumor growth by administration of killed *C. parvum, Nature* **212,** 853–854 (1966).

72. M.F.A. Woodruff and J.L. Boak, Inhibitory effect of injection of *C. parvum* on the growth of tumor transplants in isogenic hosts, *Br. J. Cancer* **20,** 345–355 (1966).

73. M.F.A. Woodruff and M.P. Inchley, Synergistic inhibition of mammary carcinoma transplants in A-strain mice by antitumor globulin and *C. parvum, Br. J. Cancer* **25,** 584–593 (1971).

74. G.H. Currie and D. Bagshawe, Active immunotherapy with *C. parvum* and chemotherapy in murine fibrosarcomas, *Br. Med. J.* **1,** 541–544 (1970).

75. B. Fisher, N. Wolmark, E. Saffer, and E.R. Fisher, Inhibitory effect of prolonged *Corynebacterium parvum* and cyclophosphamide administration on the growth of established tumors, *Cancer* **35,** 134–143 (1975).

76. L. Israel and R. Edelstein, Nonspecific immunostimulation with *C. parvum* in human cancer, in: 26th Annual Symposium on Fundamental Cancer Research at M.D. Anderson Hospital, Houston, Texas (1973), pp. 485–504.

77. L. Israel and R. Edelstein, A phase II study of daily intravenous *Corynebacterium* in 33 disseminated cancers, *Proc. Am. Assoc. Cancer Res.* **16,** 67 (1975).

78. L. Israel and B. Halpern, *C. parvum* in advanced cancers: Initial evaluation of therapeutic activity, *Nouv. Presse Med.* **1,** 19–23 (1972).

79. B. Fisher, H. Rubin, G. Sartiano, L. Ennis, and N. Wolmark, Observations following *Corynebacterium parvum* administration to patients with advanced malignancy: A phase I study, *Cancer* **38,** 119–130 (1976).

80. B. Fisher, H. Rubin, E. Saffer, and N. Wolmark, Further observations on the inhibition of tumor growth by *C. parvum* with cyclophosphamide. II. Effect of cortisone acetate, *J. Natl. Cancer Inst.* **56,** 571–574 (1976).

81. B. Fisher, N. Wolmark, H. Rubin, and E. Saffer, Further observations on the inhibition of tumor growth by *C. parvum* with cyclophosphamide: I. Variation in administration of both agents, *J. Natl. Cancer Inst.* **55,** 1147–1153 (1975).

82. B. Fisher, H. Rubin, E. Saffer, and N. Wolmark, Effect of *Corynebacterium parvum* in combination with 5-fluorouracil, L-phenylalanine mustard or methotrexate on the inhibition of tumor growth, *Cancer Res.* **36,** 2714–2719 (1976).

83. M.J.K. Harper and A.L. Walpole, A new derivative of triphenylethylene: Effect on implantation and mode of action in rats, *J. Reprod. Fertil.* **13,** 101–119 (1967).

84. J.R. Skidmore, A.L. Walpole, and J. Woodburn, Effect of some triphenylenthylenes on oestradiol binding *in vitro* to macromolecules from uterus and anterior pituitary, *J. Endocrinol.* **52,** 289–298 (1972).

85. V.C. Jordon, *Steroid Biochem.* **5,** 354 (1974), as mentioned by Band in personal communication.

86. M.P. Cole, C.T.A. Jones, and I.D.H. Todd, A new anti-oestrogenic agent in late breast cancer: An early clinical appraisal of ICI 464, *Br. J. Cancer* **25,** 270–275 (1971).

87. H.W.C. Ward, Anti-oestrogen therapy for breast cancer: A trial of tamoxifen at two dose levels, *Br. Med. J.* **1,** 13–14 (1973).

88. P. Band, H. Lerner, L. Israel, and B. Leung, Personal communication (1976).

89. O. Pearson, Personal communication (1975).

90. H.J. Tagnon, Reported at the National Conference on Breast Cancer, Montreal, Canada (1975).

4

Combination Chemotherapy for Advanced Disease

PAUL P. CARBONE AND DOUGLASS C. TORMEY

1. Introduction

1.1. Background

The chemical nonhormonal treatment of breast cancer has developed rapidly in the last three decades. In the first two decades, several reports indicated that responses could be achieved in patients with nitrogen mustard,[1] triethylenethiophosphoramide (thio-TEPA),[2] methotrexate,[3] cyclophosphamide,[4,5] and 5-fluorouracil.[6] With the demonstration in experimental animal tumors and clinically in patients with Hodgkin's disease[7] and acute lymphocytic leukemia[8] that combinations of drugs were more effective than single agents, interest in the use of multiple-drug regimens also developed for patients with breast cancer. One of the earliest reports was by Greenspan *et al.* in 1963.[9] But it was not until 1969, when Cooper[10] reported that a five-drug program produced complete responses in 90% of patients with advanced breast cancer, that the trials with combination chemotherapy became more widespread. Since then, there has been a literal explosion of combination chemotherapy programs[11] producing high response rates in the 50–60% range. In the past two years, chemotherapy has played a major role combined with surgery in the management of primary operable breast cancer.

PAUL P. CARBONE AND DOUGLASS C. TORMEY · National Cancer Institute, Bethesda, Maryland. Present address: Division of Clinical Oncology, Wisconsin Clinical Cancer Center, University of Wisconsin, Madison, Wisconsin.

During the past 30 years, chemotherapy traditionally was used as a last resort, reserved for patients who failed surgery and radiotherapy and following various hormonal maneuvers. As combination chemotherapy programs have proven to produce substantial and durable responses, there has been the realization that chemotherapy may play an important role in the management of patients before hormonal treatments. Thus, questions have arisen regarding the relative roles of chemotherapy and hormonal therapies. The reservation of systemic chemotherapy for the patient with advanced progressive hormone-refractory disease has been questioned, and more emphasis has been placed on the use of nonhormonal chemotherapy earlier in the course of the disease.[12] In this review, we plan to discuss the natural history of advanced breast cancer relative to chemotherapy, the kinetic and theoretical considerations for cancer chemotherapy, the pharmacokinetics of the important cancer drugs, the methods of clinical evaluation of anticancer drug therapy, the usefulness of combinations as compared to single agents, and the clinical results with chemotherapeutic agents. We will also discuss the potential importance of combining chemotherapy with hormonal therapy, the current status of immunotherapy in breast cancer, the changing role of chemotherapy in the treatment of primary breast cancer, and frontiers of research, particularly, ways of being more selective in the use of individual drugs.

1.2. Natural History of Advanced Breast Cancer Relative to Chemotherapy Response

While the majority of patients will eventually die of disseminated breast cancer, only 10% of patients present with advanced or Stage IV disease.[13] The median survival of patients presenting with metastatic breast cancer is 11 months, and only about 8% of patients with clinically disseminated disease will survive five years.[14] Survival is influenced by a variety of biologic characteristics of the disease. One of these factors is the extent of disease. Staging in advanced disease, while not as well defined as in primary disease, is an important prognostic feature.[15] While the age of the patient does not appear to be an important factor in prognosis, postmenopausal patients appear to have slower-progressing disease than premenopausal patients, resulting in median survivals of 12 and 8 months, respectively.[16] The ambulatory status of the patient and the organ sites of disease involvement are the two most consistent prognostic factors. Ambulatory patients survive almost twice as long as nonambulatory patients.[17] Patients with massive nodular pulmonary disease, lymphangitic pulmonary disease, intracranial metastases, or hepatic disease with abnormal function tests tend to live one-half to one-third as long as patients with other sites of involvement. [18] Bone marrow involvement, previously thought to be an unfavorable clinical feature, no longer harbors a poor prognosis with more recent active combination chemotherapy regimens. [19] However, patients with one or two different organ sites of involvement do better than patients with three or more organ sites of involvement. [20] Unlike the situation with hormone therapy, prior hormone responsiveness or the long duration of disease-free time since primary surgery are not consistently good prognostic features for chemotherapy programs.

Much of the staging evaluation can be obtained from a careful history, physical examination, and selected laboratory tests. The laboratory tests to be utilized vary with information obtained from the history and physical examination, coupled with the known frequency of various metastatic sites. Autopsy series reveal that metastases occur primarily in bone, thoracic cage, skin and subcutaneous structures, brain, adrenals, and liver (Table I). [21] This concurs with sites of first recurrence following surgery, where > 96% of metastases are found in bone, thoracic cage, skin and subcutaneous structures, and liver (Table II). [22] Brain metastases occur in fewer than 1% of patients as the first site of metastasis. It has been shown that the most useful clinical parameters to evaluate these sites include the history, physical examination, [99mTc]polyphosphate or diphosphonate bone scan, posterior–anterior and lateral chest X rays, SGOT or SGPT, and alkaline phosphatase. Liver scanning with [99mTc]sulfur colloid will detect 25% of hepatic lesions before the liver becomes clinically palpable or the liver function tests become abnormal. However, the abnormal scan precedes the abnormalities in liver size and function tests by only a few weeks and

Table I
Breast Cancer Metastases—Autopsy Data[a]

Organ	Percent	Organ	Percent
Lymph nodes	87	Kidney	13
Lungs	58–78	Diaphragm	13–14
Brain	58	Spleen	13–23
Liver	54–59	Pancreas	12–13
Bone	43–48	Skin	11–38
Adrenals	31–44	Cervix/uterus	11
Gastrointestinal tract	26	Peritoneum	9–20
Pleura	23–35	Thyroid	9
Heart	21–33	Other	12–13
Ovary	13–16		

[a]Adapted from Cutler. [21]

Table II
Site of First Recurrence in Breast Cancer
(253 patients)[a]

Site	No. of cases	Percent of cases
Nonskeletal	143	56
Operative region	48	19
Pulmonary/hilar	31	12
Supraclavicular	20	8
Pleural effusion	16	6
Opposite breast	9	4
Liver	6	2
Skin	5	2
Other	8	3
Skeletal	110	44
Pelvis	29	11
Lumbar spine	25	10
Dorsal spine	19	8
Ribs	16	6
Femur	9	4
Skull	5	2
Other	7	3

[a]Romsdahl et al. [22]

effects changes in clinical management in <1% of cases.[23,24] Thus, this procedure is usually performed for confirmation or to have a baseline for future studies. Skeletal X rays of scan-detected lesions initially provide verification in about half the cases and are superior to repeated isotope scanning for following the therapeutic course.[24] Tomography of scan-positive, X-ray-negative lesions will reveal destructive lesions in approximately half the cases. Gallium scintigraphy in breast cancer patients appears to be useful only for the detection of mediastinal lesions not visualized by plain chest X rays or tomography.[25,26] As such, it can suggest a site for biopsy by mediastinoscopy to obtain tissue for diagnosis and estrogen receptor assays.[26] Other tests such as serum calcium, blood counts, and brain scanning are obtained as a result of specific complaints or physical findings, or as a baseline for therapy.

Operative-site recurrences have been considered to be less ominous than systemic recurrences. More recently, it has been found that local recurrences should be viewed as harbingers of disseminated disease.[27,28] The time from surgery to local recurrence is the same as the time from surgery to more distant metastases.[29] Thus, these recurrences should be characterized as disseminated disease and the patient's management should include systemic as well as local treatments.

Historically, chemotherapy had been relegated to the patient with recurrent disease who had failed hormone therapy. Today, chemotherapy is being applied during the postoperative period in patients at high risk of relapse and in combination with hormone therapy (see Section 6). In many centers, the higher response rates afforded by combination chemotherapy over hormone therapy in unselected patients have led to its use prior to hormonal manipulation. This approach is based on the recurring observations in animals and in human trials that the longest survival is achieved by applying the most effective regimen first.[30-34] In patients failing their initial therapy, a regimen used as a second therapy is only 30–50% as effective as the same regimen used as a first-line therapy. As a result, survival following failure on the first therapeutic regimen is often measured in weeks or, at best, a few months. These considerations will be expanded below.

2. Experimental Background of Chemotherapy of Breast Cancer

2.1. Cell Cycle and Chemotherapy

For many years, cell division studies were mainly concerned with the events of mitosis. All other aspects of the cell cycle were characterized as interphase. The biochemical events preceding mitosis were largely unknown. In 1953, Howard and Pelc first showed that DNA synthesis did not occur continuously throughout interphase, and they defined M, G_1, S, and G_2 phases of the cell cycle.[35] Since then, much has been learned about the biochemical events in the cell cycle, as many of the antineoplastic drugs have been used to characterize these events. As a result, we have a much better understanding of the cell cycle and the mechanisms of action of the drugs.

Most of the antimetabolite anticancer drugs, either directly or after being converted to nucleotides or higher phosphates, affect the synthesis and/or functioning of the nucleic acids.[36] The cell membranes are relatively impermeable to the nucleotides and nucleic acids, whereas they readily admit purines, pyrimidines, and nucleosides. Once inside the cell, conversion to nucleotides occurs, where they can compete with naturally occurring bases and nucleosides for selected anabolic enzymes. The inhibition may occur competitively or noncompetitively. The metabolically active compounds may inhibit nucleic acid synthesis, compete with normal substrates for anabolic synthesis of nucleic acid, or be incorporated into DNA or RNA, where they interfere with nucleic acid function (Fig. 1).[37] Other antimetabolite drugs do not require metabolic activation but effectively compete with normal substrates for anabolic enzymes required for nucleic acid synthesis.

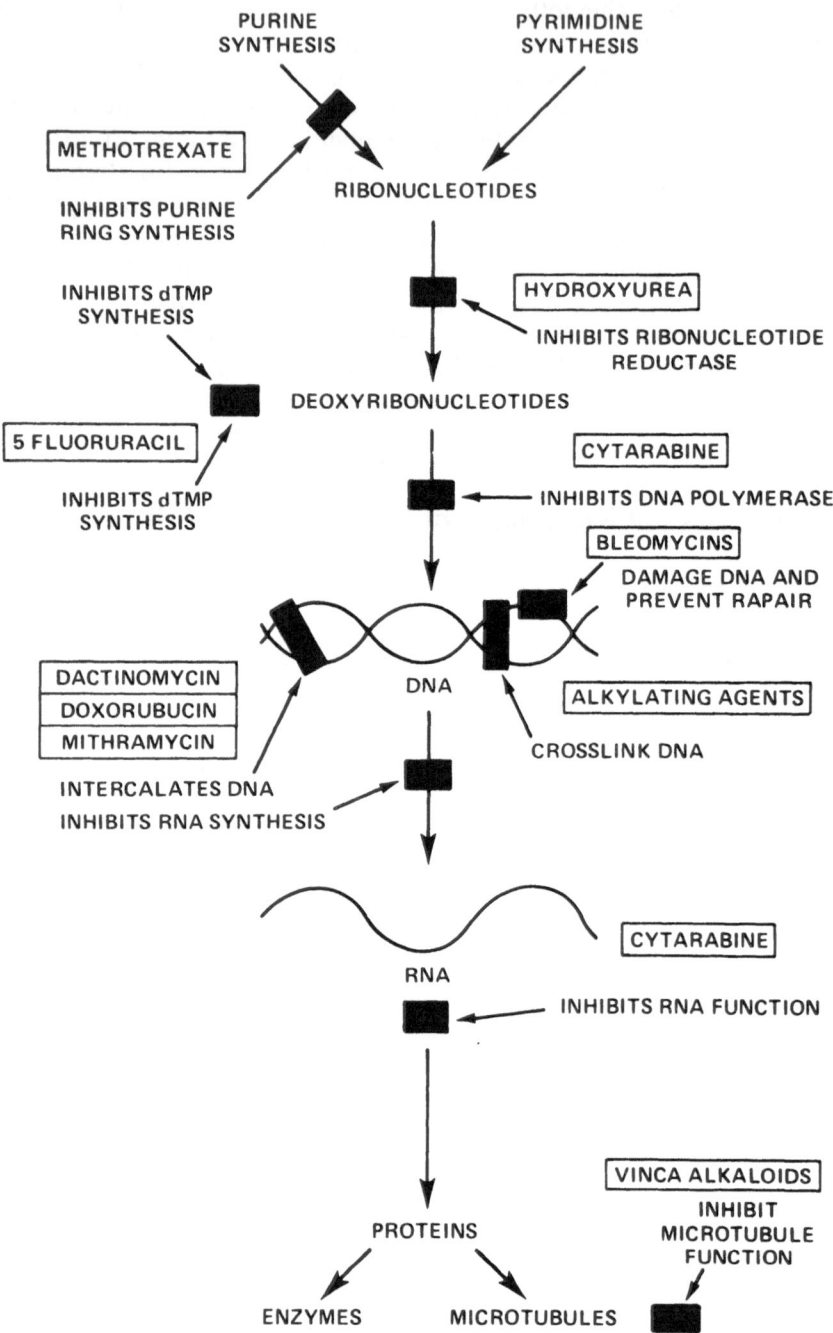

Fig. 1. Schema for drug action.[37]

The antimetabolites interfere with DNA synthesis in S phase, allowing cells in G_2 and M to proceed through G_1, where a block in further development occurs. Protein synthesis and RNA synthesis continue, leading to unbalanced growth. Other agents interfere with *de novo* synthesis of ribonucleotides and with aspects of the cell cycle that require nucleic acid synthesis. The affected cells tend to arrest in G_1. The blockade in G_1 is not as dramatic as with S-phase inhibitors. These arrests in cycle progression can result in partial synchronization of the cells and to changes in sensitivity to various chemotherapeutic agents.

Alkylating agents represent a variety of compounds drawn from different classes of chemicals such as epoxides, aziridines, alkane sulfates, or 2-chloroethylamines, which act by forming a highly reactive, positively charged alkyl radical.[38] They exert their biological effect by alkylation of nucleophilic sites within the cell. In addition to cytotoxicity, the alkylating agents are known to be more powerful mutagens and inhibit the replication of DNA viruses. These compounds tend to be more active when they are bifunctional rather than monofunctional. An important action of an alkylating agent is its binding to the N-7 position of guanine and the N-3 position of adenine in DNA. As a result of the alkylation of these two bases, slow fission of the deoxyriboside bond joining these alkylated bases to the sugar phosphate backbone occurs. Interstrand linkage also occurs, interfering with DNA replication that may lead to cell death.

At least two other major classes of agents are useful in breast cancer treatment. These are the metaphase inhibitors such as vincristine and vinblastine, which directly interfere with mitosis by binding to the microtubules of the spindle,[39] and the antitumor antibiotics, which are not easily characterized by a similar mechanism of action. In general, the latter agents may act by intercalation or binding to the DNA molecule, thereby interfering with RNA, DNA, or protein synthesis or causing DNA breaks.[40,41]

The extent of cell survival and multiplication following treatment with the antineoplastic agents can be determined by following *in vivo* and/or *in vitro* surviving fractions of normal hematopoietic cells and transplanted murine lymphoma cells[42,43] or bioassaying the neoplastic cells.[44] The shape of the curve plotting the logarithm of the surviving fraction against the concentration of the drug (Fig. 2) infers a mechanism of action for the drug.[42] When an exponential curve is obtained, the agent inhibits all phases of the cell cycle (cycle-nonspecific agents). When the curve falls rapidly and then flattens out at higher concentrations, cell-kill most likely occurs in a certain phase of the cell cycle (phase-specific drugs). An intermediate curve shape is obtained which departs clearly from either of the above, indicating multiple sites of

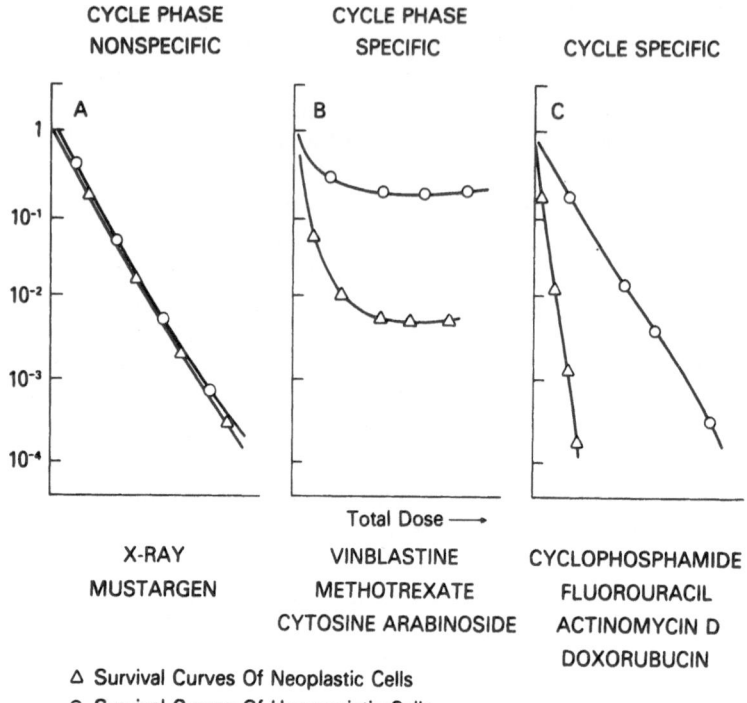

CYCLE PHASE
NONSPECIFIC

CYCLE PHASE
SPECIFIC

CYCLE SPECIFIC

X-RAY
MUSTARGEN

VINBLASTINE
METHOTREXATE
CYTOSINE ARABINOSIDE

CYCLOPHOSPHAMIDE
FLUOROURACIL
ACTINOMYCIN D
DOXORUBUCIN

△ Survival Curves Of Neoplastic Cells
○ Survival Curves Of Hemopoietic Cells

Fig. 2. Drug effects and cell survival.

lethality, but where the parts of the cell cycle are not equally sensitive
(cycle-specific).

2.2. Cell Kinetics

In addition to cell-cycle effects, since all cancer cells are not actively
proliferating, the sensitivity of tumor cells to a specific drug is a function
of the proliferating state of the tumor. The growth fraction, or proportion of proliferating cells to total cells, is particularly low in solid tumors
like breast cancer, resulting in differential sensitivity among dividing
and resting tumor cells.[45] The cycle times of tumor cells are not constant but are related to the volume of the tumor cell mass. As the tumor
increases in size, the growth rate decreases, described as a Gompertzian
function.[46] The reasons for the changes in growth rate as the tumor
increases in size are due either to lengthening in the cell-cycle times or to
a loss of the reproductive cell fraction. Furthermore, large tumors tend
to have necrotic components—due, in part, to failure of the host to
provide nutritional and/or capillary support—resulting in a relatively

nongrowing, but still viable, state. Finally, there may be other active regulatory mechanisms that limit cell growth through an immunologic control or a biologic feedback system.[47]

To develop a rational basis for chemotherapy of cancer, still other factors must be taken into account besides drug action and the cancer cell kinetics. One of these is the mechanism of cell-kill by drugs. Drugs affect tumor cells by first-order kinetics, which means that a fraction of tumor cells, rather than an absolute number, are killed with a given dose. Various analogies have been used, including that of breaking 1000 eggs by throwing bushels of nails, where each bushel of nails destroys 90% of the eggs. Therefore, 100 eggs survive the first bushel, 10 the second, 1 the third and 0.1 the fourth. Thus, after four bushels of nails, no intact eggs would be left.[48] Berenbaum has restated this analogy, implying not only fractional kill but also the concept that the tumor cells are proliferating.[49] He uses the model of eight rabbits in a field and a doubling time of three months for the rabbits, with killing accomplished by firing at random into the field a bushel of buckshot every three months. Thus, not only must one kill the rabbits in the field that are present at time zero, but also take into the account that the rabbits—i.e., tumor cells—are multiplying. If the firing were done every three months and 50% of the rabbits were killed, after three months the rabbit population would remain at eight and no decrease in the rabbit population would ever occur. Thus, in this analogy one can develop strategies related to dose and frequency of injection. Furthermore, Berenbaum postulates that the cell-kill characteristics of antimetabolites can be described as requiring a logarithmic increase in dose to cause a logarithmic increase in cell-kill. However, logarithmic increases in cell-kill by alkylating agents and radiation can be accomplished by linear increases in dose.

Into calculations of the experimental basis of chemotherapy must be taken the sensitivities and recovery times of normal host tissues, adding to the complexity.[50] Little information is available in man, although this can be done experimentally by computer model building and by the use of animal tumors, in which both normal and neoplastic tissues are studied. Important to our discussion is the concept that small tumors grow more rapidly and are more sensitive to chemotherapeutic agents. Morever, the response of the advanced "large cell mass–low growth fraction" tumor may not be predictive of the response of the exponentially growing small micrometastases.[31] Not only are the tumor cell kinetics of the small tumor more favorable for chemotherapy, but also the probabilities of drug resistance less likely when the tumor population is small, i.e., $<10^6$ tumor cells.[34] By the time the tumor reaches 1.0 cm in size, there are about one billion tumor cells and almost 30 doublings have occurred. Not only are the kinetics unfavorable for chemotherapy in this large tumor, but, in addition, the time factor increases the probability of metastases, since tumor cells are constantly being shed into the lymphatic and/or systemic circulation.[51]

2.3. Growth Rates of Human Breast Cancers

The features important to understanding the growth rate of human breast cancers include measurements of clinical doubling time (DT), estimates of G_1, G_2, S, and M, and determinations of growth fraction. Historically, the most information is available on doubling times, derived by following the growth of measurable tumor masses. Philippe and LeGal measured 78 recurrent breast cancer lesions and found a mean volume DT of about 40 days, with a range of 3 to 211 days.[52] They noted an almost bimodal distribution of DT's: a rapid group of 25 days DT and a slower group of about 93 days DT. They also noted that nonscirrhous cancers grew faster than scirrhous cancers and that only one of 16 patients with premenopausal breast cancers had a slow growth rate. After menopause, about 30% of all patients with recurrent breast cancers had slow-growing tumors. In another study by Lee and Spratt,[53] 171 metastatic sites were measured in 54 patients. They noted a mean DT of about 17 days with a 95% confidence interval of 3.4 to 86.1 days. Growth rates of simultaneously measured lesions tended to be approximately similar. They also showed that the growth rate after shrinkage following chemotherapy was about the same as before. In a study by Malaise and co-workers[54] comparing several types of tumors, adenocarcinomas, of which 75 of 122 were breast cancers, had a mean DT of 83 days (72–96 days, 95% confidence limits). In contrast, embryonal tumors had a DT of 27 days (22–32 days); hematosarcomas, 29 days (23–37 days); and squamous-cell cancers, 58 days (48–70 days). Thus, breast adenocarcinomas tend to have a wide range of DT's but, in general, are slower growing compared to other cancers (Table III).[54]

The data on labeling indices or the ability of breast tumors to take up tritiated thymidine are less readily available. The studies require analysis of the uptake of thymidine in tumor biopsy specimens. In their review, Malaise and co-workers report a relatively low labeling index of 2.1% (range 1.7–2.7) for adenocarcinomas. More recently, Schiffer and Braunschweiger have reported labeling indices of 3.5% in 14 cases of primary breast cancers and 6.8% in 6 cases of metastatic cancers.[55] As with doubling time, the relative labeling indices of the breast cancers were much slower than the other cancers measured. The embryonal tumors had values of 30%; the hematosarcomas, 29%; and squamous-cell carcinomas, 8.3%. Estimates of S time determinations (T_S) have

Table III
Certain Kinetic Parameters of Human Cancers[a]

Pathology	Labeling indices (%)	Doubling times (days)	Estimated growth fraction (%)
Embryonal tumors	30	27	90
Lymphomas	29.2	29	90
Sarcomas	3.8	41	11
Squamous-cell carcinomas	8.3	58	25
Adenocarcinomas	2.1	83	6

[a]Malaise et al. [54]

been in the range of 14 to 24 hours. Based on the calculated T_S, the cell-cycle time (T_c), and the labeling indices (LI), one can calculate growth fractions using the formula $GF = LI(T_c/T_S)$.[54] Again, adenocarcinomas are among the lowest, with a growth fraction estimate of only 6% as compared to 90% for the embryonal tumors. Thus, the data indicate that visible breast cancer lesions grow relatively slowly and have relatively high cell-loss fractions.

In collating the data on cell kinetics of breast cancer and drug action, one is left with the conclusion that the cytokinetic characteristics of the advanced breast cancer patient's tumors are highly unfavorable for achieving cell cure. Not only are the numbers of tumor cells large, in the order of 10^9 and 10^{11} cells, but the tumors are growing quite slowly. Also adversely affecting response is the feature that the large tumors, because of their bulk, areas of necrosis, and inadequate vascular supply, probably prevent adequate penetration of the active drug. Moreover, the large numbers of tumor cells not only decrease the possibility of any effective host immunologic control but also are highly likely to be associated with drug-resistant cells.[34] The resultant clinical effects, as measured by tumor shrinkage in patients, can be predicted to be small with single agents. Combinations are more likely to produce better responses, but even here the responses are not likely to be climaxed by cures. Moreover, following the first dose of drug, marked changes in the cycle time, S, and growth characteristics may occur. In general, these effects may further decrease the chances of cell-kill unless the changes are taken into account.[56] Attempts at synchronizing cells to increase their sensitivity to drugs have been made in the leukemias but not very actively in the solid tumors. As yet, most chemotherapy trials have been largely empirically based, discounting considerations of cell kinetic characteristics of the tumor. Despite this lack of theoretical basis, clinical trials in breast cancer have indicated that chemotherapy can produce substantial responses and can cause effective palliation.

A major reason for the favorable effects of chemotherapeutic agents can be attributed to the use of combinations of drugs. The principles of combination chemotherapy include the use of independently active drugs with differing mechanisms of action so that they can be combined at nearly full doses. In addition, one attempts to administer the drugs at high doses for short periods of time and intermittently to allow for host immune and stem-cell recovery. Chronic long-term schedules are less likely to produce cell cures in experimental systems.[34] Intermittent schedules allow for rational administration of immunotherapeutic stimulants as well. A critical question in the strategy of combination chemotherapy focuses around the concept of how many drugs should be included. Because most chemotherapeutic drugs affect the normal marrow and the gastrointestinal tract, marked reductions in dose of the individual agents must be made when one uses more than three or four agents. Therefore, an alternative approach has been the utilization of alternating cycles of two or three drugs in an attempt to achieve maximal cell-kill and to circumvent possible drug resistance which is likely to occur in high-volume tumors.

2.4. Animal Models

A wide variety of transplantable animal tumors are available for use in screening chemotherapeutic agents. Most of the currently available drugs for clinical use in breast cancer have not come primarily from tests in animal mammary tumors. The development of these agents is beyond the scope of this review. However, once a drug has been tested in a broad spectrum of human tumors including breast cancer and is found to cause tumor regressions clinically, specific questions can be asked of animal mammary tumors. These relate to whether there are comparable sensitivities in the animal mammary cancers to the active clinical drugs, whether the spontaneous mammary cancer carries a similar responsiveness to transplantable tumors, and how the drugs can be used together to develop optimal combinations.

One of the best characterized murine mammary tumors is the spontaneous carcinoma in the BALB/Cf C_3H × DBA/8f hybrid developed by Martin.[57] This tumor occurs in high frequency, can be transplanted, and is suitable for surgical adjuvant trials with chemoimmunotherapy. The hybrid animal host can readily tolerate extensive treatment. Most importantly, of the six major clinically active drugs in breast cancer, this tumor was sensitive to five, with methotrexate as the only false negative. Of the six tested inactive drugs in human breast cancer, none were effective against the murine tumor. Further trials with combinations of the active drugs indicate that two and three drugs combining cyclophosphamide or L-phenylalanine mustard with 5-fluorouracil and adriamycin are most effective.

A second animal mammary tumor system is the C_3H/Hen mammary tumor in mice. This tumor occurs in variable frequency but can be transplanted into hybrid mice for chemotherapy trials. Griswold was able to isolate at least ten transplantable cell lines with a wide spectrum of responses to a variety of chemotherapeutic agents.[58] As with the BALB/Cf $C_3H \times$ DBA/8f tumor, these lines were all resistant to methotrexate, had variable responses to 5-fluorouracil, and were sensitive to L-phenylalanine mustard, cyclophosphamide, and adriamycin in varying degrees. Because of the inbred strain of the parent tumor, trials in autochthonous spontaneous tumors are very difficult. Most of the studies are done in transplanted tumors.

A third well-studied tumor system is the 13762 mammary adenocarcinoma in the Fischer 344/CRB$_L$ rat. This tumor originally was induced by 7,12-dimethylbenzanthracene (DMBA) and has been transplantable for many generations. Metastases are common. Bogden and associates have treated this tumor with drugs that have clinical activity against human cancer as well as with combined modality trials. Of the active agents in humans, only methotrexate was inactive in the rat model. Combination chemotherapy programs have indicated a high degree of activity for L-phenylalanine mustard or cyclophosphamide with adriamycin and 5-fluorouracil.[59] Trials of immunostimulants and surgery plus chemotherapy have likewise been done. Noteworthy is the fact that none of the tumors described above is truly hormone-responsive to oophorectomy or exogenously administered hormones. Other tumors are hormone-dependent but have been less well characterized for chemotherapy. Thus, models for the study of hormone and chemotherapy responsiveness need to be developed.

A fourth system being evaluated currently is the use of allogeneic transplantation of human tumors into athymic or immunosuppressed mice.[60,61] Primary breast cancer transplants have been relatively difficult to grow in immunosuppressed mice, although established cell lines from pleural fluids of patients with breast cancer can be readily transplanted. Chemotherapy trials of the human tumors in these mice are being done. Some advantages can be readily appreciated in that the tissues are human, but there are also some theoretical disadvantages because the kinetics of the tumor in the mouse are probably changed and the metabolism of drugs in the mouse is not always the same as in man.

There are several possible approaches to studying the effect of drugs on breast cancer other than those in the mouse, rat, or man. These involve the use of cell culture systems; however, such approaches have not yet been extensively investigated.

In general, the important principles of combining drugs, the value of adjuvant therapy, and combining chemo- and immunotherapy have already been well demonstrated in animals. What needs to be done is to develop ways to predict the individual sensitivity of a particular patient's tumor. The answer to this problem can be visualized as a series of experiments in the animal with eventual translation to man.

3. Pharmacology

There are approximately 40 current chemotherapeutic agents that are either commercially or investigationally available. Not all of these drugs have been adequately tested in breast cancer. Table IV lists the majority of these agents and indicates the available data concerning their activity. The agents that have been tested in over 100 patients include cyclophosphamide, thio-TEPA, 5-fluorouracil, vincristine, adriamycin, methotrexate, and CCNU. Agents with apparent response rates in excess of 20% include all of these drugs except CCNU, as well as nitrogen mustard, L-phenylalanine mustard, mitomycin C, hexamethylmelamine, dibromodulcitol, and BCNU. Agents that appear to be marginally active, i.e., with response rates from 15–20%, are chlorambucil and vinblastine. Agents that appear to be inactive include cytosine arabinoside, Me-CCNU, CCNU, imidazole carboxamide, procarbazine, and 6-mercaptopurine. Agents that have not had sufficient clinical testing to warrant a judgment include 6-thioguanine, actinomycin D, mithramycin, hydroxyurea, streptonigrin, bleomycin, and daunomycin.

Representative single-agent schedules, available routes of administration, major pharmacologic properties, and toxicities are outlined in Table V for the marginally active and active agents. For further information, the reader is referred to recent reviews of the anticancer agents.[62–65] The availability of oral formulations is particularly useful for patients with poor veins or in postoperative adjunctive therapy programs. The drugs useful in this regard include cyclophosphamide, chlorambucil, L-phenylalanine mustard, methotrexate, and dibromodulcitol. Methotrexate and bleomycin can also be administered intramuscularly. The remaining drugs, as well as those mentioned above, with the exception of chlorambucil, L-phenylalanine mustard, and dibromodulcitol, require intravenous formulations.

In general, the effect of a variety of schedules of administration of these agents has not been extensively investigated in breast cancer.

Table IV
Single-Agent Response Rates in Metastatic Breast Carcinoma[a]

Drug	No. of patients evaluated	No. of patients responding	Percent response
Alkylating agents			
Nitrogen mustard (HN2)	92	32	35
Cyclophosphamide (CYT)	529	182	34
Thio-TEPA (TSPA)	162	48	30
L-Phenylalanine mustard (L-PAM)	86	20	23
Chlorambucil (CLB)	54	11	20
Antimetabolites			
Methotrexate (MTX)	356	120	34
5-Fluorouracil (5-FU)	1236	324	26
6-Mercaptopurine	44	6	14
Hydroxyurea	16	2	12
Cytosine arabinoside	64	6	9
Mitotic inhibitors			
Vincristine (VCR)	226	47	21
Vinblastine (VBL)	95	19	20
Antibiotics			
Mitomycin C (Mito C)	60	23	38
Adriamycin (ADR)	221	81	37
Others	99	13	13
(actinomycin D, mithramycin, streptonigrin, bleomycin, daunomycin)			
Synthetics			
Hexamethylmelamine (HXM)	39	11	28
Dibromodulcitol (DBD)	22	6	27
BCNU[b]	76	16	21
CCNU[b]	155	18	12
Imidazole carboxamide	29	2	7
MCCNU[b]	33	2	6
Procarbazine	21	1	5

[a]Modified from Broder and Tormey.[11]
[b]Abbreviations: BCNU = 1,3-bis(2-chloroethyl)-1-nitrosourea; CCNU = 1-(2-chloroethyl)-3-cyclohexyl-1-nitrosourea; MCCNU = 1-(2-chloroethyl)-3-(4-methylcyclohexyl)-1-nitrosourea.

However, there is evidence to suggest that 5-fluorouracil is most active in an intermittent loading dose schedule and methotrexate on a once to twice per week schedule. For either theoretical or ease of administration reasons, the following drugs are usually administered in intermittent regimens: mitomycin C, cyclophosphamide, adriamycin, and BCNU.

Table V
Single-Agent Characteristics

Drug	Common schedules/routes[a]	Pharmacologic principles	Common major toxicity
Nitrogen mustard	17–24 mg/M² i.v. every 3 wk 0.2–0.4 mg/kg i.c.	Plasma $T_{1/2}$ = 30–60 sec; renal clearance: 50% within 24 hr; metabolites inactive	Nausea, emesis, leukopenia, thrombocytopenia
Cyclophosphamide	500–800 mg/M² i.v. weekly 2–2.5 mg/kg per day p.o.	Plasma $T_{1/2}$ = 3.8–5.5 hr; renal clearance: 65% in 48 hr, 32% of which is active drug; oral route: 17–31% excreted in stool as active drug	Nausea, emesis, alopecia in 50%, leukopenia, thrombocytopenia, hemorrhagic cystitis in 1–4%, fever to 101°F
Thio-TEPA	30–60 mg i.v. every 1–4 wk	90% plasma clearance within 3 hr; most of drug excreted in urine as active form within 48 hr	Leukopenia, thrombocytopenia
L-Phenylalanine mustard	6 mg/M² p.o. on day 1–5 every 4–6 wk	Cleared from plasma within 6 hr; renal excretion of metabolites	Leukopenia, thrombocytopenia, mucosal ulceration
Chlorambucil	0.1–0.2 mg/kg per day p.o.	—	Leukopenia

Methotrexate	15–30 mg/M^2 i.v., i.m., p.o. twice weekly	Plasma $T_{1/2}$ = 3.5 hr; renal clearance: 90% as active form within 12 hr (p.o.) or 6 hr (i.v.); 50% bound to albumin and displaceable by sulfa or aspirin; cerebrospinal fluid concentration: 10% that of plasma; effects reversible by citrovorum factor for up to 72 hr	Leukopenia, mucosal ulcers, hepatic damage, pneumonitis
5-Fluorouracil	15 mg/kg per week, i.v. 15 mg/kg on day 1–5 → 7.5 mg/kg on day 7, 9	Plasma clearance rapid for 3 hr, then slow for 24 hr; renal clearance: 10–30% as active drug in 1 hr, most of the rest expired as CO_2	Mucosal ulcers, diarrhea, nausea, emesis, leukopenia, thrombocytopenia, alopecia, sun-exposure dermatitis, cerebellar ataxia
Vincristine	1–2 mg/M^2 per week i.v.	Plasma $T_{1/2}$ = 30 min; excretion almost totally by liver into bile, small portion directly into gastrointestinal tract	Constipation → paralytic ileus, peripheral neuropathy, alopecia
Vinblastine	0.1–0.3 mg/kg per week i.v.	Similar to vincristine	Leukopenia, alopecia, areflexia, paresthesia, mucosal ulcers
Mitomycin C	0.5 mg/kg i.v. every 4–6 wk	Rapid plasma clearance; 33% of intact drug in urine within a few hours	Leukopenia, thrombocytopenia

Continued

Table V-Continued

Drug	Common schedules/routes[a]	Pharmacologic principles	Common major toxicity
Adriamycin	60–75 mg/M² i.v. every 3 wk	Plasma $T_{1/2}$ = 27 hr; metabolites excreted in bile and urine	Leukopenia, thrombocytopenia, myocardial damage, mucositis, alopecia
Hexamethylmelamine	4–8 mg/kg per day in divided doses	Renal excretion: 19% in first 24 hr increasing to 50–65% with daily administration; still present in urine 7 days after stopping drug	Leukopenia, thrombocytopenia, nausea, emesis, diarrhea, central and peripheral neuropathia
Dibromodulcitol	4–12 mg/kg per day p.o. in divided doses 180–210 mg/M² per day × 10 every 4 wk	Renal excretion: 35% of dose within 12 hr, of which one-half is intact drug; cerebrospinal fluid concentration: 50% that of plasma	Leukopenia, thrombocytopenia, hepatic damage
BCNU	100–150 mg/M² i.v. every 4–8 wk	Plasma $T_{1/2}$ = <5 min; for metabolites, $T_{1/2}$ = 60–70 hr; renal clearance: 62% within 48 hr; cerebrospinal fluid concentration: 18% of plasma level in 1 min, 60–70% in 6 hr	Leukopenia, thrombocytopenia, nausea, emesis

[a] i.c. = intracavitary; i.m. = intramuscular; i.v. = intravenous; p.o. = oral.

The pharmacokinetics of the agents enter into a consideration of optimal scheduling, either when used alone or in combination. Thus, the long plasma half-lives of drugs like cyclophosphamide and adriamycin, coupled with their steep dose–response curves, suggests that high-dose intermittent schedules would be superior to low-dose, 1–7 times/week schedules. Alternatively, the short plasma half-lives of drugs like methotrexate, coupled with very shallow dose–response curves in the clinically tolerable dose range, suggest that chronic low-dose exposure would be superior to high-dose intermittent schedules. The ability to reverse toxic effects of this drug with citrovorum factor makes it possible to achieve 1–2 log drug dose increments for short intervals, which may be superior to the older low-dose chronic schedules. 5-Fluorouracil is an example of an intermediate drug in that the dose–response curve is reasonably steep, providing a rationale for high-dose, 5–7-day-course type of therapy despite a short plasma half-life. The utilization of pharmacokinetic parameters in the treatment strategy of breast cancer has been reviewed recently.[66] Surprisingly little attention is afforded these parameters in the design of clinical trials.

Another aspect of drug pharmacokinetics that is utilized in the development of optimal drug schedules as single agents and in combinations is the cell-cycle specificity (see Section 2.1). Similarly, it is useful to attempt to combine agents with widely different partition coefficients in polar:nonpolar solvent mixtures. Highly nonpolar agents like BCNU and dibromodulcitol have the capability to more readily cross membrane structures and enter relatively inaccessible sites like the central nervous system and the cerebral spinal fluid. In general terms, with all else being equal, a combination of adriamycin instead of methotrexate with cyclophosphamide and 5-flourouracil would be expected to be more effective, since its partition coefficient is more disparate from the other two drugs than is that of methotrexate.

Most of the agents in Table V are myelosuppressive. The major exceptions are bleomycin and vincristine; however, vincristine will frequently enhance the myelosuppressive capability of simultaneously administered agents. Vinblastine and cyclophosphamide bone marrow toxicity is primarily leukopenia, whereas that of adriamycin is leukopenia and thrombocytopenia. Adriamycin and the antimetabolites can exhibit major gastroenteric toxicity in the form of mucositis and mucosal ulcerations. Vincristine causes peripheral neurotoxicity which can be incapacitating. Skin toxicities are unusual except for bleomycin, which also produces pulmonary fibrosis. Adriamycin has progressive, refractory, congestive heart failure as a major complication. Although it has occurred at total cumulative doses as low as 240 mg/M^2, it is most unusual below cumulative doses of 500 mg/M^2. It has been suggested that the dose limit in patients who have received radiotherapy to the chest should be dropped to 450 mg/M^2. This toxicity has been the subject of a recent study,[67] and predictive tests to estimate when the drug should be stopped in an individual patient are under investigation.[67,68]

4. Clinical Evaluation of Drugs

The development of new chemotherapeutic drugs for patients with breast cancer traditionally involves three phases. The first phase is not usually carried out exclusively in patients with breast cancer but rather in a broad spectrum of tumor patients, and is designed to determine optimal doses and limiting drug toxicities. The patients, although treated for therapeutic intent, may not have evaluable parameters to estimate tumor response. Once the initial dose finding has been accomplished, the drug enters into a Phase II trial.

Phase II trials attempt to determine if the drug has any antitumor activity in a variety of cancers. Since breast cancer is a relatively common problem, usually 15 to 30 such patients are treated on a specific Phase II protocol. In the past, the focus of the Phase II trial was on the drug, and the characteristics of the patients entering the trial were not defined specifically except to require a certain degree of marrow function, ambulatory status, and/or measurable disease. Since breast cancer treatment with chemotherapy has many options prior to the use of an experimental agent, the patients are usually late in their clinical course and have had considerable previous treatment. Particularly with the advent of combination chemotherapy programs, the patients have been exposed to a broad spectrum of active agents prior to entering the Phase II trial, and the new drug would therefore have to be very active to show any degree of activity. Moreover, since there may be several drugs of interest, selection of patients to receive one drug and not another could easily occur. For example, if there were two drugs to be tested and one required intravenous administration as an inpatient, the tendency would be to use the more ill patients requiring hospitalization for that drug, whereas the better performance status patients would be treated as outpatients. To circumvent this problem, as well as to give the drugs a more effective trial, some protocol studies have incorporated a special master protocol clearly defining the patient characteristics and a randomization between two options. Thus, the element of patient selection is decreased. Ideally, one would also want to incorporate a standard treatment as well. However, in a study by Ahmann and co-workers, it was observed that exposure of patients to an ineffective new agent prejudiced the subsequent response and survival to an effective regimen.[69]

Another problem raised by a Phase II drug-oriented trial is that whereas in lung cancer or renal cell cancer, little effectiveness has been demonstrated for any agent, for breast cancer there are many active drugs. Therefore, one might want to examine all drugs for activity against lung and renal cell cancer but be more selective in breast cancer patients. The objectives of Phase II trials in breast cancer might be best directed toward defining new and novel chemical structures or drugs that are not myelotoxic.[70] In breast cancer, Phase II trials may also include the development of combination chemotherapy programs or regimens that contain immunotherapy or hormonal drugs. Once the drug has been shown to be active in a Phase II trial, it is then ready to enter into a Phase III study. The objective here is to determine specific answers concerning the drug's usefulness in a comparative way with a standard regimen as a control. Phase III trials require large numbers of patients and strict attention to tumor and host parameters that might influence response.

In considering any effect of drugs on the tumor, one must first define what one implies by response. In breast cancer patients undergoing chemotherapy for their metastatic disease, we know that the tumor may be present in the bones, liver, or lung, as well as in the skin and lymph nodes. Pleural effusions are also relatively common. Moreover, the skin lesions may be relatively easily measured or indistinct. Bone lesions notoriously have several different characteristics, including lytic and/or blastic. Therefore, in evaluating response, one must clarify response in terms of the measurability of the lesions. The lesions may be either clearly bidimensionally definable, measurable only in one dimension (such as flat skin lesions or liver involvement), or evaluable only, such as brain symptoms or lymphangitic pulmonary disease. Therefore, one defines response in terms of all the lesions that the patient has by means of serial measurements, X rays, scans, or photographs.

Through experience, a time element has also been added to response. Serial measurements are taken at defined intervals, usually every one to four weeks. While no general agreement exists as to a single time period, the definitions of response usually require a decrease in size by a certain percentage for at least a month and some for six months. To qualify for a response, most investigators have required not only proof of shrinkage but also the demonstration that no progression has developed in any known area of involvement and that no new areas of disease have appeared. This requires that the patient be subjected to a complete reevaluation at regular intervals, usually at three or six months.

Since shrinkage of tumor masses must be quantitated, the question arises as to how much shrinkage is necessary to qualify for a response.

We know from animal studies that the actual cell-kill in a tumor is greater than the apparent shrinkage of the tumor.[71] In the animal tumors, these measurements can be checked by bioassay techniques. Clinically, most investigators have required that tumors shrink by a certain percentage (≥50%). There is no agreed defined way of coming up with these numbers. Investigators have used the sum of the products of the diameters of all the bidimensional lesions, the product of a single indicator-lesion's diameters, or a decrease in the size of the liver or a unidimensional lesion by a certain percentage. For nonmeasurable lesions, one usually requires a change by complete or almost complete clearing.

Because of these difficulties in definitions of response, the Breast Cancer Task Force of the United States assembled a group of investigators to set up a standard set of definitions. The ultimate outcome of these deliberations was the establishment of the response definitions listed in Table VI. Complete response is easy to define if all tumor disappears and the bone lesions return to normal. This rarely occurs, however, and more often the tumor has mixed responses, where some lesions improve but others remain static. In general, for a partial response one must have at least a 50% decrease in tumor size with either no change or progression in any other lesion. Progression is defined as the growth of lesions while on treatment, regrowth of an originally defined responsive lesion, or the development of a new lesion. The

Table VI
Response Definitions[a]

Measurable lesions: unidimensional or bidimensional measurements
    Complete response: complete disappearance of all known disease for at least four weeks
    Partial response: ≥50% decrease in tumor measurements with no increase ≥25% in any single lesion
    No change: ≤50% decrease or ≤25% increase in measurable disease
    Increasing disease: appearance of new lesion or ≥25% increase in existent lesions
Nonmeasurable lesions and bone disease
    Complete response: complete disappearance of all lesions for at least four weeks, including normalization of bone X rays and/or scans
    Partial response: partial decrease (≥50%) in lesions for at least four weeks or blastic changes in previous lytic lesions or decreased density of blastic lesions for at least eight weeks
    No change: no significant change in lesions for at least four weeks or in bone lesions for eight weeks
    Increasing disease: appearance of new lesions or estimated ≥25% increase in existent lesions

[a] Hoogstraten *et al.*, National Cancer Institute Breast Cancer Task Force Report on Combination Chemotherapy, 1976. Available from Dr. Mary Sears, Executive Secretary, Breast Cancer Task Force Treatment Committee, National Cancer Institute, Bethesda, Maryland 20014.

ultimate goal of the Phase III trial is to show improved survival. There has been a consistent relationship between response and improved survival as compared to nonresponders.

5. Combinations

5.1. Relative Activity Compared to Single Agents

Table IV shows the relative activity of single agents in advanced breast cancer patients. In general, the more active agents produce remissions in 20–37% of patients. Phase III trials comparing various single agents have demonstrated approximate equivalency between cyclophosphamide, 5-fluorouracil, and methotrexate, with response rates near 20–25%.[72,73] Adriamycin has been tested in Phase III trials against combination chemotherapy regimens and produced responses in 43% of patients.[74] In these trials, the patients had not been previously exposed to other chemotherapy. This is an important consideration, since response rates drop by a factor of approximately two when a drug program is used as a second-line regimen. Two of the more commonly used combinations are cyclophosphamide, methotrexate, and 5-fluorouracil, or adriamycin and vincristine. Both combinations induce remissions in approximately 50–55% of previously untreated patients. However, when patients failing one of these combinations are then treated with the other regimen, the response rate decreases to 25–30% for both regimens.

Most of the current major clinically used combinations induce remissions in 50% or more of patients with advanced disease. The variety of combinations utilized has recently been the subject of two reviews.[11,14] If the results of those trials and the single-agent data in previously untreated patients are plotted as a function of the number of drugs used, it is seen that the response rate tends to level off at three- to four-drug combinations (Fig. 3). Direct Phase III comparisons of combinations against single agents have also been performed and the data summarized elsewhere.[11,14] Investigators at the Mayo Clinic compared a variety of single agents to a combination of cyclophosphamide, 5-fluorouracil, and prednisone, with and without vincristine.[69] The combinations tended to be associated with higher response rates, response durations, and survival. The Eastern Cooperative Oncology Group compared L-phenylalanine mustard to a combination of cyclophosphamide, methotrexate, and 5-fluorouracil.[75] The response rate was 53% to the combination (15% complete responses) and 19% to the single agent (5% complete responses). The combination was also associated with a longer response duration and survival. Similar trials by

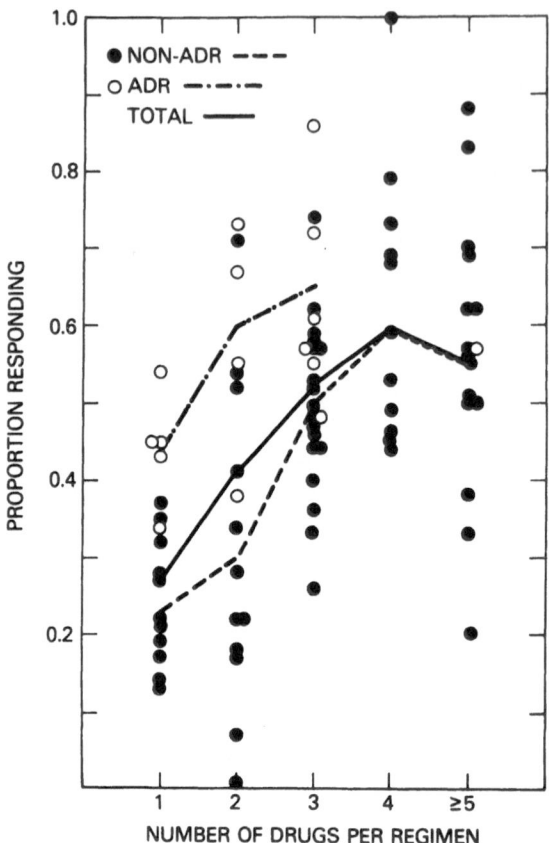

Fig. 3. The mean proportion of patients responding to chemotherapy as a function of the number of drugs used in the chemotherapy regimen. Only chemotherapy regimens used in patients who were not previously treated with chemotherapy are included. ADR and NON-ADR refer to adriamycin and non-adriamycin-containing regimens, respectively. Total includes both adriamycin and non-adriamycin-containing regimens.[14]

three other cooperative groups have led to a similar conclusion.[14] Only one trial does not fit this pattern,[76] but that trial was performed with a combination which was probably inferior to those used in the other studies.[11] Thus, there is little question that effective combination regimens are superior to the use of single agents.

5.2. Maximizing Effects of Combinations

The principles inherent in developing an effective combination have been discussed above. In general, it is desirable to develop combinations using the drugs that are most active as single agents and have the fewest overlapping toxicities, and to use each agent on its optimal single agent schedule. Other considerations that enter into the developmental phase include the drug's pharmacology, biochemical and cell-cycle mechanisms of action, partition coefficients, and interactions, both therapeutic and toxic, with the other drugs proposed for the combination. By judicious selection and scheduling of each agent, it is frequently possible to employ each drug at from 40 to 80% of its full dose when used as a single agent. The relative dose proportion of each drug in the regimen is a compromise between the factors mentioned above and each drug's relative activity against the disease. For example, combinations employing adriamycin tend to maximize this drug because of its marked single-agent activity.

5.3. The Concept of Alternating Combinations

The classic approach with either single-agent or combination chemotherapy treatment is to treat the patient until failure on the regimen. The patient is then treated with the next best therapy. Using this approach, those combinations with response rates between 50 and 80% tend to be associated uniformly with response durations of approximately eight to ten months. This observation has led to the suggestion that the maximal effect of any single combination has been reached by four to five months and that further treatment, while perhaps slowing net tumor growth, will not further decrease the tumor burden. This hypothesis assumes that cells resistant to the combination are responsible for ultimate failure. Since most patients with advanced disease will have 10^{10} to 10^{11} cells, it is not unlikely that at least one resistant clone of cells will be present. Other hypotheses for these observations include the possibility that the kinetics of the tumor have changed so it is no longer reached adequately by the drugs, or that the decreased drug dose delivered after several months of therapy due to cumulative toxicity falls below the therapeutic threshold. At the present time, there is little evidence for either of the latter hypotheses.

The clinical extrapolation of the cell-resistance hypothesis is to utilize fixed rotational sequences of two or more non-cross-resistant combination regimens. Thus, a patient would be treated for one to three months with combination A, then switch to combination B for an equivalent time, then return to combination A, etc., until disease progression or cure. This approach is currently being tested in several Phase III trials, but as yet, no results are available. If the approach is correct, then new drug testing should search for additional agents which are not only more active than current drugs but are also not cross-resistant with them. If the approach fails, then detailed kinetic and biologic studies will be needed to evaluate the other hypotheses.

5.4. Useful Combinations

There have been a large number of combination regimens studied in patients with breast cancer.[11,14] Some of the more commonly used effective programs with their associated response rates are listed in Table VII. All except the adriamycin–vincristine regimens are derivatives of the cyclophosphamide, methotrexate, 5-fluorouracil, vincristine, and prednisone program reported by Cooper in 1969.[10] The original regimen was not an intermittent program, but similar intermittent regimens devised by several cooperative oncology groups have been found to be equally active and better accepted by the patients.[11,14] One cooperative group deleted vincristine and another deleted prednisone, and found no loss of activity when compared to the full five drugs. Similarly, deletion of both 5-fluorouracil and vincristine were equally as effective as the complete five-drug program; however, deletion of cyclophosphamide and methotrexate led to an inferior regimen. Substitution of adriamycin for methotrexate in the five-drug program has provided a regimen that is at least as active as the parent combination. Another trial substituted adriamycin for methotrexate, deleted vincristine and prednisone, and compared the resulting cyclophosphamide, adriamycin, and 5-fluorouracil regimen to the parent five-drug regimen. The response rate to the adriamycin regimen was superior. We have found a similar cyclophosphamide, adriamycin, and 5-fluorouracil regimen to be superior to a cyclophosphamide, methotrexate, and 5-fluorouracil regimen.

The addition of prednisone to cyclophosphamide, methotrexate, and 5-fluorouracil may provide a slight therapeutic advantage, as may the addition of fluoxymesterone after the first six months of therapy.[77] This observation would make the three-drug regimen slightly inferior to the parent five-drug program, since the latter has already been found equivalent to the four-drug prednisone-containing regimen. The cyclophosphamide, methotrexate, and 5-fluorouracil regimen has also been found to be equivalent to a cyclophosphamide, 5-fluorouracil, and prednisone program[11]; however, the addition of vincristine to the latter program gave an inferior result.[69] Similarly, no difference has yet been observed between regimens containing cyclophosphamide, 5-fluorouracil, and prednisone, and those containing cyclophosphamide and adriamycin.[78]

The interrelationships of these various trials are depicted in Fig. 4. A study of these results suggests that the most active and simplest current

Table VII
Current Combination-Regimen Response Rates[a]

Regimen	No. of responses/total	Percent response
Every 21–28 days, courses of CYT 200 mg/M² i.v. on day 3–6 ADR 40 mg/M² i.v. on day 1	40/55	74
Every 21 days, courses of ADR 60 mg/M² i.v. on day 1 VCR 1.2 mg/M² i.v. on day 1	37/67[b]	79
Every 28 days, courses of CYT 100 mg/M² p.o. on day 1–14 ADR 30 mg/M² i.v. on day 1, 8 5-FU 500 mg/M² i.v. on day 1, 8	69/93[b]	74
Every 28 days, courses of CYT 100 mg/M² p.o. on day 1–14 MTX 30–40 mg/M² i.v. on day 1, 8 5-FU 500–600 mg/M² i.v. on day 1, 8	147/274[b]	75
Every 28–35 days, courses of CYT 4 mg/kg i.v. on day 1–5 5-FU 8 mg/kg i.v. on day 1–5 Prednisone 30 mg/day on day 1–14, then taper to 10 mg/day	68/121	69

[a]Modified from Tormey and Neifeld.[14]
[b]Also includes data using same drugs on other schedules.

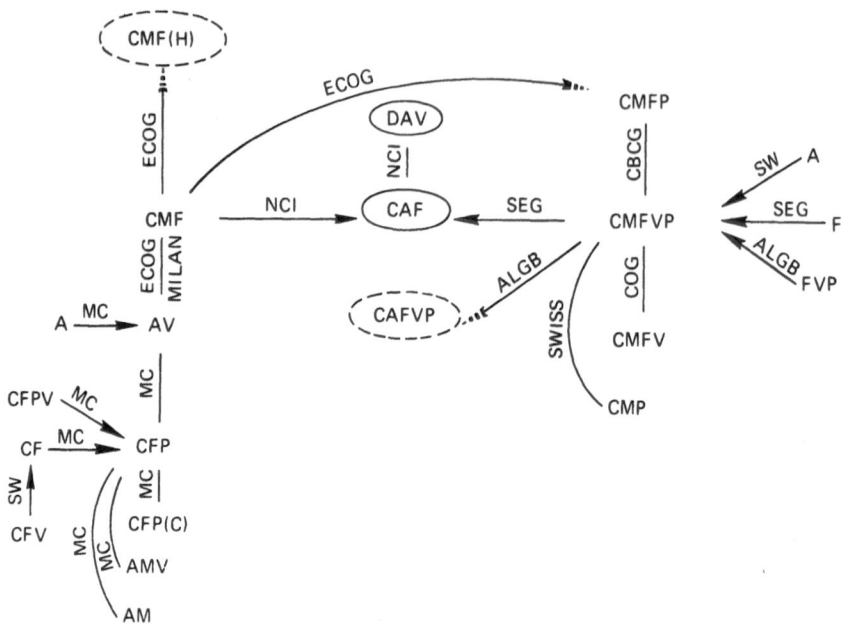

Fig. 4. Relative efficacy of chemotherapy regimens in advanced disease. The assignments are based upon results from randomized clinical trials reviewed by Broder and Tormey[11] and Tormey and Niefeld.[14] The arrows point to the more effective regimen based on response rate and/or response duration analyses. A broken arrow indicates possible, but as yet not proven, superiority. ⬭ = apparently most effective regimen; ⬚ = regimens which may be as effective as the ⬭ regimens; C = cyclophosphamide; M = methotrexate; F = 5-fluorouracil; V = vincristine; P = prednisone; A = adriamycin; D = dibromodulcitol; (H) = fluoxymesterone; (C) = calasterone; SEG = Southeastern Oncology Group; SW = Southwestern Oncology Group; ALGB = Cancer and Acute Leukemia Group B; COG = Central Oncology Group; CBCG = Cooperative Breast Cancer Group; SWISS = Swiss Cooperative Oncology Group; NCI = National Cancer Institute; ECOG = Eastern Cooperative Oncology Group; MILAN = National Cancer Institute, Milan; MC = Mayo Clinic.

regimen is cyclophosphamide, adriamycin, and 5-fluorouracil. There are no direct data available to indicate whether or not vincristine and prednisone add to this regimen, but by analogy with the results of the parent five-drug regimen, at least one of these two drugs are probably not necessary. It is also unclear whether or not fluoxymesterone added to the cyclophosphamide, methotrexate, and 5-fluorouracil ± prednisone regimen after six months of induction might provide an equivalent or superior regimen to the three- to five-drug adriamycin regimens.

5.5. The Role of Adriamycin in Combinations

The integration of adriamycin into the parent five-drug regimens derived from Cooper's program has provided a therapeutic advantage in terms of response rate. As will be discussed below, it has not altered the response durations; however, by placing more patients in a responding category, the net result is an improved time spent free of disease progression for more patients. It is anticipated that this will translate into a survival advantage, since the median survival of responders is in excess of eighteen months, compared to only six months for patients who do not respond.[79]

A second major advantage that has accrued as a result of the development of adriamycin is the ability to test the concept of fixed rotational therapy by using two non-cross-resistant combinations. The studies currently in progress are rotating therapy between either (1) dibromodulcitol, adriamycin, and vincristine, or adriamycin and

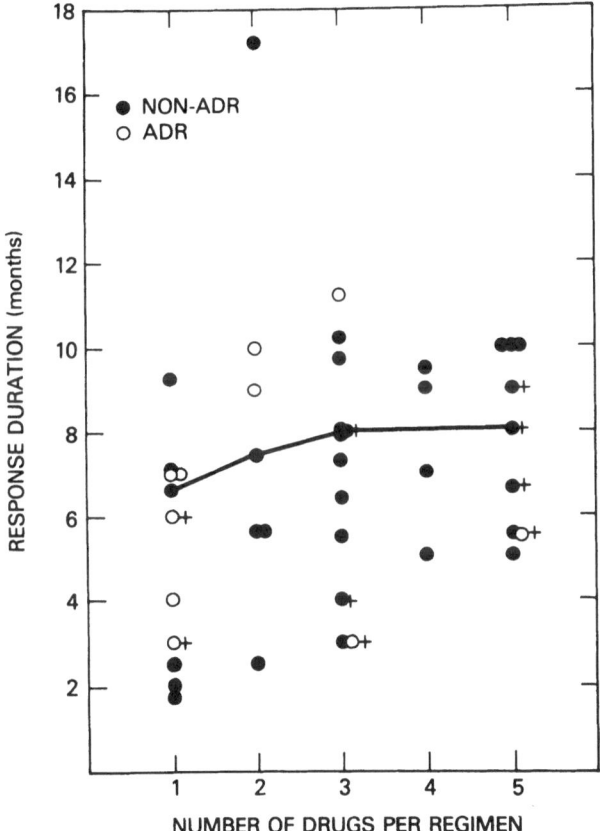

Fig. 5. The median response duration for patients responding to chemotherapy related to the number of drugs used in the chemotherapy regimen. Only chemotherapy regimens used in patients who were not previously treated with chemotherapy are included. ADR and NON-ADR refer to adriamycin and non-adriamycin-containing regimens, respectively.[14]

vincristine with cyclophosphamide, methotrexate, and 5-fluorouracil; or (2) adriamycin and L-phenylalanine mustard with cyclophosphamide, 5-fluorouracil, and prednisone.

5.6. Response Duration and Survival

Response durations with single agents tend to be no more than four to six months. The duration rises with two and three combinations to reach a median of nine to ten months (Fig. 5). This slight gain in the median response duration must also be viewed in the context that the proportion of patients entering the response curves has increased from 25–30% with single agents to 50–80% with combinations.

It has already been discussed that survival with combination regimens is superior to that with single-agent therapy, and also that responders to combinations have a median survival that is at least threefold longer than the six months observed for nonresponders.

6. Chemotherapy and Hormonal Therapy

The experimental mammary cancers induced by DMBA in rats have clearly been shown to be hormone-dependent. They regress following oophorectomy and hypophysectomy and can be stimulated to grow by adding prolactin. Simpson-Herren and Griswold have shown that these tumors have a marked decrease in their labeling indices with tritiated thymidine by almost 99.9% following oophorectomy.[80] As the tumors recur or are stimulated by hormones, the DNA synthetic rate increases dramatically. Experimental studies of combined chemotherapy and hormonal therapy have not been done as frequently as separate chemotherapy or hormone studies. In one study, the addition of cyclophosphamide to androgens did not increase the effectiveness of the hormonal therapy alone.[81]

In humans, the combining of chemotherapy and hormonal therapies has been done for at least three reasons. One is to enhance the effect of the two therapies by combining the two modalities with their different modes of action and toxicities. Secondly, at least one study was done attempting to stimulate the growth of the breast cancer by giving estrogens and then adding chemotherapy to take advantage of the increased DNA synthesis.[17] A third approach has been to add androgens, primarily to improve the anabolic state of the host and stimulate the regrowth of marrow elements. The latter approach has not been fully evaluated as yet.

Table VIII
Hormonal Chemotherapy—Ongoing Trials[a]

1. Oophorectomy ± CYT/MTX/5-FU	Eastern Cooperative Oncology Group
2. Oophorectomy ± Cytoxan or CYT/MTX/5-FU/VCR/prednisone	Cancer and Acute Leukemia Group B
3. Oophorectomy ± CYT/5-FU/prednisone	Mayo Clinic
4. Estrogen ± CYT/MTX/5-FU	National Cancer Institute Breast Cancer Service
5. Estrogen ± CYT/ADR/5-FU	Emory University, Miami
6. Estrogen ± CYT/5-FU	University of Minnesota
7. (ADR VCR) (CYT/MTX/5-FU) ± progesterone	Guy's Hospital
8. Adrenalectomy ± FU	Harvard

[a]For a summary of reported trials, see Tormey and Neifeld.[14]

Chemotherapy has been added to estrogens, oophorectomy, adrenalectomy, androgens, thyroid hormones, and progesterone in an attempt to enhance the effectiveness of the hormone procedure. The use of physiologic estrogen doses plus chemotherapy was tested by Taylor and co-workers with the idea that one might stimulate the growth of the breast cancer cells and then take advantage of the proliferating tumor cells' increased sensitivity to chemotherapy. The results of this trial were negative.[17]

The use of adrenalectomy combined with chemotherapy was tested by Moore and colleagues, and their trials, though not controlled, indicated that 5-fluorouracil combined with adrenalectomy improve the disease response duration.[82] Van Dyk and Falkson showed that cyclophosphamide added to oophorectomy prolonged the remission duration of patients undergoing oophorectomy alone.[32] The use of progesterone and thyroid hormone added to chemotherapy has been tested both in controlled and uncontrolled trials with no obvious benefit.[83,84]

Greenspan and associates first reported the addition of androgens to combination chemotherapy in breast cancer, and their experience indicated that there was some benefit in terms of nonspecific feeling of well-being and healing of bone lesions.[9,85] However, since their trials were not controlled, no clear-cut definition of the role of androgens in combination chemotherapy programs can be derived.

In more recent times, several trials have been undertaken testing the efficacy of hormonal therapies added to chemotherapy (Table VIII). The studies have been designed as simultaneous administration or sequential addition of the two treatments. Data are not available on these studies, although there is good evidence to indicate that adrenalectomy[86] and oophorectomy[87] responses are not as frequent as those achieved by combination chemotherapy programs.

The ultimate roles of hormonal therapy and chemotherapy should not be looked on as ones of mutual exclusion. With the better definition of hormone-responsive tumors by using the estrogen receptor assay, one can select those patients who have little, if any, chance to respond to hormonal therapies. Those patients should undergo treatment with chemotherapy-based regimens. For patients who can be shown to be hormone-responsive, the problem remains of how to best use both modalities. A simple addition may not be the answer.

7. Immunotherapy

Tumor-specific antigens in breast cancer have been demonstrated by intracutaneous injection of autologous and allogeneic tumor cells,[88,89] leukocyte-migration inhibition,[90,91] reaction of breast cancer cells or their extracts against the patient's lymphocytes,[92] and skin-window techniques.[93] In addition to tumor-specific immunity, much emphasis has been placed on studying the host's immunity to nonspecific challenges. In general, these studies have shown that one can demonstrate reactivity of the patients to breast tumor cells that indicate some degree of specificity as well as common shared antigens for other breast cancers. The patient's general immunity to nonspecific stimuli has been shown to be relatively normal in the early stages of disease, but clear evidence of anergy develops as the disease progresses to advanced stages. The loss of nonspecific delayed immunity has been correlated with early relapse.[94] Histologically, evidence for immunity to breast cancer has been postulated to be associated with sinus histiocytosis,[95] with enlargement of contralateral nonneoplastic axillary lymph nodes,[96] and with lymphocytic infiltration in the tumor.[95]

In attempting to use immunologic mechanisms to treat advanced metastatic disease, one is immediately faced with the issue that the high number of tumor cells would not be favorable for the use of immunotherapy in the therapeutic regimen unless the bulk of the disease is first diminished by excision and/or chemotherapy. Using Martin's $CD8F_1$ model, Stolfi and associates demonstrated the effectiveness of immunostimulation combined with chemotherapy and surgery in the control of murine mammary cancer.[97] Martin postulates that immunotherapy would be able to accomplish the killing of the last few cells that chemotherapy, because of the first-order kinetics of its lethality, would not be able to eliminate. Moreover, immune stimulation would be able to overcome the immunosuppressive effects of chemotherapy. Bogden and co-workers likewise have shown that a methanol-soluble fraction of *Mycobacterium butyricum* (MSF-MB) would enhance the effect of surgery, chemotherapy, and radiotherapy in a syngeneic transplantable rat tumor.[59] Fisher and co-workers have demonstrated that *Corynebacterium parvum* administration, when combined with cyclophosphamide, was capable of causing tumor regressions in a C_3H mammary tumor system.[98]

While immunostimulation has been employed regularly in the clinical treatment of malignant melanoma and acute leukemia, the use of immunostimulation or specific immunotherapy in patients with advanced breast cancer has been rather limited. Israel reported the effects of *Corynebacterium parvum* added to a five-drug combination chemotherapy program compared to the chemotherapy alone in patients with beast cancer.[99] The group treated with the *Corynebacterium parvum* combination chemotherapy program had much better survival at 18 months ($P = <0.0005$) than did the group treated with drugs only.

Gutterman and co-workers have examined the role of bacillus Calmette–Guérin (BCG) added to a three-drug regimen of 5-fluorouracil, cyclophosphamide, and adriamycin. The preliminary results indicate a prolongation of the remission duration and survival for the BCG-treated group. [100] In a proposed Eastern Cooperative Group study, *Corynebacterium parvum* will be added to the three-drug regimen of cyclophosphamide, methotrexate, and 5-fluorouracil by one of two routes. An attempt will be made not only to evaluate the additive effects of *Corynebacterium parvum* to chemotherapy but also to see if immunotherapy has any protective effect for marrow function.

Several trials are under way evaluating various immunostimulants and chemotherapy in the treatment of patients with Stage II breast cancer, but these are beyond the scope of this chapter. However, Rojas and co-workers have published the results of an interesting study of Stage III breast cancer in which patients were randomly allocated to levamisole or nothing after radiotherapy.[101] The report indicates a significant prolongation of the levamisole-treated group's disease-free survival (median 29 months versus 9 months). The use of this immunostimulant alone appears surprisingly effective considering that these patients have a very high tumor burden following local treatment only.

8. The Changing Role of Chemotherapy in Breast Cancer Treatment

In the past five years, the use of combination chemotherapy has played a significant role in the treatment of patients with metastatic breast cancer. The relegation of chemotherapy to end-stage hormone-resistant patients has been replaced by an aggressive use of combination chemotherapy even prior to hormonal therapy. The latter application of chemotherapy is particularly likely to occur when the patient presents with rapidly progressive liver or lung disease as the first sign of metastatic disease. When the premenopausal patient presents in this manner, very often chemotherapy is administered as the first treatment or immediately following a surgical- or radiation-induced oophorectomy, without waiting for an evaluation of the ablative procedure. In postmenopausal women, combination chemotherapy is most likely to be used as the first treatment upon recurrence, unless the patient is more than ten years postmenopausal and/or the disease is limited to soft-tissue sites. Although several chemotherapy regimens have been used in combination with hormones and/or ablative procedures, as pointed out earlier, the best method of combining these modalities has not been determined.

Not only has the concept of the use of chemotherapy changed, but our concept of metastatic disease has also been modified. Heretofore, the approach to treatment of Stage I and II breast cancer has been the application of local therapies only, i.e., radiation therapy and/or surgery. More than 50% of these patients eventually relapse by five years with local treatment only. With the greater appreciation of tumor cell kinetics and the concepts of micrometastatic disease, more emphasis has been placed on using chemotherapy before the patient develops gross metastatic disease. Several studies have reported beneficial effects of these programs in the combined modality approach.[102,103] Moreover, as Schabel has indicated, the effectiveness of chemotherapy is enhanced when used against micrometastatic foci; in human breast cancer, the results in the more favorable micrometastatic situation also appear to be accentuated compared to the gross metastatic disease.[31] Of particular interest was the testing of L-phenylalanine mustard in patients with advanced disease, where it produced responses in only 19% of patients,[75] compared to the effectiveness of this drug in reducing the early recurrence rate by 50% in the Stage II patient. Likewise, the cyclophosphamide, methotrexate, and 5-fluorouracil combination, which in advanced disease produced a 53% response rate, was able to decrease early recurrences by 80% in the adjuvant situation. This has stimulated other trials adding or subtracting drugs in an attempt to define the most effective chemotherapy regimen with the least toxicity.

As a result, the use of chemotherapy in the postsurgical situation has unique consequences for those patients who eventually recur. As yet, we do not know what fraction of patients will recur following postsurgical chemotherapy, but some undoubtedly will. We thus can visualize that those patients who have been previously treated will need some form of systemic therapy. We do not know whether they will still be hormonally responsive, allowing the application of various hormone-additive or -ablative approaches. Attempts are being made to develop a variety of other combinations which are less likely to be used in the adjuvant situation. Some of these are listed in Table IX.

For those 10% of patients who first present with metastatic disease, the strategy of treatment likewise should be reevaluated. Unlike the results in acute lymphocytic leukemia of childhood or advanced Hodgkin's disease, where cures can be achieved in systemic cancers, patients with breast cancer who are treated with intensive chemotherapy have not developed a high proportion of complete remission or long-term survival. Obviously, aggressive combined trials are important to attempt cell-cure of advanced disease, but one must be skeptical that any single chemotherapy program alone is able to rid the patient of 10^{10} or 10^{11} tumor cells. An approach more likely to be successful will

Table IX
Additional Combination Chemotherapy Programs for Breast Cancer

Cytoxan	2 mg/kg per day p.o.[a]	
Methotrexate	0.12 mg/kg p.o. on day 1–3 every week	
Prednisone	1 mg/kg per day × 14 → taper to 10–15 mg/day	
Dibromodulcitol	150 mg/M² p.o. on day 1–10[b]	Every 28 days
Adriamycin	45 mg/M² i.v. on day 1	
BCNU	1.5 mg/kg i.v. on day 1[c]	
Dacarbazine (DTIC)	3 mg/kg i.v. on day 1, 2	
Vincristine	0.025 mg/kg i.v. on day 1	Every month
FU	10 mg/kg i.v. on day 1–5	
6-Methylprednisone	48 mg on day 1–10	
BCNU	100 mg/M² i.v. on day 1[d]	
Cytoxan	400 mg/M² i.v. on day 1	Every month
Adriamycin	40 mg/M² i.v. on day 2	
Dibromodulcitol	150 mg/M² p.o. on day 1–10[e]	
Adriamycin	45 mg/M² i.v. on day 1	Every 28 days
Vincristine	1.2 mg/M² i.v. on day 1, 8	
Hexamethylmelamine	100 mg p.o. on day 1–14[f]	
Vincristine	1.4 mg/M² i.v. on day 1, 8	Every 28 days
Methotrexate	40 mg/M² i.v. on day 1, 8	

[a]Brunner et al.[104]
[b]Tormey et al.[105]
[c]van Eden et al.[106]
[d]Presant et al.[107]
[e]Tormey.[108]
[f]Longacre et al.[109]

be to combine some type of surgery or radiotherapy—to rid the patient of bulky tumor—followed by intensive chemotherapy or chemotherapy combined with immunotherapy or hormonal therapy.

Patients with Stage III breast cancers belong to a group with intermediate tumor loads. Here, patients have primary tumors that are not amenable to cure by surgery and radiotherapy, both of which have been able to control local growth with only moderate success.[110] Stage III patients make up about 10 to 25% of all presenting breast cancers, depending on the type of population seen at the clinic or center. Despite treatment with a variety of surgical and radiotherapeutic techniques, their survival is only about 50% at three years. Two relatively new studies are worth mentioning. Rojas and colleagues have employed levamisole (see Section 7) with what appear to be early promising results.[101] DeLena and colleagues have attempted to use preradiotherapy chemotherapy with adriamycin and vincristine given for three cycles, followed by intensive radiotherapy. They subsequently administered continued chemotherapy. Following the induction chemotherapy, they noted that about 76% of the patients experienced some beneficial effects on tumor size. After radiotherapy, about 80% of the patients had what was classified as complete disappearance of local disease. Maintenance chemotherapy was associated with prolonged local and systemic control as compared to nonmaintenance.[111] Several other studies are under way following these leads.

9. Special Problems

9.1. Hypercalcemia

Approximately 30% of breast cancer patients with advanced disease will develop hypercalcemia during their course. The usual therapeutic procedures for managing this complication in the cancer patient are well known. When it becomes refractory to simpler measures, many oncologists utilize mithramycin over prednisone for this condition. More recently, it has been suggested that breast cancer cells produce an osteolytic-stimulating activity.[112] This activity may be interfered with by acetylsalicylic acid and/or indomethacin.[113] A clinical trial to evaluate the effect of these agents in preventing both bone metastases and hypercalcemia is under way in England.[114]

A special circumstance is the development of hypercalcemia within the first two weeks of initiating therapy with exogenous androgens or estrogens. In this setting, the hormone should be withdrawn until normocalcemia is obtained, after which it may be reinstated at lower dosage, i.e., one-third the full dose, and the dose escalated in 25–30% increments every three to seven days until therapeutic levels are obtained.

9.2. Central Nervous System (Brain, Meninges)

Metastatic involvement of the brain occurs in approximately 20% of patients with breast carcinoma. The symptoms are those of generalized increased intracranial pressure with or without associated neurologic deficits, the nature of which depends on the location of the metastatic lesion. Because of the high proportion of multiple brain lesions in these patients, and since the presence of brain disease is almost invariably associated with dissemination to other organ sites, craniotomy with resection of the metastatic tumor mass is generally not indicated. Treatment usually involves the use of osmotic diuretics, high-dose glucocorticoids (e.g., 8–12 mg dexamethasone daily in divided doses), cranial radiotherapy (4000–6000 rads), and the use of systemic chemotherapy, including agents that cross the blood–brain barrier.

Diffuse involvement of the leptomeninges with tumor occurs in approximately 10% of patients with metastatic breast carcinoma. The most common initial symptoms of meningeal carcinomatosis are headache, low back pain, and dysesthesias of the legs. Lower extremity weakness, depressed tendon reflexes, sensory abnormalities, and sphincter dysfunction are also commonly seen. Cranial nerve involvement and deterioration of mental function are generally late stages in the course of the syndrome.

The early peripheral symptoms of carcinomatous meningitis are similar to those of spinal epidural compression from metastatic breast carcinoma. It is important to differentiate between these two entities, since the latter is quite amenable to radiotherapy of the involved spinal segments. Myelography is the only means of establishing a diagnosis of epidural compression, and must be performed in suspected cases. Isolated spinal epidural compression generally occurs adjacent to roentgenographically involved vertebral bodies.

Forty percent of the patients with carcinomatous meningitis have histologic involvement of the spinal leptomeninges and cauda equina. Isolated forms of meningeal carcinomatosis involving the spine alone have been reported. Coexisting mass lesions in the brain are seen in 25% of patients with meningeal carcinomatosis. The "classic" cerebrospinal fluid findings of high protein, low sugar, mononuclear pleocytosis, and tumor cells on cytological examination are seen in only 30% of the patients. In the presence of suggestive symptomatology, therefore, repeat lumbar punctures with cerebrospinal fluid examinations for malignant cells are often necessary to establish a diagnosis. The prognosis for patients with meningeal carcinomatosis is poor. In recent series, the median survival for patients with breast cancer was less than six weeks from the time of diagnosis of the meningeal involvement. Currently used treatment modalities involve the use of craniospinal radiotherapy, inthrathecal methotrexate, or a combination of the two approaches. The diagnosis, clinical course, and treatment of carcinomatous meningitis have recently been reviewed.[115,116]

9.3. Pulmonary

Pulmonary metastases are seen in approximately 50–70% of autopsied patients with metastatic breast carcinoma and can be nodular and/or lymphangitic. Metastases may be so small as to be undetectable on routine chest X-ray examination; in such cases, whole-lung tomograms may disclose metastatic foci. The presence of a single isolated pulmonary lesion does not preclude its surgical removal, especially in patients with a long disease-free interval since mastectomy (more than five years). However, the disseminated nature of the disease at the time of the discovery of an apparently isolated metastatic focus, plus recent advances in adjuvant chemotherapy, would argue in favor of systemic treatment for these patients following resection of the lesion.

Lymphangitic carcinomatosis of the lungs is secondary to a rapid growth and dissemination of tumor cells through the peribronchial and perivascular lymphatics that penetrate the pleural lymphatic network, and is particularly common in patients with prior pleural or mediastinal tumor involvement. Its diagnosis is often heralded by the appearance of Kerley B-lines on chest roentgenograms and/or by frequent coughing. Its clinical appearance can be abrupt and rapidly progressive, with chest pain, cough, and severe dyspnea with hypoxia. Symptomatic treatment should include the use of oxygen, nebulizers, and intermittent-positive-pressure breathing (IPPB). Because there is often an associated damage to the pulmonary microvascular and lymphatic network with pulmonary edema, diuresis may improve the hypoxia. Digitalization has been of no therapeutic value in the absence of overt congestive heart failure. Because of the rapidly progressive nature of lymphangitic pulmonary carcinomatosis, combination chemotherapy is generally the initial antitumor treatment of choice. Some authors have recommended the addition of prednisone in doses up to 70 mg daily to the other chemotherapeutic agents, although there has not been a randomized trial attesting to its efficacy.

9.4. Bone Marrow Failure

Myelosuppression in patients with breast cancer may be acute or chronic, selective for one or more blood components or pancytopenic. The major causes of bone marrow failure may be the result of (1) the administration of myelotoxic chemotherapeutic agents, (2) the aftereffects of extensive radiotherapy to marrow-bearing bones, and (3) the infiltration and replacement of the functioning marrow with tumor cells. The etiology of marrow failure can be inferred from knowledge of the patient's previous therapy, evaluation of the peripheral blood hemogram, and performance of a bone marrow biopsy. Characteristically, the patients who have marrow replacement and peripheral cytopenia may have marked leukoerythroblastosis or even tumor cells in the peripheral blood, and a bone marrow that is densely infiltrated with tumor cells. While bone lesions are common metastatic sites, and marrow biopsies may indicate infiltration with tumor cells in about 30 to 50% of patients with bone lesions, the marked pretreatment abnormalities associated with leukoerythroblastosis rarely occur. Therapy may be endocrine manipulation or combination chemotherapy programs.[117]

The more common causes of bone marrow failure are more likely a result of treatment with chemotherapy and/or radiotherapy. The degree and persistence of the cytopenias may be transient (acute) or persistent (chronic). In general, one expects a certain degree of myelotoxicity that is usually recoverable within one or two weeks without undue complications. Occasionally, because of underlying renal failure, liver dysfunction, or unsuspected synergism between nonanticancer drugs such as Zyloprim and phenobarbital, the drug pharmacodynamics may become altered, and persistent severe life-threatening myelotoxicity may occur. In these circumstances, one needs to monitor the patient frequently for signs and symptoms of infection or bleeding and/or institute prophylactic platelet or white cell transfusions. Reverse isolation and barrier nursing may be helpful in preventing exposure of the patient to exogenous organisms, but more important hazards associated with endogenous microbes are not affected by these measures. Institution of broad-spectrum antibiosis and blood-component replacement therapy are more likely to be beneficial. The only known specific antidote to major chemotherapeutic agents is citrovorum factor following methotrexate administration. However, this is of value only during the phase when methotrexate is still in the circulatory system.

Persistent or chronic bone marrow failure is a more common problem. The patient may or may not have clinically significant bleeding or dangerously low granulocyte levels ($<500/mm^3$). However, the patient may have extreme sensitivity to further therapy, which prohibits the administration of further antineoplastic treatment. Androgens are known to stimulate red cells, white cells and platelets,[118] while vincristine may cause thrombocytosis.[119] However, the role of androgens in overcoming marrow toxicity of myelotoxic agents and/or radiotherapy has not been conclusively proven. Likewise, the use of *Corynebacterium parvum* as an immunostimulant may be associated with some marrow-sparing.[120] However, the best way to manage marrow failure is probably to avoid it. One should use radiation therapy for specific indications to rather limited fields and regulate the dose of chemotherapy carefully. Long-term low-dose administration, particularly of alkylating agents, may be severely marrow-depressing. The use of short, high-dose, intermittent courses may be more marrow-sparing in the long run. The judicious use of nonmyelotoxic agents, particularly hormonal therapies, and the use of nonmyelotoxic agents such as vincristine and prednisone may be possible alternative therapeutic modalities in these patients.

9.5. Effusions

Pleural effusions are common in patients with metastatic breast cancer and may result from blockage of venous and lymphatic outflow or from tumor involvement of the serosal surfaces, either abdominal or thoracic. The etiology can be inferred from careful examination of the aspirated pleural fluid using chemical and cytological, pleural biopsy, and radiographic studies.[121] In breast cancer, pleural effusions are usually indications of widespread disease. When there is no other evidence of disease, however, the diagnosis should be aggressively approached, since other nonneoplastic causes may be present.

If the fluid is found not to contain tumor cells but is associated with outflow obstruction of lymphatics, then conservative measures such as diuresis and salt restriction combined with systemic chemotherapy and/or directed radiotherapy should be taken. If the effusion is found to be serosal in etiology, then one should decrease fluid formation by drainage or by the instillation of chemotherapeutic agents, thereby obliterating the pleural space. Intrapleural administration of radioisotopes ^{198}An and ^{90}Y has been utilized, but it produces delayed results and is an associated radiation hazard to others. Intrapleural administration of chemotherapeutic agents such as nitrogen mustard, thio-TEPA, and 5-FU is a frequently used treatment because such agents are effective, less expensive, and pose no radiation hazard to others. In general, one should tap the pleural space dry, instill the drug, and then attempt to maintain the pleural surfaces in contact with each other by repeated tapping or underwater external drainage.[122] These materials are undoubtedly absorbed systemically and may produce myelotoxicity. Nonspecific sclerosing agents such as quinicrine, tetracycline,[123] and talc have also been used. While systemic myelosuppression does not occur, fever and pleuritic chest pain as well as other systemic effects may occur.

Ascites is less common in breast cancer but may occur. Intraperitoneal instillation of chemotherapeutic agents is most useful, as well as attempts to decrease fluid production by diuretics and salt restriction. 5-FU or 5-FUDR (fluoxyuridine) as well as thio-TEPA are the most useful agents for intraperitoneal administration.

Malignant pericardial effusions are relatively commonly caused by breast cancer. Because of their life-threatening and insidious nature, prompt diagnosis and treatment by aspiration are important. Recurrent effusions may be managed by instillation of thio-TEPA, external radiation, and surgically by a pleuropericardial window for drainage.

9.6. Inflammatory Cancer

Inflammatory carcinoma of the breast is an uncommon clinical presentation of breast malignancy, occurring in 1 to 2% of patients with breast carcinoma.[124] It is seen most frequently in women with large, pendulous breasts, and is often initially mistaken for a breast abscess. Yonemoto has established the following criteria for making a diagnosis of inflammatory breast carcinoma: (1) erythema and edema involving greater than one-third of the skin overlying the breast; (2) skin changes not due to direct extension of a growing breast mass; (3) skin thickening on mammography; and (4) presence of tumor cells in dermal lymphatic ducts.[125] Although some pathologists have attempted to define inflammatory breast carcinoma histologically, it remains primarily a clinical diagnosis. The causative factors leading to this presentation are not well understood. Corall and Dao have demonstrated delayed hypersensitivity reactions in patients with inflammatory breast carcinoma to extracts of their own tumors.[126]

The tumor has a poor prognosis with early nodal and distant metastases. Five-year survivals have been less than 5% in most series. Simple or radical mastectomy has not been effective in controlling the disease, and for this reason, many physicians consider inflammatory breast carcinoma as a contraindication for mastectomy. Radiotherapy has caused transient tumor regression in approximately one-half of the patients, but five-year survivals are less than 2%.[127] Oophorectomy combined with bilateral adrenalectomy appears to be the most effective palliative treatment.[127–129] Responses have been seen with combination chemotherapy, but its ultimate therapeutic role has not been adequately assessed.[111]

9.7. Long-Term Effects of Chemotherapy

Many of the anticancer chemotherapy drugs are carcinogens and/or cocarcinogens in animals.[130] Alkylating agents are particularly potent carcinogens, acting very much like radiation. In addition, cancer drugs may affect the normal immune mechanisms that may be responsible for suppression of tumorigenesis. However, the fact that carcinomas can be induced in animals and the occurrence of second clinical cancers in patients treated with chemotherapy may not be too relevant. Most carcinogen experiments in animals are designed to enhance carcinogenesis, while therapeutic trials in patients with breast cancer usually are carried out in older patients with limited life spans. Moreover, many patients also receive radiotherapy during their clinical course. Breast cancers characteristically are associated with the development of other tumors, particularly in the ovary, colon, uterus, and opposite breast. However, acute leukemias have been reported by Penn in at least four patients treated with methotrexate and cyclophosphamide. [131] Combination chemotherapy programs that can produce damage to DNA and RNA through multiple mechanisms may produce more problems than single agents.

Besides induction of cancers, other long-term problems associated with chemotherapy include hepatic damage (methotrexate), pulmonary fibrosis (bleomycin), cardiac toxicity (adriamycin), cerebellar ataxia (5-fluorouracil), paresthesias and peripheral neurological deficits (vincristine), hemorrhagic cystitis (cyclophosphamide), renal damage (methotrexate), and osteoporosis (myeleran and methotrexate). Of particular concern in breast cancer is the possible effect of chemotherapy on gonadal function. A persistent chemical oophorectomy may occur secondary to the drugs. In addition, one may postulate that oocyte damage may occur, leading to subsequent fetal malformation or fetal wastage. Ross, in a review of the effects in women with choriocarcinoma who were cured and subsequently became pregnant, noted no striking increase in congenital abnormalities. [132] Thus, chemotherapy has possible potential side effects that may produce long-term effects which, as yet, have not been completely evaluated. As more and more patients with early breast cancer are treated with chemotherapy, careful follow-up with appropriate controls must be done to document the true incidence of these long-term hazards.

10. The Future of Chemotherapy

10.1. New Drugs

As discussed above, there is a pressing need for new agents. At the present time, about five to six new agents enter the clinic for Phase I and II testing each year. Not only is it desirable to have drugs with higher activity, but even more important to develop active agents that are bone-marrow-sparing with a high therapeutic index for other normal structures as well. An enhanced specificity for the breast cancer cell would provide a potentially more powerful therapeutic tool. Although we are still a long way from developing specific physiologic therapies or genetic-modulation approaches, these still remain the ultimate goal for treatment of all cancers that are not prevented.

10.2. Developing Approaches

We have discussed the newer approaches that are now under clinical test, namely, the integration of chemotherapy with hormonal and immunotherapies, and their application to patients at the time of first diagnosis. We have also discussed the concept of rotating therapy with non-cross-resistant therapeutic regimens. All of these approaches would benefit greatly from a more detailed understanding of drug–drug interactions with the biochemistry and kinetics of both the tumor and normal cells. Although an enormous amount of work has already gone into these areas, we are only now beginning to understand some of these interactions. The appropriate dosing and timing of therapeutic modalities will continue to improve as more information is obtained about these parameters.

An approach which has not been adequately tested in advanced disease is how best to combine systemic and local approaches. In this regard, the potential for systemic radiotherapy should not be overlooked. The ability of surgery and radiotherapy to dramatically reduce the tumor burden has not been seriously applied as an adjunct to systemic therapy.

10.3. Selectivity

Just as the development of the estrophillin assay has enabled greater selectivity in segregating for or against hormonal therapy for the individual patient, similar assays are needed for chemotherapy. Approaches to this problem are currently under way and range from in vitro assays with the drugs of interest, to assaying for specific biochemical pathways, to statistical characterizations of the tumor's enzyme profiles, to statistical evaluation of patient characteristics relative to specific therapies. At the present time, none of these approaches has been exploited extensively enough to develop specific recommendations.

10.4. Monitoring

In addition to the usual monitoring of patients by current clinical techniques, new approaches are being pursued. A wide variety of tests of immunologic functions are being investigated in an attempt to identify those features which predict success or failure to both immunologic and chemotherapeutic approaches. This approach is similar to the development of biochemical markers such as carcinoembryonic antigen. Biochemical markers are now under extensive exploration and, in some cases, may predict success or failure to chemotherapy within two to three days[133,134] or predict relapse from a remission status up to three months before current conventional techniques.[135] Current research is geared toward solidifying these observations and developing new and more breast-cancer-specific markers.

11. References

1. C. Rhoads, Report on a cooperative study of nitrogen mustard (HN₂) therapy of neoplastic disease, *Trans. Assoc. Am. Physicians* **60**, 110–117 (1948).
2. C.G. Zubrod, M. Schneiderman, E. Frei, III, C. Brindley, G.L. Gold, B. Shnider, R. Oviedo, J. Gorman, R. Jones, Jr., U. Jonsson, J. Colsky, T. Chalmers, B. Ferguson, M. Dederick, J. Holland, O. Selawry, W. Regelson, L. Lasagna, and A.H. Owens, Jr., Appraisal of methods for the study of chemotherapy of cancer in man: Comparative therapeutic trial of nitrogen mustard and triethylenethiophosphoramide, *J. Chronic Dis.* **11**, 7–33 (1960).
3. E.B. Schoenbach, J. Colsky, and E.M. Greenspan, Observations on the effects of the folic acid antagonists, aminopterin and amethopterin, in patients with advanced neoplasms, *Cancer* **5**, 1201–1220 (1952).
4. R.W. Rundles, J. Laszlo, F.E. Garrison, and J.B. Hobson, The antitumor spectrum of cyclophosphamide, *Cancer Chemother. Rep.* **16**, 407–411 (1962).
5. H. Atkins, H.G. Gregg, and G.A. Hyman, Clinical appraisal of cyclophosphamide in malignant neoplasms, *Cancer* **15**, 1076–1080 (1962).
6. F. Ansfield, J. Schroeder, and A. Curreri, Five years clinical experience with 5-fluorouracil, *J. Am. Med. Assoc.* **181**, 295–299 (1962).
7. V.T. DeVita, A.A. Serpick, and P.P. Carbone, Combination chemotherapy in the treatment of advanced Hodgkin's disease, *Ann. Intern. Med.* **73**, 881–895 (1970).
8. J. Simone, R.A.J. Aur, H.O. Hustu, and D. Pinkel, Total therapy studies of acute lymphocytic leukemia in children, *Cancer* **30**, 1488–1494 (1972).
9. E.M. Greenspan, M. Fieber, G. Lesnick, and S. Edelman, Response of advanced breast carcinoma to the combination of the antimetabolite, methotrexate, and the alkylating atent, thio-TEPA, *J. Mt. Sinai Hosp. N.Y.* **30**, 246–267 (1963).
10. R.J. Cooper, Combination chemotherapy in hormone resistant breast cancer, *Proc. Am. Assoc. Cancer Res.* **10**, 15 (1969).
11. L. Broder and D.C. Tormey, Combination chemotherapy of carcinoma of the breast: A review, *Cancer Treat. Rev.* **1**, 183–203 (1974).
12. P.P. Carbone, The role of chemotherapy in treatment for breast cancer, in: *Cancer Chemotherapy—Fundamental Concepts and Recent Advances* (M.D. Anderson Hospital, ed.), pp. 311-322, Year Book Medical Publishers, Inc., Chicago (1975).
13. L.M. Axtell and M.H. Myers, Recent trends in survival of cancer patients 1960–1971, End Results in Cancer Report #4, DHEW Publication (NIH) (1975), #767.
14. D.C. Tormey and J.P. Neifeld, Chemotherapeutic approaches to disseminated breast cancer, in: *Breast Cancer Management—Early and Late* (B.A. Stoll, ed.) (1977), in press.
15. S.J. Cutler, Classification of extent of disease in breast cancer, *Semin. Oncol.* **1**, 91–96 (1974).
16. B. Fisher, R.G. Ravdin, and R.K. Ausman, Surgical adjuvant chemotherapy in cancer of the breast: Results of a decade of cooperative investigation, *Ann. Surg.* **168**, 337–356 (1968).
17. S.G. Taylor, III, S.J. Pocock, B.I. Shnider, J. Colsky, and T.C. Hall, Clinical studies of

5-fluorouracil + premarin in the treatment of breast cancer, *Med. Pediatr. Oncol.* **1**, 113–121 (1975).

18. D.C. Tormey, P. Band, and M. Bauer for the Eastern Cooperative Oncology Group, Results of analyses of combination chemotherapy trials (1976) (unpublished).
19. J. Ingle, D.C. Tormey, and J. Bull. Bone marrow involvement in breast cancer, *Proc. Am. Soc. Clin. Oncol.* **16**, 245 (1975).
20. S.J. Cutler, A.J. Asire, and S.G. Taylor, III, Classification of Patients with disseminated cancer of the breast, *Cancer* **24**, 861–869 (1969).
21. M. Cutler, Local extension and distant metastases, in: *Tumors of the Breast*, pp. 124–147, J.B. Lippincott Co., Philadelphia (1962).
22. M.M. Romsdahl, M.E. Sears, and N.E. Eckles, Post treatment evaluation of breast cancer, in: *Breast Cancer: Early and Late* (M.D. Anderson Hospital, ed.), pp. 291–299, Year Book Medical Publishers, Inc., Chicago (1970).
23. S.M. Levenson, J.J. Ingle, S.D. Richman, R.S. Frankel, D.C. Tormey, A.E. Jones, and G.S. Johnston, Liver scanning in metastatic carcinoma of the breast, *J. Nucl. Med.* **16**, 545 (1975).
24. D.C. Tormey and J.N. Ingle, Diagnostic considerations in breast cancer, in: *Breast Cancer Diagnosis* (G.S. Johnston and A.E. Jones, eds.), pp. 1–17, Plenum Medical Book Co., New York (1975).
25. S.D. Richman, J.N. Ingle, S.M. Levenson, J.P. Neifeld, D.C. Tormey, A.E. Jones, and G.S. Johnston, The usefulness of gallium scintigraphy in primary and metastatic breast carcinoma, *J. Nucl. Med.* **16**, 996–1001 (1975).
26. J.A. Neifeld, J.N. Ingle, D.C. Tormey, M.E. Lippman, S.D. Richman, and L.L. Michaelis, Mediastinoscopy: A diagnostic aid in metastatic carcinoma of the breast, *Cancer* **37**, 1973–1976 (1976).
27. T.L. Dao and T. Nemoto, The clinical significance of skin recurrence after radical mastectomy in women with cancer of the breast, *Surg. Gynecol. Obstet.* **117**, 447–453 (1963).
28. A.N. Papaioannou, F.J. Tanz, and H. Volk, Fate of patients with recurrent carcinoma of the breast; recurrence five or more years after initial treatment, *Cancer* **20**, 371–376 (1967).
29. J. Bruce, D.C. Carter, and J. Fraser, Patterns of recurrent disease in breast cancer, *Lancet* **1**, 433–435 (1970).
30. D.S. Martin and R.A. Fugmann, Clinical implications of the interrelationship of tumor size and chemotherapeutic response, *Ann. Surg.* **151**, 97–100 (1960).
31. F.M. Schabel, Jr., Concepts for systemic treatment of micrometastases, *Cancer* **35**, 15–24 (1975).
32. J.J. van Dyk and G. Falkson, Extended survival and remission rates in metastatic breast cancer, *Cancer* **27**, 300–303 (1971).
33. R.V. Smalley, S. Murphy, Y.K. Chan, and C.M. Huguley, Comparison of two five-drug regimes vs. sequential chemotherapy in metastatic breast carcinoma, *Cancer Chemother. Rep.* **57**, 110 (1973).
34. H.E. Skipper and F.M. Schabel, Jr., Quantitative and cytokinetic studies in experimental tumor systems, in: *Cancer Medicine* (J. Holland and E. Frei, III, eds.), 2nd Edition, Lea and Febiger, Philadelphia (1977), in press.
35. A. Howard and S.R. Pelc, Synthesis of deoxyribonucleic acid in normal and irradiated cells and its relationship to chromosome breakage, *Heredity* **6** (Suppl.), 261–273 (1953).
36. G.P. Wheeler and L. Simpson-Herren, Effects of purines, pyrimidines, nucleosides and chemically related compounds on the cell cycle, in: *Drugs and the Cell Cycle* (A.M.

Zimmerman, G.M. Padilla, and I.L. Cameron, eds.), pp. 250–306, Academic Press, New York (1973).

37. P. Calabresi and R.E. Parks, Chemotherapy of neoplastic diseases, in: *The Pharmacological Basis of Therapeutics* (L.S. Goodman and A. Gilman, eds.), 4th ed., pp. 1348–1396, Macmillan, London (1970).

38. P. Brookes, Reaction of alkylating agents with nucleic acids, in: *Chemotherapy of Cancer* (P.A. Plattner, ed.), pp. 32–43, Elsevier, Amsterdam (1964).

39. J.S. Johnson, J.G. Armstrong, M. Gorman, and J.P. Burnett, The vinca alkaloids: a new class of oncolytic agents, *Cancer Res.* **23**, 1390–1427 (1963).

40. S.K. Carter and M. Slavik, Chemotherapy of cancer, *Annu. Rev. Pharmacol.* **14**, 157–183 (1974).

41. H. Umezawa, M. Ishizuka, K. Maeda, and T. Takeuchi, Studies on bleomycin, *Cancer* **20**, 891–895 (1967).

42. W.R. Bruce, B.E. Meeker, and F.A. Valeriote, Comparison of the sensitivity of normal hematopoietic and transplanted lymphoma colony forming cells to chemotherapeutic agents administered *in vivo*, *J. Natl. Cancer Inst.* **37**, 233–245 (1966).

43. F. Valeriote and L. van Putten, Proliferation-dependent cytotoxicity of anticancer agents: A review, *Cancer Res.* **35**, 2619–2630 (1975).

44. W.S. Wilcox, D.R. Griswold, W.R. Laster, Jr., F.M. Schabel, Jr., and H.E. Skipper, Experimental evaluation of potential anticancer agents. XVII. Kinetics of growth and regression after treatment of certain solid tumors, *Cancer Chemother. Rep.* **47**, 27–39 (1965).

45. H.E. Skipper, Kinetics of mammary tumor cell growth and implications for therapy, *Cancer* **28**, 1479–1499 (1971).

46. G.G. Steel, Cytokinetics of neoplasia, in: *Cancer Medicine* (J. Holland and E. Frei, III, eds.), pp. 125–139, Lea and Febiger, Philadelphia (1973).

47. A.K. Laird, Dynamics of tumor growth, *Br. J. Cancer* **18**, 490–502 (1964).

48. W.S. Wilcox, The last surviving cancer cell: the changes of killing it, *Cancer Chemother. Rep.* **50**, 541–542 (1966).

49. M.C. Berenbaum, The last surviving cancer cell: the changes of killing it, *Cancer Chemother. Rep.* **52**, 539–541 (1968).

50. M.C. Berenbaum, Dose–response curves for agents that impair cell reproductive integrity. The relation between dose–response curves and the design of selective regimens in cancer chemotherapy, *Br. J. Cancer* **23**, 434–445 (1969).

51. A.A. Sandberg and G.E. Moore, Examination of blood for tumor cells, *J. Natl. Cancer Inst.* **19**, 1–11 (1957).

52. E. Philippe and Y. LeGal, Growth of seventy-eight recurrent mammary cancers; quantitative study, *Cancer*, **21**, 461–467 (1968).

53. Y.N. Lee and J.S. Spratt, Rate of growth of soft tissue metastases of breast cancer, *Cancer* **29**, 344–348 (1972).

54. E.P. Malaise, N. Chavaudra, A. Charbit, and M. Tubiana, Relationship between the growth rate of human metastases, survival and pathological type, *Eur. J. Cancer* **10**, 451–459 (1974).

55. L.M. Schiffer and P.G. Braunschweiger, Cytokinetics of human breast cancer, primary vs. metastatic lesions, *Proc. Am. Assoc. Cancer Res.* **17**, 238 (1976).

56. R.C. Young and V.T. DeVita, The effect of chemotherapy on the growth characteristics and cellular kinetics of leukemia L1210, *Cancer Res.* **30**, 1789–1794 (1970).

57. D.S. Martin, R.A. Fugmann, R.L. Stolfi, and P.E. Hayworth, Solid tumor animal model therapeutically predictive for human breast cancer, *Cancer Chemother. Rep.* **5**, 89–110 (1975).

58. D.P. Griswold, Jr., The potential for murine tumor models in surgical adjuvant chemotherapy, *Cancer Chemother. Rep.* **5**, 187–204 (1975).

59. A.E. Bogden, H.J. Esber, D.J. Taylor, and J.H. Gray, Comparative study on the effects of surgery, chemotherapy and immunotherapy, alone and in combination, on metastases of the 13762 mammary adenocarcinoma, *Cancer Res.* **34**, 1627–1631, (1974).

60. S.I. Detre, A.J.S. Davies, and T.A. Connors, New models for cancer chemotherapy, *Cancer Chemother. Rep.* **5**, 133–144 (1975).

61. B.C. Giovanella, J.S. Stehlin, and L.J. Williams, Jr., Heterotransplantation of human malignant tumor in nude thymusless mice. II. Malignant tumors induced by injection of cell cultures derived from human solid tumors, *J. Natl. Cancer Inst.* **52**, 921–930 (1974).

62. E.S. Greenwald, *Cancer Chemotherapy*, 2nd ed., pp. 28–346, Medical Outline Series, Medical Examination Publishing Co., Inc., New York (1973).

63. B.A. Chabner, C.E. Myers, C.N. Coleman, and D.G. Johns, The clinical pharmacology of antineoplastic agents, *N. Engl. J. Med.* **292**, 1107–1113 and 1159–1168 (1975).

64. E. Mihich, Pharmacologic principles and the basis of selectivity of drug action, in: *Cancer Medicine* (J. Holland and E. Frei, III, eds.), pp. 650–674, Lea and Febiger, Philadelphia (1973).

65. P.R. Bergevin, D.C. Tormey, and J. Blom, Guide to the use of cancer chemotherapeutic agents, *Mod. Treat.* **9**, 185–273 (1972).

66. L.E. Broder and P.P. Carbone, Pharmacokinetic considerations in the design of optimal chemotherapeutic regimens for the treatment of breast carcinoma: a conceptual approach, *Med. Pediatr. Oncol.* **2**, 11–27 (1976).

67. R.A. Minow, R.S. Benjamin, and J.A. Gottlieb, Adriamycin (NSC 123127) cardiomyopathy—an overview with determination of risk factors, *Cancer Chemother. Rep.* **6**, 195–201 (1975).

68. J.J. Rinehart, R.P. Lewis, and S.P. Balcerzak, Adriamycin cardiotoxicity in man, *Ann. Intern. Med.* **81**, 475–478 (1974).

69. D.L. Ahmann, H.F. Bisel, R.G. Hahn, R.T. Eagan, J.H. Edmonson, J.L. Steinfeld, D.C. Tormey, and W.F. Taylor, An analysis of a multiple drug program in the treatment of patients with advanced breast cancer utilizing 5-fluorouracil, cyclophosphamide and prednisone with or without vincristine, *Cancer* **36**, 1925–1935 (1975).

70. S.K. Carter, Study design principles for the clinical evaluation of new drugs as developed by the chemotherapy program of the NCI, in: *The Design of Clinical Trials* (M. Staquet, ed.), pp. 242–291, Futura Publishing Co., Mt. Kisco, New York (1972).

71. H.E. Skipper, Kinetic considerations associated with therapy of solid tumors, in: *The Proliferation and Spread of Neoplastic Cells* (University of Texas, M.D. Anderson Symposium, 1967), pp. 213–234, Williams and Wilkins, Baltimore (1968).

72. R.W. Talley, V.K. Vaitkevicius, and G.A. Leighton, Comparison of cyclophosphamide and 5-fluorouracil in the treatment of patients with metastatic breast cancer, *Clin. Pharmacol. Ther.* **6**, 740–748 (1965).

73. Eastern Cooperative Group in Solid Tumor Chemotherapy, Comparison of antimetabolites in the treatment of breast and colon cancer, *J. Am. Med. Assoc.* **200**, 770–778 (1967).

74. D.C. Tormey, Adriamycin in breast cancer: an overview of studies, *Cancer Chemother. Rep.* **6**, 319–327 (1975).

75. S.G. Taylor, G.P. Canellos, P. Band, and S. Pocock, Combination chemotherapy for advanced breast cancer: Randomized comparison with single drug therapy, *Proc. Am. Soc. Clin. Oncol.* **15**, 175 (1974).

76. L.M. Baker, C.B. Vaughn, M. Al-Sarrof, M.L. Reed, and V.K. Vaitkevicius, Evaluation of combination vs. sequential cytotoxic chemotherapy in the treatment of advanced breast cancer, *Cancer* **33**, 513–518 (1974).

77. P. Band, D. Tormey, and M. Bauer, Unpublished observations from Eastern Cooperative Oncology Group trials (1976).

78. D. Ahmann, T. Dao, and J. Horton, Personal communication (1976).

79. M. DeLena, C. Brambilla, A. Morabito, and G. Bonadonna, Adriamycin plus vincristine compared to and combined with cyclophosphamide, methotrexate and 5-fluorouracil for advanced breast cancer, Cancer 35, 1108–1115 (1975).

80. L. Simpson-Herren and D.P. Griswold, Jr., Studies of the cell population kinetics of induced and transplanted mammary adenocarcinoma in rats, Cancer Res. 33, 2415–2424 (1973).

81. I.S. Goldenberg, N. Sedransk, H. Volk, A. Segaloff, R.M. Kelley, and C.R. Haines, Combined androgen and antimetabolite therapy of advanced female breast cancer; a report of the Cooperative Breast Cancer Group, Cancer 36, 308–310 (1975).

82. F.D. Moore, S.B. Vandevanter, C.M. Boyden, J. Lokich, and R.E. Wilson, Adrenalectomy with chemotherapy in the treatment of advanced breast cancer: Objective and subjective response rates; duration and quality of life, Surgery 76, 376–388 (1974).

83. I.S. Goldenberg, Secondary chemotherapy of advanced breast cancer, Cancer 31, 660–663 (1973).

84. P.B. Stott, L. Zelkowitz, and W.G. Tucker, Combination chemohormonal therapy for disseminated breast carcinoma, Cancer Chemother. Rep. 57, 106 (1973).

85. E.M. Greenspan, Regression of metastatic hepatomegaly from mammary carcinoma. Cytotoxic combination chemotherapy with 5-FU, N.Y. State J. Med. 64, 2442–2449 (1964).

86. T. Nemoto, J. Horton, T. Cunningham, R. Sponzo, D. Rosner, R. Diaz, and T.L. Dao, Update report. Comparison of combination chemotherapy vs. adriamycin vs. adrenalectomy in breast cancer, Proc. Am. Assoc. Cancer Res. 16, 46 (1975).

87. G. Falkson and L. Leone, Personal communication (1976).

88. C. Alford, A.C. Hollinshead, and R.B. Herberman, Delayed cutaneous hypersensitivity reactions to extracts of malignant and normal human breast cells, Ann. Surg. 178, 20–24 (1973).

89. A.C. Hollinshead, W.T. Jaffurs, L.K. Alpert, J.E. Harris, and R.B. Herberman, Isolation and identification of soluble skin reactive membrane antigens of malignant and normal breast cells, Cancer Res. 34, 2961–2968 (1974).

90. M.M. Black, H.P. Leis, Jr., B. Shore, and R.E. Zachrau, Cellular hypersensitivity to breast cancer; assessment by a leukocyte migration procedure, Cancer 33, 952–958 (1974).

91. R.B. Herberman, Cellular immunity to human tumor associated antigens, Isr. J. Med. Sci. 9, 300–307 (1973).

92. J.H. Dean, J.S. Silva, J.L. McCoy, C.M. Leonard, M. Middleton, G.B. Cannon, and R.B. Herberman, Lymphocyte blastogenesis induced by potassium chloride extracts of allogeneic breast carcinoma and lymphoid cells, J. Natl. Cancer Inst. 54, 1295–1298 (1975).

93. M.M. Black and H.P. Leis, Jr., Human breast carcinoma. Part III. Cellular responses to autologous breast cancer: Skin-window procedure, N.Y. State J. Med. 70, 2583–2589 (1970).

94. T.J. Cunningham, D. Daut, P.E. Wolfgang, M. Mellyn, S. Maciolek, R.W. Sponzo, and J. Horton, A correlation of DNCB-induced delayed cutaneous hypersensitivity reactions and the course of disease in patients with recurrent breast cancer, Cancer 37, 1696–1700 (1976).

95. M.M. Black and H.P. Leis, Jr., Cellular responses to autologous breast cancer tissue; correlation with stage and lymphoreticuloendothelial reactivity, Cancer 28, 263–273 (1971).

96. S.J. Cutler, C. Zippin, and A.J. Asire, The prognostic significance of palpable lymph nodes in cancer of the breast, *Cancer* **23**, 243–250 (1969).

97. R.L. Stolfi, R.A. Fugmann, L.M. Stolfi, and D.S. Martin, Synergism between host anti-tumor immunity and combined modality therapy against murine breast cancer, *Int. J. Cancer* **13**, 389–403 (1974).

98. B. Fisher, N. Wolmark, E. Saffer, and E.R. Fisher, Inhibitory effect of prolonged *Corynebacterium parvum* and cyclophosphamide administration on the growth of established tumors, *Cancer* **35**, 134–143 (1975).

99. L. Israel, A randomized study of chemotherapy versus chemotherapy with *Corynebacterium parvum* in advanced breast cancer, in: *Proceedings XI International Cancer Congress* (P. Bucalossi, U. Veronesi, and N. Cascinelli, eds.), Vol. 6, pp. 77–79, Excerpta Medica, Amsterdam (1975).

100. J.U. Gutterman, G.R. Blumenschein, G. Hortobagyi, G. Mavligit, and E.M. Hersh, Immunotherapy for breast cancer, *Breast, Diseases of the Breast* **2**, 29–34 (1976).

101. A.F. Rojas, E. Mickiewicz, J.N. Feierstein, H. Glait, and A.J. Olivari, Levamisole in advanced human breast cancer, *Lancet* **1**, 211–215 (1976).

102. B. Fisher, P.P. Carbone, S.G. Economou, R. Frelick, A. Glass, H. Lerner, C. Redmond, M. Zelen, D.L. Katrych, N. Wolmark, P. Band, and E.R. Fisher, L-Phenylalanine mustard (L-PAM) in the management of primary breast cancer: A report of early findings. *N. Engl. J. Med.* **292**, 117–122 (1975).

103. G. Bonadonna, P. Valagussa, and U. Veronesi, Results of ongoing trials with adjuvant therapy in operable breast cancer, in: *Breast Cancer: Trends in Research and Treatment; A Monograph of the European Organization for Research on Treatment of Cancer* (J.C. Heuson, W.H. Matthiem, and M. Rozencweig, eds.), pp. 239–258, Raven Press, New York (1976).

104. K.W. Brunner, R.W. Sonntag, G. Martz, H.J. Senn, P. Obrecht, and P. Alberto, A controlled study in the use of combined drug therapy for metastatic breast cancer, *Cancer* **36**, 1208–2119 (1975).

105. D.C. Tormey, J. Bull, C. Falkson, P. Band, and J. Blom, Adriamycin and dibromodulcitol in metastatic breast cancer, *Proc. Am. Assoc. Cancer Res.* **16**, 129 (1975).

106. E.B. van Eden, G. Falkson, A.M. van der Merwe, J.J. Van Dyk, and H.C. Falkson, FIVB—A new combination of drugs in the treatment of cancer, *S. Afr. Med. J.* **47**, 982–984 (1973).

107. C.A. Presant, J.F. Kolhouse, and C. Klahr, Adriamycin, 1,3-bis(2-chloroethyl)-1-nitrosourea (BCNU-NSC 409462) and cyclophosphamide in refractory adenocarcinoma of the breast and other tumors, *Cancer* **37**, 620–628 (1976).

108. D.C. Tormey, Unpublished data (1976).

109. P. Longacre, T. Cunningham, K. Olson, J. Horton, and R. Sponzo, HOM chemotherapy in advanced neoplasms, *Proc. Am. Assoc. Cancer Res.* **17**, 99 (1976).

110. R. Zucali, C. Uslenghi, R. Kenda, and G. Bonadonna, Natural history and survival of inoperable breast cancer treated with radiotherapy and radiotherapy followed by radical mastectomy, *Cancer* **37**, 1422–1431 (1976).

111. M. DeLena, L. Brugnatelli, C. Uslenghi, R. Zucali, and G. Bonadonna, Combined chemotherapy and radiotherapy in inoperable (T3$_b$T4) breast cancer, *Proc. Am. Assoc. Cancer Res.* **16**, 273 (1975).

112. A. Bennett, A.M. McDonald, J.S. Simpson, and I.F. Stamford, Breast cancer, prostaglandins and bone metastases, *Lancet* **1**, 1218–1220 (1975).

113. T.J. Powles, S.A. Clark, D.M. Easty, G.C. Easty, and A.M. Neville, The inhibition by aspirin and indomethacin of osteolytic tumour deposits and hypercalcaemia in rats with Walker tumour and its possible application to human breast cancer, *Br. J. Cancer* **28**, 316–321 (1973).

114. T. Powles, Personal communication (1975).
115. J.R. Little, A.J.D. Dale, and H. Okazuki, Meningeal carcinomatosis: clinical manifestations, *Arch. Neurol.* **30**, 138–143 (1974).
116. M.E. Olson, N.L. Chernik, and J.B. Posner, Infiltration of the leptomeninges by systemic cancer—a clinical and pathologic study, *Arch. Neurol.* **30**, 122–137 (1974).
117. S. Kaufman and M. Goldstein, Combination chemotherapy in disseminated carcinoma of the breast, *Surg. Gynecol. Obstet.* **137**, 83–86 (1973).
118. B.J. Kennedy and A.S. Gilbertson, Increased erythropoiesis induced by androgenic hormone therapy, *N. Engl. J. Med.* **256**, 719–726 (1957).
119. P.P. Carbone, V. Bono, E. Frei, and C.O. Brindley, Clinical studies with vincristine, *Blood* **21**, 640–647 (1963).
120. N.V. Dimitrov, S. Andre, G. Eliopoulos, and B. Halpern, Effect of *Corynebacterium parvum* on animal and human bone marrow cultures, *Proc. Am. Assoc. Cancer Res.* **16**, 151 (1975).
121. J.M. Baron and J.E. Ultmann, The management of malignant serous effusions, in: *Chemotherapy of Malignant Neoplasms* (F.J. Ansfield, ed.), pp. 126–145, Charles C. Thomas, Springfield, Illinois (1973).
122. C.B. Anderson, G.W. Philpott, and T.B. Ferguson, The treatment of malignant pleural effusions, *Cancer* **33**, 916–922 (1974).
123. R.M. Rubinson and H. Bolooki, Intrapleural tetracycline for control of malignant pleural effusion: A preliminary report, *South. Med. J.* **65**, 847–849 (1972).
124. G.F. Robbins, J. Shah, P. Rosen, F. Chu, and J. Taylor, Inflammatory carcinoma of the breast, *Surg. Clin. North Am.* **54**, 801–810 (1974).
125. D.L. Ellis and S.L. Teitelbaum, Inflammatory carcinoma of the breast; a pathological definition, *Cancer* **33**, 1045–1047 (1974).
126. J.T. Corall and T.L. Dao, The etiology of inflammatory reactions in breast carcinoma, *Surg. Forum* **9**, 611–614 (1958).
127. C.C. Wang, Management of inflammatory carcinoma of the breast, *J. Am. Med. Assoc.* **201**, 533 (1967).
128. R.M. Yonemoto, J.L. Keating, R.L. Byron, and D.M. Reihiwaki, Inflammatory carcinoma of the breast treated by bilateral adrenalectomy, *Surgery* **68**, 461–467 (1970).
129. T.L. Dao and J.D. McCarthy, Treatment of inflammatory carcinoma of the breast, *Surg. Gynecol. Obstet.* **105**, 289–294 (1957).
130. C.C. Harris, The carcinogenicity of anticancer drugs: A hazard in man, *Cancer* **37**, 1014–1023 (1976).
131. I. Penn, Second malignant neoplasms associated with immunosuppressive medications, *Cancer* **37**, 1024–1032 (1976).
132. G.T. Ross, Congenital anomalies among children born of mothers receiving chemotherapy for gestational trophoblastic neoplasms, *Cancer* **37**, 1043–1047 (1976).
133. D.H. Russell, B.G.M. Durie, and S.E. Salmon, Polyamines as predictors of success and failure in cancer chemotherapy, *Lancet* **2**, 797–799 (1975).
134. T.P. Waalkes, C.W. Gehrke, W.A. Bleyer, R.W. Zumwalt, C.L.M. Olweny, K.C. Kao, D.B. Lakings, and S.A. Jacobs, Potential biologic markers in Burkitt's lymphoma, *Cancer Chemother. Rep.* **59**, 721–727 (1975).
135. D.C. Tormey and T.P. Waalkes, Biochemical markers in cancer of the breast, *Recent Results Cancer Res.* **57**, 78–94 (1976).

5

Physiological Principles Underlying Endocrine Therapy of Breast Cancer

WILLIAM LEO McGUIRE

1. Introduction

The subject of endocrine therapy for advanced breast cancer is certainly not new. The first demonstration of hormonal control of breast cancer was made 81 years ago when regression of metastatic tumor was produced by ovariectomy.[1] Since then, adrenalectomy and hypophysectomy have been used to achieve similar results. These ablative procedures serve to remove sources of circulating hormones which stimulate or support breast tumor growth. Alternatively, breast cancer regression can be achieved by administering large pharmacological doses of estrogen, androgen, progestin, or glucocorticoid. Historically, the choice of endocrine therapy for an individual patient has been in large part empirical, guided by certain clinical features such as menopausal status, free interval, site of the dominant lesion, and the response to any previous endocrine therapy. Since the empirical approach has been extensively reviewed in the literature, I will not dwell upon it further in this chapter. Instead, I refer the reader to several excellent books and chapters on the subject.[2-4]

Regardless of the type of endocrine therapy employed, objective tumor regression occurs in only 20–40% of breast cancer patients. With the recent success of combination chemotherapy achieving objective remission in perhaps 60% of patients (see other chapters in this volume),

WILLIAM LEO McGUIRE · Department of Medicine, University of Texas Health Science Center, San Antonio, Texas. Observations from the author's laboratory were supported in part by the USPHS CA-11378, CB-23862, and the American Cancer Society BC-23.

clinicians are understandably reluctant to routinely recommend ablative endocrine surgery as the therapy of choice. However, a renewal of interest in endocrine therapy is resulting from basic investigations which have led to the development of assays that can determine with considerable confidence those breast cancer patients who will or will not respond to endocrine therapy. This advance is largely the result of a major effort in the past few years to understand the subcellular biochemical pathways of hormone action in both normal and neoplastic cells. At present, the most well-defined and clinically relevant studies have focused on hormone receptors.

Normal target tissues, including mammary glands, contain specific receptors for hormones—cytoplasmic proteins for the steroids and cell surface receptors for polypeptides. These receptor sites are responsible for the initial interaction between the hormone and the cell, and function to trigger the biochemical chain of events characteristic for the particular hormone. Hormone-dependent tumors also contain receptors, but it now appears that independent, or autonomous, tumors often may not. [5]

Consequently, it has been proposed that when malignant transformation occurs, the cell may retain all or only part of the normal population of receptor sites. If the cell retains the receptor sites, its growth and function, like those of the normal cell, are potentially capable of being regulated by its hormonal environment. If the cell loses the receptors as a consequence of its malignant transformation, it is no longer recognized as a target cell by circulating hormones and endocrine control is abolished.

This implies that the presence of specific receptors in mammary tumor tissue may indicate hormone dependence, and thereby identify the 20–40% of breast cancer patients who will actually benefit from endocrine therapy.

In this chapter, I will review the role of several hormones and their receptors in breast cancer tissues and examine mechanisms of control, as well as provide pathophysiological correlation whenever possible. Many of the studies on hormone-dependent breast carcinoma employ animal models, particularly carcinogen-induced rat mammary tumors which regress after endocrine ablative surgery. The relevance of these animal models to the clinical problem of human breast cancer will be demonstrated. It is therefore my purpose in this chapter to illustrate the physiological principles of hormone action in breast cancer tissue so that an appreciation of the mechanism of endocrine-induced breast tumor regression will develop. Such an understanding should lead to a more rational approach for selecting or rejecting endocrine therapy for advanced breast cancer patients.

2. Prolactin

2.1. Rat Mammary Tumors

Prolactin may be the single most important hormone in rat mammary tumor growth[6-8]:

1. Procedures or agents which stimulate prolactin secretion enhance tumor growth: (a) Prolactin alone is able to reactivate tumor growth, at least for a short term, after ablation of the ovaries, adrenals, and pituitary gland.[9,10] (b) Administration of the tranquilizer perphenazine, which stimulates prolactin secretion in tumor-bearing rats,[11] increases the number and size of tumors in adrenalectomized–ovariectomized rats.[9] (c) Lesions in the median eminence of the tuber cinereum stimulate release of prolactin and inhibit release of all other pituitary hormones.[12] Such lesions cause a considerable increase in the size and number of tumors.[13,14] Estradiol benzoate implants into the median eminence of tumor-bearing rats also raise blood prolactin levels over controls and significantly increase the size and number of tumors.[15] These effects of prolactin have been reviewed.[16]

2. Procedures or agents which diminish prolactin secretion or effectiveness inhibit tumor growth: (a) Daily administration of antiprolactin antiserum causes tumor regression in 50% of dimethylbenzanthracene (DMBA)-induced tumor-bearing rats, whereas treatment with normal rabbit serum results in only a 13% tumor regression.[17] Similar results have been reported with antiadenohypophysis serum.[18] (b) Ergot alkaloids inhibit prolactin secretion, probably by direct action on both pituitary and hypothalamus.[18,20] Growth of DMBA-induced mammary tumors is inhibited in rats treated with ergot alkaloids,[21-23] as is the growth of spontaneous mammary tumors.[24] Complete remissions have been obtained in 62% of these induced rat tumors, and a majority of the regressed tumors fail to recur after cessation of treatment.[25] A combination of ergocornine and reserpine designed to induce panhyopituitarism was found to be as effective as hypophysectomy in causing remission of DMBA tumors.[26] Other agents which depress serum prolactin (pargyline, L-dopa, and lysergic acid diethylamide) inhibit DMBA-tumor growth, whereas haloperidol and methyldopa, which elevate serum prolactin, stimulate tumor growth.[27,28] An excellent review of the effect of ergot alkaloids on prolactin secretion and prolactin-dependent processes is available.[29]

Although prolactin is undoubtedly important in stimulating DMBA-tumor growth, other experiments suggest that prolactin may not be solely responsible for hormone dependence. First, growth hormone is also able to stimulate mammary tumor induction in carcinogen-fed hypophysectomized rats[30] and promote growth of established tumors following hypophysectomy.[31] Second, if DMBA-tumor-bearing rats are ovariectomized and simultaneous lesions are placed in the median eminence to increase prolactin release, the tumors grow at an accelerated pace for only 10–12 days and then regress, even though prolactin levels remain elevated.[13,32] The ovarian factor responsible for maintaining tumor growth under these circumstances has not been identified. Third, pregnancy stimulates the growth of experimental tumors,[33–35] while parturition and weaning are followed by regression of a large number of these tumors. The tumor growth-promoting factor of pregnancy is probably placental lactogen.[36] Since the maintenance of tumor size or growth during lactation depends upon the suckling stimulus, and tumors regress if suckling is prevented,[37,38] prolactin would appear to be responsible. The true situation is more complex, however, since ovariectomy blocks the stimulatory effects of endogenous or exogenous prolactin on tumor growth and injection of progesterone removes this block.[37] One interpretation would be that prolactin stimulation of tumor growth under these circumstances is dependent on progesterone, or, alternatively, that the high levels of progesterone which are under prolactin control in the lactating rat[39] are responsible for the tumor growth.

Finally, the recent demonstration that prolactin can alter steroid metabolism inside DMBA-tumor cells provides additional evidence that part of the action of prolactin may be to modulate the direct effects of steroids on tumor cell growth and function.[40]

2.2. Human Breast Cancer

It may be concluded from animal-tumor studies that simple raising or lowering of blood prolactin levels is insufficient to explain breast tumor growth and regression, and this conclusion is supported by studies in human breast cancer. There is no doubt that hypophysectomy causes regression of metastatic tumor.[41] This could be explained by elimination of pituitary prolactin and/or growth hormone, which might be directly supporting tumor growth, or by the removal of gonadotropins and consequent lowering of estrogen and progesterone production by the ovaries, or even by the elimination of adrenocorticotropin, leading to reduced adrenal synthesis of estrogen precursors, progesterone, and glucocorticoids. Early attempts to unravel these possibilities led to conflicting results. Pearson *et al.*[42] correlated the degree of hypercalcuria with the growth rate of osteolytic metastases in patients with breast cancer, and using this as an index of hormonal stimulation of tumor growth, reported that bovine growth hormone[43] and human growth hormone[44] stimulated metastatic mammary carcinoma. This conclusion was not supported by Lipsett and Bergenstal,[45] who found that neither human growth hormone nor ovine prolactin stimulated calcium excretion in breast cancer patients more than in control patients. But both groups[44,45] emphasized an important observation: following regrowth after hypophysectomy, further remissions of breast cancer are not obtained with pharmacologic estrogen or androgen therapy. Furthermore, physiologic doses of estrogen do not exacerbate the disease in those hypophysectomized patients who are in remission. These results suggest a central role for the pituitary in human breast tumor growth and in the response to endocrine therapy. However, in other studies, the role of prolactin is less clear.

L-Dopa, which suppresses serum prolactin levels,[46-48] has been administered to patients with metastatic breast cancer with variable results.[49-54] Most agree that L-dopa can acutely lower prolactin levels and that relief of bone pain is frequent in patients with bone metastases. Objective tumor regression is infrequent, however, due perhaps to the incomplete or temporary nature of the prolactin suppression. It has been proposed that the relief of bone pain during L-dopa therapy be used as a simple test to predict which patients will respond to surgical endocrine ablation, but this proposal has not yet been tested in a controlled study.

Ergot derivatives also effectively suppress prolactin levels in humans.[55-58] Unfortunately, objective tumor regressions with these agents are rarely seen.[59-61]

The possibility that patients with breast cancer might have higher average blood levels of prolactin has been refuted in at least four studies.[62-65] Nevertheless, two series did report higher prolactin levels in families with a high frequency of breast cancer.[64,66] It has been reported that women taking reserpine (which stimulates prolactin secretion in humans) have a higher than normal incidence of breast cancer.[67-69] This has been challenged by two recent studies.[70,71] It should be noted that peak prolactin secretion occurs at night.[72,73] so that studies of patient population at risk for breast cancer or with established disease may be of limited value if only random daytime prolactin levels are measured.

Finally, the most disconcerting data regarding a primary role for prolactin in human breast cancer growth concern the high prolactin levels accompanying tumor regressions after pituitary-stalk section. Ehni and Eckles[74] noticed that four patients who had undergone stalk section for metastatic breast cancer lactated after the operation, though all four experienced some degree of objective tumor regression. Many years later, these important clinical observations were confirmed by actual measurement of blood levels of prolactin in patients treated with pituitary-stalk section for metastatic breast cancer.[75] Of eleven such patients, eight experienced objective remissions for periods ranging from seven months to twelve years, and five of these had elevated prolactin levels during the period of remission. Among the three who showed no objective remission, two had elevated prolactin levels. Thus, in humans as well as in animal models, the biochemical mechanism of mammary tumor regression following endocrine ablation involves more than simple alterations of the blood prolactin level.

2.3. Mechanism of Prolactin Dependence

Although claims of a singular role for prolactin in hormone dependence may be exaggerated, there is little doubt of prolactin's importance in stimulating several biochemical processes in mammary tissues. These processes have been extensively studied, especially with the organ culture technique, and have been reviewed.[76] They do not provide any direct clues about the mechanism of hormone dependence.

Other pituitary polypeptide hormones act on their respective target cells through binding to surface membrane receptors. This interaction sets off a chain of events involving generation of cyclic AMP and activation of protein kinase ultimately resulting in target cell function.[77] It was reasonable to postulate that mammary cell surfaces also have specific receptor sites to recognize prolactin. Turkington[78] showed that prolactin covalently linked to sepharose (so that it theoretically could not enter cells) could still stimulate RNA synthesis in isolated mammary cells. After *in vivo* injection, radioactive prolactin was located on the surface of mammary and other target cells.[79,80] Direct measurement of [^{125}I]prolactin binding to membrane particles from rabbit and mouse mammary gland followed.[81–85]

These findings suggested a possible explanation for hormone dependence or autonomy in breast cancer cells: the hormone-dependent tumor cell, like the normal mammary cell, has retained the surface receptor, whereas the autonomous cell has lost the receptor and hence, the ability to recognize and be regulated by prolactin.[86–89] We examined this possibility by comparing prolactin receptors in normal rat mammary tissues and in both hormone-dependent and autonomous rat mammary tumors.

Binding of [^{125}I]prolactin was first determined in tissue slices to avoid the recovery problems inherent in membrane purification procedures. Lactating mammary gland had high-affinity (K_d 2×10^{-9} M) saturable binding to approximately 3000 prolactin receptor sites per cell. Only rat or ovine prolactin competed for binding.[90,91]

We then studied two sublines of the transplantable rat mammary carcinoma MTW9. One of the sublines, MTW9-MD, is hormone-dependent. It grows in intact rats but regresses promptly following ovariectomy. This tumor has the same number of prolactin receptor sites as the normal mammary gland and has appreciable numbers of receptor sites for estrogen (ER). In contrast, the autonomous subline MTW9-MA, which grows in hypophysectomized or ovariectomized rats, contained only one-sixth of the receptor sites for prolactin and estrogen found in the hormone-dependent MTW9-MD.[86] These data demonstrate that receptors for prolactin can be either retained or lost during the process of malignant transformation and subsequent mammary tumor growth.

Unfortunately, tumors are not absolutely positive or negative for prolactin receptors. In DMBA tumors a wide range is seen,[87,88,92,93] and this has led to proposals utilizing both prolactin receptor and ER data to predict hormone responsiveness.[88] In fact, there is much experimental data which link estrogen and prolactin action. Prolactin increases the uptake of estradiol into mammary gland explants *in vitro*[94] Furthermore, Vignon and Rochefort[95,96] have shown a prompt fall of ER in DMBA tumors regressing after ovariectomy. Prolactin injections not only stimulated the tumor to resume growth, but restored the concentration of ER. The authors conclude that prolactin sensitizes the mammary tumor to estradiol by stimulating estrogen receptor sites. The most intriguing new development is the report of a conversion of an ovarian-nonresponsive to an ovarian-responsive mammary tumor strain by chronic stimulation of endogenous prolactin.[97] It will be very important to determine whether the new tumors have acquired additional receptor sites for either estrogen or prolactin.

A recent development which may bear on the question of prolactin receptor regulation in mammary tumors comes from studies in rat liver. Independent observations show that prolactin receptors rapidly decrease in liver cells following hypophysectomy and can be restored by prolactin.[98-100] Ovariectomy and thyroidectomy achive a similar decrease in liver-cell prolactin receptors, which can be restored by estradiol and thyroid hormone.[101] Such a hormonal regulatory system has not yet been demonstrated for prolactin in mammary tumors, but it has been suggested that placental lactogen may increase prolactin receptors in the pregnant rat mammary gland.[91]

The possible causal relationship between the loss of prolactin receptors and the loss of hormone dependence in experimental breast cancer is also complicated by the following observation. The R3230AC transplantable rat mammary carcinoma grows well in ovariectomized female rats and is therefore considered not to be dependent upon hormones for growth, yet the tumor can respond to prolactin injections by synthesizing enzymes and specific mRNA's concerned with milk protein synthesis.[89,102-104] We found a normal complement of prolactin receptor sites in this tumor.[90] Clearly, in this case, growth autonomy arose in the presence of normal prolactin receptors and prolactin responses. One possible explanation of R3230AC's autonomy is suggested by its marked deficiency in estrogen receptor as compared to hormone-dependent tumors.[105,106] Another explanation is that malignant transformation might sometimes unmask occluded receptors on the mammary cell surface, thereby exposing the tumor cells to stimulation by hormones which do not affect growth of normal mammary tissue. In this case, the tumors might appear autonomous to prolactin manipulation while they are in fact hormone-dependent but on different hormones. This situation has actually been reported in certain adrenal tumors.[107]

In summary, prolactin can clearly be implicated in the growth of experimental rat mammary tumors. Its role in regulating the growth of human mammary cancer demands further study.

3. Estrogen

Estrogen acts directly on the normal mammary gland to promote growth and differentiation.[108-111] However, estrogen also stimulates the release of pituitary prolactin, which likewise acts upon the mammary cell.[112] Since estrogen cannot support mammary tumor growth in the absence of a pituitary,[113] whereas prolactin reportedly supports both normal mammary gland and mammary tumor growth in the absence of ovaries and adrenals,[9,10] estrogen is considered by many to play only a secondary role in tumor growth and regression.[114] Prolactin stimulation of tumor growth in the absence of ovarian steroids is of brief duration, however. If DMBA-tumor-bearing rats are ovariectomized and simultaneous lesions are placed in the median eminence to increase prolactin release, the tumors grow at an accelerated pace for only 10–12 days and then regress, even though prolactin levels remain elevated.[13,32] Furthermore, the transplantation survival of the MTW9 rat mammary tumor appears to depend on ovarian hormones,[115] and growth of MTW9 tumors is impaired in rats immunized with estradiol–BSA conjugates.[116] One might summarize the role of physiologic estrogen levels as follows: estrogens are probably essential, but not sufficient, for growth of certain mammary tumors.

On the other hand, estrogens in pharmacologic doses cause regression of mammary tumors.[117] This paradoxical effect of estrogen may involve interference with the prolactin stimulation of growth, since the effect can be overcome by increasing endogenous[118] or exogenous[119] prolactin.

There is considerable current information on portions of the intracellular estrogen response mechanism in both rate mammary tumor systems and human breast cancer. We will now examine aspects of this mechanism and its role in endocrine control over mammary cancer cells.

3.1. Localization of Estrogens in Responsive Tumors

In 1959, two laboratories reported that radioactively labeled estrogen injected *in vivo* into experimental animals was localized in those organs which either respond to estrogen or excrete it.[120,121] Soon after, breast cancer patients scheduled for adrenalectomy to remove the source of circulating estrogens were given tritiated hexestrol just prior to surgery. It was discovered that the tumor metastases of the patients responding to the adrenalectomy concentrated a larger fraction of [³H] hexestrol than those of patients who failed to respond,[122] as if only responsive tumors behaved as estrogen target tissues. Other investigators studying the uptake of radioactive estrogens into human mammary tissue[123–126] found a correlation between the uptake of estrogen by malignant breast tissue and the response to endocrine therapy, but this correlation was not sufficiently strong to be useful for predicting response in an individual patient.

Similar results were obtained in experimental mammary carcinomas, and hormone-dependent tumors *in vitro* also took up more estrogen than did autonomous tumors.[127–134] This *in vitro* uptake could be completely inhibited by synthetic estrogen analogues, whereas the relatively low uptake in other tissues such as muscle could not be inhibited, indicating specificity of the uptake into tumors. From these results, Jensen proposed that the *in vitro* technique might be extended to human tumor tissue samples to predict the response to adrenalectomy. By this time, estrogen receptor had been discovered in target tissues including tumors[135–139] and appeared to be responsible for the specific uptake of estrogen by these tissues. Direct studies of the presence and role of receptor in mammary tumors followed, and raised the possibility of using the presence of the receptor to predict hormone dependence.

3.2. Measurement of Estrogen Receptor

There are now several procedures for measurement of ER in cytosols of target tissues.[140,141] The receptor can be quantitated by demonstration of specific 8 S and 4 S binding of [³H]estradiol on sucrose density gradients (SDG). The dextran-coated-charcoal method (DCC) is equally quantitative and less expensive. Non-receptor-bound [³H]estradiol is removed from specific estradiol-bound receptor by charcoal. The binding data obtained from incubating cytosol with increasing concentrations of hormone can be plotted by the method of Scatchard to determine both the number and affinity of estrogen binding sites.

Assays based on protamine precipitation of receptor have recently been developed to measure both free and hormone-bound receptor from cytoplasmic[142] and nuclear[143] extracts. The receptor is precipitated with protamine, and the solid-phase protamine–receptor complex is then incubated with radioactive estradiol. Incubation at 30° or 37° permits exchange of any previously bound nonradioactive ligand, while at 4° only unoccupied receptor is radiolabeled. The combination of these assays has the unique advantage of using only one basic technique to assess both free and bound estrogen receptor sites in tumor cytosol and nuclei. This procedure could prove particularly useful where premenopausal cancer patients might have high levels of plasma estrogens that would transfer cytoplasmic ER to nuclear sites, making them inaccessible to assay by SDG or DCC. Since the presence of free cytoplasmic ER in tumors now has prognostic value in helping to predict the proper type of treatment for breast cancer patients (see below), those premenopausal women who have ER masked by endogenous estrogens might otherwise be denied beneficial treatment.

3.3. Rat Mammary Tumors as a Model System

Because of their many similarities to human breast cancer, DMBA-induced rat mammary tumors have been extensively studied to provide insight into the mechanism of hormonal influence in tumor growth. These tumors have complex hormonal requirements for growth[114,144] and have ER values which range widely.[88,144,145] Absent or low levels of tumor ER are associated with a failure to regress after ovariectomy, whereas the majority of ER-positive tumors regress following endocrine ablative procedures. The finding of ER-positive DMBA tumors which do not respond is similar to the situation in human breast cancer, and demands further study. It has been suggested[146] that the receptor might be defective in nonresponding tumors, but nuclear translocation of ER is normal in autonomous DMBA rat tumors.[147] In addition, chromatin from autonomous rat mammary tumors is capable of binding ER under cell-free conditions.[106,148] It is fair to summarize that in DMBA-induced rat mammary tumors, ER may be essential to hormonally regulated growth and regression, but the mere presence of ER in a tumor does not guarantee that the tumor will behave in a hormone-dependent fashion.

3.4. Estrogen Receptor in Human Breast Tumors

The properties of the ER found in hormone-dependent rat tumors have now been demonstrated in human mammary tumors as well.[149] In ER-positive tumors, Scatchard plots of the binding data from either DCC or protamine assays usually reveal a single class of receptor sites with a very-high-affinity binding component (K_d 10^{-10} M).[150,151] The receptor sediments primarily at 8 S in low-salt sucrose gradients and at 4 S in high-salt gradients.[149]

Values of ER in primary tumors range from 0 to almost 1000 fmol/mg of cytosol protein.[152] The wide range of values may be due to a combination of factors. First, since tumors commonly exhibit cellular heterogeneity, the ER content might vary directly with the proportion of those cells that contain cytoplasmic ER. Early reports indicated no obvious correlation between the histology of a tumor and its ability to bind estrogen.[140] More recently, a strong association between ER and invasive lobular carcinoma has been described, while a low frequency of ER is seen in tumors with a prominent local lymphocyte reaction.[153] Second, one might suppose that contamination of a tumor specimen by normal mammary cells containing ER would give variable assay results. But this is not the case, since ER cannot be readily detected in nonlactating human breast cells.[154-156] This last point has been confirmed in animal studies in which estrogen uptake or actual ER levels are very low in virgin or pregnant mammary glands but then markedly increase during lactation.[157-160] Finally, the amount of endogenous estrogen secreted by the patient must be considered, since endogenous estrogen would occupy ER sites and make them unavailable for assay using conventional techniques. This may at least partially explain why the highest values for tumor ER are seen in postmenopausal patients. Exchange techniques for measuring ER occupied by endogenous estrogen are now available.[142,143,161-163]

Jensen's original suggestion that the presence of ER in a human breast tumor might indicate that the tumor is hormone-dependent and will regress with appropriate endocrine manipulation[133] has now been evaluated. A number of laboratories using a variety of techniques have assayed ER in breast tumor specimens and data on clinical response to endocrine therapy are now available in many of these cases. On July 18 and 19, 1974, an international workshop was held in Bethesda, Maryland, to correlate these data.[140] Details of both ER assay procedures and clinical evaluation criteria were examined, and 436 treatment trials in 380 patients were ultimately accepted. The general pattern of results was the same for all investigators, and the collective data are summarized below:

Surgical Ablation (Castration, Adrenalectomy, Hypophysectomy). Thirty-three percent of 211 treatment trials yielded objective tumor regression. Of the 94 trials in patients with negative tumor-ER values, only 8 (8%) were successful, whereas 59 (55%) of the 107 trials in patients with positive tumor-ER values succeeded. Patients with borderline tumor-ER values had a 30% response rate.

Additive Therapy (Pharmacological Doses of Estrogens, Androgens, and Glucocorticoids). Thirty-four percent of 170 trials yielded objective tumor regressions. Of the 82 trials in patients with negative tumor-ER values, 7 (8%) were successful, whereas 51 (60%) of the 85 trials in patients with positive tumor-ER values succeeded.

Miscellaneous Therapy. Twenty-seven percent of 55 trials yielded responses to a variety of endocrine therapies including antiestrogens, aminoglutethimide, etc. Of 32 trials in patients with negative tumor-ER values, 5 (16%) were successful, whereas 10 (43%) of 23 trials in patients with positive-ER values succeeded.

There remains little doubt that ER values can be helpful in predicting the results of endocrine therapy for metastatic breast cancer. It is clear that if a patient has a negative tumor-ER value, the chances of tumor regression in response to endocrine therapy are minimal. A large number of patients can thus be spared unrewarding major endocrine ablative therapy if ER assays are performed routinely. When the tumor-ER value is positive, the response to endocrine therapy is 55–60%. This single piece of evidence, when coupled with available clinical prognostic factors such as menopausal status, disease-free interval, site of dominant lesion, and, especially, response to previous hormonal therapies, should permit the practicing oncologist to select or reject endocrine therapy with considerable confidence.

Why did 45% of the patients with positive tumor-ER values not respond to endocrine therapy? Several possible reasons have been discussed. (1) The role of other hormone receptors must be considered, since ER is only one part of the complex hormonal control system which influences mammary cell growth and function. The mechanism(s) by which these other hormones affect breast tumor growth must be equally important, since receptors for prolactin, progestins, androgens, and glucocorticoids have also been identified in breast tumors[164]; these are discussed elsewhere in this chapter. Perhaps simultaneous analysis of these receptor proteins in addition to ER will be helpful in eliminating the 45% of those patients who have positive tumor-ER values but do not respond to any type of hormonal manipulation.[165] (2) Tumors might contain a heterogeneous population of hormone-dependent and autonomous cell types and therefore express a mixed response to hormone therapy. Such conditions could explain why some ER-positive tumors show only partial or short-term remission before progressing to a completely autonomous condition. (3) Tumors might contain defective cytoplasmic receptor proteins which prevent the induction of the incompletely known sequence of biochemical events ultimately leading to tumor regression upon hormone therapy. Defective receptor proteins have in fact been demonstrated in several experimental systems,[146,147] but no correlations to human tumor responses have yet been made. (4) It has been reported that specific nuclear acceptor sites for receptor are required for hormone action,[166] and it is possible that absent or defective sites would lead to insensitivity to ER. The evidence for such sites remains controversial.[167-170] (5) We have recently discovered a human breast cancer cell line in which the majority of the cellular ER is in the nucleus even in the absence of estrogen in the environment.[171] We are investigating the possibility that free nuclear ER may be stimulating cell proliferation under these circumstances. Biologically active free nuclear receptors would continue to stimulate cell growth even after ovariectomy or adrenalectomy and such tumors would be considered autonomous. An important consideration is that they might regress following antiestrogen therapy.

3.5. Antiestrogens

The discovery that certain estrogen analogues could antagonize estrogen stimulation of target tissues was promptly applied to the problem of breast cancer. Growth of DMBA tumors could be inhibited by clomiphene,[172] nafoxidine,[173,174] or tamoxifen,[175] though there exists one report of tumor growth-promoting activity of these agents.[176] Tumor induction was also prevented by nafoxidine.[177] The ability of tamoxifen to cause regression of a DMBA tumor was highly correlated with the presence of estrogen receptor in a biopsy of that tumor.[178]

The positive results of these experiments led to clinical trials of antiestrogens for therapy of breast cancer patients. Tamoxifen was used successfully,[179-181] as was nafoxidine[182-184] and clomiphene.[185] The remission rates were reported to be around 30%, the same as those achieved by other endocrine therapies. And as with other endocrine therapies, success was correlated with the presence of estrogen receptor in the patient's tumor,[140] though the correlation did not appear to be quite as good as with other endocrine therapies.

The mechanism of action of antiestrogens has been studied principally in the rat uterus. They have been found not only to bind to the estrogen receptor,[186,187] but also to translocate this receptor into the nucleus[188] and even to initiate early estrogenic responses.[189] A complete response does not develop, however, and the cells remain for a time refractory to the action of active estrogens. Because some antiestrogens retain receptor in the nucleus for many days, in contrast to several hours for active estrogens,[188] this retention was at first thought to be an essential feature of their effect. More recent work has shown that some do not share this property, though apparently all fail to replenish receptor in the cytoplasm,[190] which may explain insensitivity to later estrogen action. Nothing is yet known of the differences between receptor–estrogen and receptor–antiestrogen complexes in the nucleus which might account for the differences in their activity.

Even less is known of antiestrogen action in human breast cancer, beyond the fact that antiestrogens bind to tumor estrogen receptor[191,192] and decrease DNA synthesis in a human breast cancer cell line.[193] It has been suggested that a principal effect may be the reduction of estrogen-stimulated prolactin levels,[177,194,195] but this effect does not seem to be sufficient to account for the response in rat DMBA tumors.[175] It is also possible that antiestrogens inhibit ovarian synthesis of estradiol. These questions are under active investigation.

Because of the protective effect of early pregnancy against development of breast cancer, combined with the increased estradiol excretion seen during pregnancy[196,197] and low urinary excretion of estriol in breast cancer patients,[198] it has been proposed that estriol has significant anticarcinogenic properties by acting as an antiestrogen, competing with estradiol for the cytoplasmic receptor sites in mammary tissues.[199-202] This possibility now seems unlikely, because the relatively weak binding of estriol to the receptor compared to estradiol would require large amounts of estriol to compete successfully,[203] whereas it has recently been shown that there is actually more unconjugated estradiol than estriol present during pregnancy.[204-205] In addition, estriol itself is able to enter target cell nuclei and to induce the synthesis of an estrogen-specific protein in the rat uterus; the degree of stimulation is proportional to the amount estriol bound to the cytoplasmic receptor and to the amount of estriol found in the nucleus.[206] Finally, estriol has now been shown to be carcinogenic in mice.[207] Although it is easy to criticize parts of the estriol hypothesis on theoretical grounds, the very important observations regarding the protective effect of early pregnancy on the subsequent development of breast cancer should not be ignored. With a few exceptions,[208] new approaches to understanding the relevance of this observation are notably lacking.

3.6. Systemic Approaches to Reducing Estrogen Production

In castrated premenopausal or in postmenopausal breast cancer patients, estrogen precursors are secreted by the adrenal gland and converted to estrogens by peripheral tissues.[209-213] This has been the rationale for surgical adrenalectomy in these patients. One alternative to surgical removal of the adrenals has been to administer pharmacologic doses of glucocorticoid, thus inhibiting ACTH release and producing adrenal atrophy. This pharmacologic approach results in an overall remission rate of 25%,[214] which may be somewhat less than that achieved by surgical adrenalectomy.[2] This fact, coupled with the severe side effects of high doses of glucocorticoids, has prompted another approach to adrenal suppression. The anticonvulsive drug aminoglutethimide (AG) produces a block in steroidogenesis at an early step in the biosynthetic pathway.[215,216] However, reduction in cortisol production by AG causes a large compensatory increase in ACTH production, leading to adrenal hypertrophy which tends to override the drug-induced blockage of adrenal steroidogenesis. The logical attempt to inhibit this AG-induced rise in ACTH by adding physiological amounts of dexamethasone (Dex) to the regimen met with only limited success[217,218] until it was discovered that AG accelerates Dex metabolism. Using higher doses of Dex with AG,[219] complete adrenal suppression has been achieved for as long as 19 months, and objective tumor regression occurred in 8 of 22 patients without producing Cushing-like side effects.

Combined AG/Dex treatment thus appears to achieve an effective nonsurgical adrenalectomy for postmenopausal breast cancer patients. The treatment also seems likely, at least in theory, to provide an alternative to ovariectomy for premenopausal patients when administered along with antiestrogens or with a gonadotropin inhibitor.

4. Progesterone

4.1. Clinical Effects in Breast Cancer

Because of the cyclic changes of blood estrogen and progesterone levels which occur in females, and these hormones' interrelationships in regulating target tissue development and growth, it was inevitable that progesterone would be studied for its effect on breast cancer. Although progesterone itself is not a carcinogen, it may be a potent target-specific cocarcinogen for induction of mammary tumors by viral or chemical agents.[220] The hormone has also been implicated in both tumor enhancement and tumor suppression.

That progesterone plays a role in stimulating tumor growth is suggested by the pioneering studies of Huggins et al.[34,221,222] They showed that pregnancy promoted the growth of DMBA-induced rat mammary tumors. Administration of progesterone to intact rats accelerated the appearance of tumors, increased the number of tumors, and augmented the growth rate of established tumors.

Parturition and weaning are followed by regression of a large number of pregnancy-stimulated tumors.[33,35] The principal tumor growth-promoting factors of pregnancy and lactation are probably placental lactogen[36] and prolactin,[37,38] as noted previously. Ovariectomy, however, blocks the stimulatory effects of endogenous or exogenous prolactin on tumor growth, and injection of progesterone removes this block.[37] Either prolactin stimulation of tumors under these circumstances is dependent upon progesterone, or, alternatively, the high levels of circulating progesterone stimulated by prolactin in the lactating rat[39] are responsible for the tumor growth. This does not mean that progesterone alone is responsible for maintaining rat mammary tumor growth, since in these experiments the animals had both high prolactin levels and intact adrenal glands. On the other hand, these studies do suggest that progesterone plays an important physiological role in stimulating tumor growth.

In contrast to the stimulatory effects of progesterone described above, progesterone can induce rat mammary tumor regression or prevent tumor appearance, at least when combined with moderate to large doses of estrogen.[34,223] In humans, too, the percentage of breast tumor regressions in response to a progesterone–estrogen combination is generally higher than with progesterone alone.[224] Postmenopausal patients with endogenous estrogen levels (presumably of adrenal origin) sufficient to cornify the vaginal mucosa have a 29% tumor-remission rate with progesterone therapy, whereas patients with an atrophic vaginal smear experience only 6% remission rate with progesterone alone.[225] These data would support a requirement for estrogen in progesterone-mediated tumor regression, and may be due to estrogen stimulation of progesterone receptor (PgR) synthesis (see below). In fact, since moderate to large doses of estrogens alone can cause mammary tumor regression in rats[117–119] and humans,[226] it is necessary to ask whether addition of the progestational agent accomplishes more than the estrogen alone. The answer would seem to be yes, at least in some cases, because patients whose tumors have failed to regress following treatment with high-dose estrogen alone have responded to a combination of estrogen–progesterone.[227–229]

The mechanism by which progesterone promotes tumor regression is not clear. Large doses of synthetic progestins can cause significant lowering of serum LH and cortisol levels, suggesting that alteration of pituitary function may be involved,[230] but at least four previously hypophysectomized patients are reported to have had breast tumor regression following combinations of estrogen–progesterone.[231,232] This is in contrast to the lack of tumor response to estrogens alone in hypophysectomized patients.[44,45,233]

In summary, the specific mechanisms involved in progesterone-mediated breast tumor growth and regression are poorly understood. However, the hormone's metabolism, its binding to specific receptor proteins, and its effect on the actions of other steroid hormones have been extensively studied in several target tissues.

4.2. Subcellular Metabolism of Progesterone

Progesterone is a precursor common to estrogens, androgens, and adrenal hormones. The uptake and metabolic fates of progesterone have been extensively investigated in the uterus,[234–240] mammary gland,[241,242] and other target tissues.[243–246] The results and interpretations of these studies have often been quite contradictory, for the following reasons. They have been performed in a variety of different tissues from different species under *in vivo, in vitro,* or cell-free conditions. In some cases, the progesterone concentration has been high, and in others, low. Certain studies deal with normal animals, others with pseudopregnant or pregnant animals. Metabolic patterns differ in estrogen-treated versus castrated animals. It is perhaps understandable, then, that a simple representative metabolic scheme cannot be presented. Despite these limitations, certain observations are pertinent to the present discussion.

Although studies of progesterone metabolism and excretion in breast cancer patients reveal no major differences from control patients, the intracellular metabolism of progesterone by the tumor itself may be quite important. It has been shown that certain human breast tumors can synthesize progesterone from pregnenolone, which means that the tumor itself can control intracellular hormone concentration.[247]

In contrast to estrogens, where intracellular metabolism does not seem to play an important regulatory role, progesterone can be extensively metabolized in a manner analogous to androgens, where testosterone is converted intracellularly to an active metabolite, dihydrotestosterone, and an inactive product, androstanediol.[248,249] Lawson and Pearlman[241] administered [^{3}H]progesterone as a continuous infusion and found that the mammary gland of the pregnant rat was able to concentrate tritium above plasma levels. In addition to progesterone, small amounts of 20α-hydroxypregn-4-ene-3-one (20α-OHPg) were found. The pattern of metabolites varied with the endocrine status of the gland: 20α-OHPg dominated the pregnant gland, whereas ring-A reduction to dihydroprogesterone (5α-DHPg) was higher in the lactating gland.[242,250] Since estrogen priming is required for full functional expression of progesterone activity, its effect on formation of metabolites may provide a clue to their physiological role. Saffran et al. [251] have shown that at physiological progesterone concentrations, the effect of estrogen is to inhibit reductase activity. At high progesterone concentrations, the effect is reversed. Progesterone concentration does not affect 20α-OH steroid dehydrogenase activity, which is increased by estrogen at low or high progesterone levels.

Thus, the role of estrogen on progesterone metabolism appears to be twofold. First, it increases PgR (see Section 4.3) and thereby reduces progesterone metabolism because the hormone is protected by receptor binding. Second, it increases the concentration of reducing enzymes, particularly 20α-OH steroid dehydrogenase, thereby increasing metabolism. The net effect of estrogen treatment is balanced between increased binding and increased degradation, and the concentration of progesterone determines which effect predominates.

One serious problem in the earlier studies was that the presence and importance of an intracellular receptor for progesterone had not been appreciated. Although it is perhaps incorrect to assume that all progesterone effects must operate through a receptor mechanism, a good place to begin would be to see which metabolites in a given tissue can bind to the progesterone receptor or perhaps to some other receptor, and whether this binding correlates with biological activity. This could give insight as to whether a certain metabolic pathway is critical to the action of the hormone or whether the pathway is primarily a means of degradation and excretion. In mammalian tissues, [^{3}H]5α-DHPg does not bind to a receptor, the unlabeled hormone does not compete for progesterone binding to PgR, and neither 5α-DHPg nor 3α-hydroxy-5α-pregnan-20-one possess progestational activity. [252,253] Therefore, it appears that these metabolites serve little biological function in mammals.

Strott [254] has studied the chick oviduct to show which metabolites can bind to PgR in this tissue and whether this binding correlates with biological activity. In unstimulated oviducts, essentially no bound progesterone can be found. In marked contrast to this, after estrogen stimulation, 70% of protein-bound hormone is unmetabolized progesterone. Therefore, in estrogen-primed chicks, as in mammals, progesterone is the major bound hormone, though some 5α-DHPg is also bound. The biological activity of 5α-DHPg in the chick, unlike that in the mammal, may reside in its ability to compete for progesterone binding to PgR. [255]

In the absence of evidence for a functional role of progesterone metabolites in mammals, their significance remains to be determined, and their formation may simply serve to terminate the action of progesterone. One must conclude that the capacity to elicit a progestational effect resides in the progesterone molecule itself, and that it acts without metabolic transformation, as supported by the demonstration of specific progesterone-binding proteins in a variety of target tissues and cells.

4.3. Progesterone Receptors

We now turn to studies of progesterone receptor (PgR) and its dependence on estrogen priming. Extensive investigations using guinea pig uterus unequivocally demonstrated PgR in a mammal.[256-262] The receptor migrates at 6-8 S in sucrose gradients and does not bind glucocorticoids. Uterine levels of PgR are maximum at proestrus and fall progressively during estrus and proestrus to a 16-fold lower level in diestrus. Injection of estrogen causes an 8-fold rise in PgR within 24 hours, which can be prevented by inhibition of protein or RNA synthesis. The normal half-life of PgR is approximately three to five days, but an injection of progesterone will deplete the uterine cytoplasm of PgR within three hours. Evidence for nuclear translocation of PgR is available from direct biochemical and autoradiographic studies. Similar conclusions have been reached about PgR in the hamster,[252,263] rabbit,[264-266] mouse,[267,268] rat,[264,267-270] and human.[271-273] In the latter two species, PgR has been difficult to demonstrate reproducibly because the majority of radioactive progesterone binds in the 4 S region of the sucrose gradient, making it difficult to distinguish PgR from the corticosteroid-binding globulin. With incorporation of glycerol into buffers or gradients, the receptor complex is stabilized,[273] and a specific, high-affinity (K_d 3-8 × 10^{-9} M) 7 S binding component is seen occasionally in myometria from women treated with estrogen,[271] in endometrium obtained from proliferative (estrogen-dominated) tissues,[273,274] in hyperplastic endometrium,[275] and in endometrial carcinoma.[274]

The receptor is precipitated by ammonium sulfate,[276] and this property has been used in its purification.[277] The pure receptor (which migrates as a single band of mol. wt. 110,000 on SDS polyacrylamide gels) sediments at 3.7 S on sucrose gradients (after elution with hypertonic salt), has a $K_d \sim 10^{-9}$ M, and does not bind hydrocortisone. The purified receptor–hormone complex will bind to nuclei; the nuclear-bound form also sediments at 3.7 S.

The most exhaustive studies of PgR have been done using the estrogen-primed chick oviduct. In this tissue, administration of a single dose of progesterone *in vivo* stimulates chromatin template capacity, DNA-dependent RNA polymerase activity, and synthesis of a specific messenger RNA, culminating with induction of the specific protein avidin.[245] Unlabeled progesterone, its active metabolites, and testosterone (a good inducer of avidin) block [³H]progesterone binding to the receptor. [278] Progesterone receptor concentration is increased 20-fold by estradiol. [279] The receptor has been purified to homogeneity and found to consist of two similar subunits which have distinctly different affinities for DNA and chromatin. [280]

Although the normal breast is also a target of progesterone action, virtually no information about receptor binding of the hormone exists. After injection, an apparent selective accumulation of progesterone by human breast tissue has been described [281]; this property was reported to be lost in neoplastic tissue. [124] Terenius [282] used charcoal-resistant radioactivity of cytosols containing [³H]progesterone and excess hydrocortisone to indicate the presence of a progesterone binder in human and rat mammary carcinomas. Attempts to demonstrate directly receptors in normal mammary tissue using progesterone have been unsuccessful, despite the fact that glucocorticoid receptors (which are often difficult to distinguish from PgR) are present. [283,284] Recent demonstration of PgR in human breast cancer will be discussed in Section 4.5.

This survey of PgR in various tissues fails to explain progesterone-induced regression and stimulation of experimental and human breast cancers, but it may provide important clues about the estrogen requirement for progesterone effects. Most important is the stimulation of PgR following estrogen priming. Estrogen modulation of PgR levels is probably a direct effect on the target cell and not mediated by the pituitary, since in ovariectomized, adrenalectomized, and hypophysectomized rats, uterine PgR levels are restored by estradiol, but not by prolactin, injections. [285] In addition to controlling PgR levels, the estrogen requirement for progesterone action may be due to estrogen's role in regulating progesterone metabolism.

4.4. Progesterone Interrelationship with Other Steroid Hormones

Progesterone may control breast tumor growth or regression in several ways. The simplest mechanism involves a direct effect of the hormones on the tumor. However progesterone can also modify the actions of the other steroid hormones which influence the mammary gland, and this may form the basis for interhormonal control mechanisms.

4.4.1. Estrogens

The ability of progesterone to antagonize and/or modify the action of estrogen is well documented. [286,287] Tamoxifen and nafoxidine, two widely used antiestrogens, exhibit progesterone-like effects. [288–290] Hsueh et al. [290] have shown that after depletion of cytoplasmic ER by high-dose estrogen treatment, progesterone blocks the overshoot of ER seen during replenishment. They propose that this reduction of ER is correlated with reduced sensitivity of the uterus to estrogen. There is no evidence, however, that progesterone affects replenishment of ER after physiological estrogen treatments or alters basal ER levels. In summary, estrogen and progesterone may exert feedback control on each other in the target tissue. Estradiol pretreatment enhances tissue sensitivity to progesterone through increased PgR levels. Progesterone, in turn, may modify cytoplasmic ER and redirect the cell's ability to respond to estradiol.

4.4.2. Androgens

The androgenic properties of progestins are well known, and fetal virilization can result from their use in man.[291] Progestins can masculinize the reproductive tract of rat fetuses,[292] and can mimic androgen effects in several organs.[293-296] Recently, Bullock et al.[295] and Mowszowicz et al.[293] have demonstrated that progestins can be either synandrogenic (by potentiating androgen effects) or antiandrogenic (by inhibiting these effects), depending on the steroid structure, dose, and tissue. If androgens have similar modifying effects on progesterone actions, it may be one reason why they are effective in treatment of hormone-dependent breast cancer. Although the mechanism of androgen-induced regression of breast tumors is not known, androgens cause regression of fetal mammary buds[297] and may have similar effects on dedifferentiated malignant cells. It is possible that progestin-induced tumor regression is a reflection of the progestins' androgenic properties.

4.4.3. Glucocorticoids

By far the most familiar model for the interaction of two differing steroids is that proposed by Rousseau et al.[298] to explain the inhibitory effects of progestins and the stimulatory effects of glucocorticoids on tyrosine aminotransferase production in rat hepatoma tissue culture (HTC) cells. Competition by progestins for glucocorticoid binding has also been demonstrated in mammary carcinomas[299,300] and lactating mammary glands.[283,284] Since glucocorticoids are involved in mammary gland maturation, it is possible that progestins may affect mammary tumors by modifying glucocorticoid action.

We have recently shown that MCF-7, a stable cell line derived from a human mammary carcinoma, contains receptors for progestins, androgens, glucocorticoids, and estrogens. These cells may prove useful for studying interrelationships between the binding and biological actions of these four steroids and their role in tumor endocrine response.[164]

4.5. Progesterone Receptors in Human Breast Cancer

As discussed previously, around 40% of human breast cancers fail to respond to endocrine therapy in spite of the presence of ER. However, since binding to receptors is only an early step in hormone action, it is possible that in ER+ tumors where endocrine manipulations fail, the lesion is at a later step. An ideal marker of an endocrine-responsive tumor would, therefore, be a measurable product of hormone action rather than the initial binding step.

Because in estrogen target tissues the synthesis of PgR depends on the action of estrogen,[260] we investigated the possibility that PgR might be such a marker. If so, it would be expected that PgR would be rare in tumors that lack ER. The presence of PgR in tumors containing ER would indicate that the tumor is capable of synthesizing at least one end product under estrogen regulation, and that the tumor remains endocrine-responsive. Conversely, the prospect of a successful response to therapy would be low in tumors with ER but no PgR.

We have used 8 S binding of the synthetic progestin [³H]R5020[267] to identify PgR in human breast cancer tissue.[164,301] We have now determined PgR and ER in more than 500 human mammary tumors. In primary tumors, 20% are ER⁻, PgR⁻; 3% ER⁻, PgR⁺; 18% ER⁺, PgR⁻; 59% ER⁺, PgR⁺. In metastatic tumors, 33% are ER⁻, PgR⁻; 1% ER⁻, PgR⁺0 27% ER⁺, PgR⁻; 39% ER⁺, PgR⁺. PgR is more frequently found in tumors with high ER content. The usefulness of PgR measurements requires direct correlation of the presence of PgR with objectively defined clinical remission. Our preliminary data are encouraging. We find that in cases where ER is positive and PgR negative, success response rate is much lower than if both receptors are present. However, these are preliminary data on only 65 treatment trials, and a much larger case series will be required to determine if PgR measurements are of value.

Many questions remain unsolved. How does one interpret contradictory responses to one or more therapeutic trials? What is the effect of previous therapy on receptor levels in multiple biopsies or metastases? How does menopausal status or menstrual cycle affect PgR levels in biopsies? Is measurement of only cytoplasmic receptors an adequate representation of the total receptor content of the cell? And, in considering cytoplasmic receptors, what constitutes a positive assay for PgR? How are we to interpret the tumors that have no 8 S binding but considerable suppressible 4 S? Finally, we have shown that human breast tumor cells can contain receptors for at least four steroid hormones. How are we to incorporate androgen and glucocorticoid receptor data in estimating the response potential of a tumor?

5. Glucocorticoids

Glucocorticoids affect a wide variety of normal tissues. In the rat mammary gland, they are required along with prolactin to support lactation,[76] and their availability limits the rate of milk production.[302,303] Experiments with mammary gland explants have indicated that proliferation and maintenance of rough endoplasmic reticulum is a primary direct effect of the glucocorticoids in lactation.[304] Spermidine may mediate these effects, since Takumi and Perry[305] recently showed that spermidine is increased by glucocorticoids and can replace them in inducing casein and α-lactalbumin synthesis in explants; the glucocorticoid effect is abolished by specific inhibition of spermidine synthesis.

A specific receptor protein for glucocorticoids has been described in a number of target tissues. Like other steroid receptors, it appears to be localized in the cytoplasm and to be translocated to the cell nucleus after interaction with glucocorticoids.[306] There is little definite information on its mechanism of action. Though specific acceptor sites for binding the receptor in the nucleus have been proposed to be on the DNA of hepatoma cells,[307] receptor binding to DNA was not found to be saturable,[308] so that other components must also be involved if such acceptor sites are actually present. A glucocorticoid binder found among the nonhistone proteins of liver nuclei has properties similar to those of the cytoplasmic receptor, suggesting that it may not be a separate component.[309] The action of glucocorticoid receptor as studied in hepatoma cells has been reviewed recently.[310]

In liver and hepatoma tissue, the action of the hormone–receptor complex is largely inductive, while in lymphocytes and lymphoma cells, its action is inhibitory and ultimately leads to cell death.[311] Most glucocorticoid-resistant cells derived from established lymphoma lines and isolated resistant human leukemic lymphoblasts are found to have lost their cytoplasmic receptors.[312–314] It is interesting, however, that about 10% of resistant cell lines contain an altered receptor which cannot enter the nuclei, while another 10% have another type of nonfunctional receptor.[315–317] Clearly, more than one lesion can exist in the pathway from hormone binding to response.

Glucocorticoids have been used extensively in the treatment of human cancer, especially in malignancies of lymphatic origin. They have also been found to inhibit mammary tumor growth in a number of animal models including the R3230AC,[318,319] though, paradoxically, they may also be required to permit tumor induction by chemical carcinogens[320] and appear to induce mouse mammary tumor virus as well.[321,322] The effectiveness of glucocorticoids in treatment of human breast cancer was discussed earlier. It should be noted that in a recent investigation by Pihl et al.,[323] regressions due to prednisone treatment occurred only when tumors contained ER. This would suggest that glucocorticoid therapy has features in common with ablative and other hormone therapies.

The actual mechanism of glucocorticoid-induced remission is not known. Some have assumed that the high doses normally used inhibit ACTH production and therefore stop adrenal synthesis of estrogen precursors.[323] It has also been suggested that there may be a differential effect on cellular versus humoral immune mechanisms, such that less blocking antibody is produced to interfere with cell-mediated destruction of tumor.[324] Glucocorticoids may also act directly on mammary tumor cells, since specific glucocorticoid receptors have recently been found in several animal mammary tumors[299,300] as well as in normal lactating mammary tissue.[283,284,325,326] Both DMBA and R3230AC rat tumors have receptor levels similar to those of the lactating rat, and much more receptor than virgin or pregnant gland.[284] These rat receptors all share the same sedimentation properties, relative steroid affinities, and ability to translocate to cell nuclei.[327] Virus-induced mouse mammary tumors have less receptor than does lactating mouse mammary gland, but again, the receptors are qualitatively similar.[328] In human breast cancer, the occurrence and distribution of glucocorticoid receptors is not yet known, nor has any correlation yet been shown between the presence of receptors and glucocorticoid-induced remission. An exciting new development, however, is the discovery of glucocorticoid receptor in the MCF-7 cell line, which was derived from a hormone-dependent human breast tumor. Since MCF-7 cells also possess substantial levels of the receptors for estrogens, progestins, and androgens, they may prove valuable in establishing both the significance of glucocorticoid receptor and its relationship to other hormone effects in mammary cancer cells of human origin.[164]

6. Androgens

Androgens affect their target cells through a receptor mechanism similar in many ways to that described earlier for the other steroids.[306] Although testosterone (T) is the primary circulating androgen, there is now abundant evidence that in a number of target tissues including the prostate, T must be converted by the enzyme 5α-reductase (Δ^4-3-ketosteroid-5α-reductase) to dihydrotestosterone (DHT) in order to bind the androgen receptor and enter the nuclei. DHT is in turn metabolized by 3-ketosteroid oxidoreductase) to androstanediols, which do not bind to DHT receptor. It has been suggested on the basis of different *in vitro* actions of DHT and androstanediols that the two, operating through distinct mechanisms, may both be physiologically important.[329] No separate receptor for androstanediols has been identified, however. On the other hand, some tissues may possess a different receptor specific for T itself; the mouse kidney has very little 5α-reductase activity, so that [^{3}H]T is translocated largely unchanged to the nuclei, where it presumably is the active androgen.[330] DHT is rapidly converted to androstanediols in mouse kidney cytosol, even at 4°C, so that affinity of the receptor for DHT has been difficult to evaluate.[330] The 3-ketoreductase reaction is reversible *in vivo*, so that the biological activity of androstanediols in mouse kidney may be due to their conversion back to DHT.[331]

The importance of T metabolism for at least some androgenic activities is emphasized by two congenital defects. The testicular feminization syndrome described in mice, rats, and humans appears to be due to a deficiency of DHT receptors[332-334] conversion of T to DHT by 5α-reductase appears normal in these cases.[335] Another form of inherited male pseudohermaphroditism in man has been described in which 5α-reductase is deficient while T production is normal.[336] However, considerable male development of these patients at about age 12, together with the observations that 5α-reductase is very low in adult animal tissues[337] and that DHT receptor levels fall with age,[338] suggest that conversion of T to DHT may be less significant after development is completed.

The level of DHT receptors in the rat prostate falls rapidly after castration.[339] They are restored after several days, however, even in adrenalectomized or hypophysectomized animals, so some factor other than a steroid or pituitary hormone may be involved in the control of receptor levels.[340] Another study did not find receptor restoration seven days after castration[341]; however, prostate nuclei were able to take up DHT, although cytoplasmic receptor was not demonstrable. A component appearing in prostate cytosol after castration was found to interfere with DHT binding to receptor, suggesting that the observations of receptor loss after castration may, at least in part, be apparent rather than real.

Analogues that function as antiandrogens have been described. Two classes can be distinguished: one in which compounds possess progestational activity, represented by cyproterone acetate and medroxyprogesterone acetate, and a second in which there is no progestational activity, represented by flutamide, BOMT, and unesterified cyproterone. Members of both classes directly inhibit DHT binding to its receptor.[342,343] Progestational antiandrogens bind to PgR as well,[344] which may provide a mechanism for their apparent synergism with androgens in some tissues at doses lower than those required for androgen atagonism.[293]

6.1. Androgens in Mammary Carcinoma

Androgens cause regression of a large percentage of carcinogen-induced rat mammary tumors,[345,346] though this effect is reversed at extremely high androgen doses.[347] A number of androgens and androgen derivatives have proved effective in treatment of human breast cancer.[348-350] Like other endocrine therapies, androgen administration appears to be particularly useful against tumors possessing receptors for estrogen.[351] The actual mechanism of androgen-induced regression is not known, but from existing data at least five different hypotheses can be proposed:

1. Androgens could act directly on tumors through an androgen receptor. There is no evidence that androgen receptors are required for normal female functions, and in fact, Tfm/0 mice deficient in these receptors reproduce normally except for somewhat premature aging of the ovaries.[352,353] Nevertheless, androgens cause regression of mammary buds or mammary bud explants of fetuses of either sex.[297] The action is prevented by cyproterone acetate,[354,355] consistent with mediation by DHT receptor. Both DHT receptors[164,356-359] and androgen-metabolizing enzymes, including 5α-reductase,[360-363] have been described in human breast tumors, so that it is possible that tumor regression might also involve the DHT receptor system. An *androgen-dependent* transplantable mouse mammary tumor, the Shionogi 115, has been shown to possess androgen receptor[364] and to metabolize T to DHT,[365] although T is the principal intranuclear steroid following injections of [^{3}H]T. Since two of the seven autonomous sublines of the same tumor also possessed androgen receptor and since T is translocated to the nucleus,[366] it would seem that the presence of androgen receptor may be necessary, but not sufficient, for androgen-dependent growth behavior. In tissue culture lines derived from the Shionogi tumor, DHT was more effective in growth-promoting activity than T, but unmetabolized T was still translocated.[367-369]

2. Quadri et al.[370] have found that high doses of prolactin can override testosterone suppression of DMBA-induced mammary tumor growth. Since T treatment has been reported not to reduce circulating levels of prolactin,[371] it was hypothesized that androgen might somehow reduce tumor responsiveness to prolactin, perhaps by an effect on

prolactin receptors. Evidence from our laboratory reveals that pharmacologic androgen administration does reduce prolactin receptor content of DMBA mammary tumor.[92] It is not clear whether this is a cause or a result of the androgen-induced tumor regression.

3. Androgens could induce mammary tumor regression by conversion to estrogens. Pharmacologic doses of estrogens do reverse tumor growth, and conversion of only 2% of the standard 1-mg testosterone propionate injection to rats would produce sufficient estradiol to induce such a regression.[119] In particular, it has been shown that both breast adipose tissue and breast tumors can aromatize various steroid precursors to active estrogens.[372,373] Further, both androgen- and estrogen-induced regressions share the property of being reversed by large doses of prolactin,[119,370] suggesting a parallelism in their mechanisms.

4. Alternatively, androgens may block estrogen production. Though androgen suppression of gonadotropin production and consequent cessation of ovarian function is probable, this mechanism seems unlikely to be effective in postmenopausal women. More likely would be androgen inhibition of peripheral conversion of adrenal precursors to active estrogens. Such a mechanism would be consistent with the activity of several androgens that probably cannot be converted to estrogens, and of at least one, Δ^1-testololactone, that has no known hormonal activity at all.[350] This mechanism might also allow one to explain the observation that very high doses of testosterone propionate are less effective than lower doses in causing regression of DMBA tumors[347], perhaps the intermediate doses serve to block conversion of adrenal precursors, while the very high doses permit conversion of very small amounts of the injected T itself, yielding just enough estrogen to stimulate tumor growth.

5. Of particular interest is the possible direct influence of androgens on ER. Because tumors lacking ER fail to respond to androgen treatment,[351] it has been suggested that androgens may affect ER directly. At extremely high concentrations in vitro, T and DHT have been reported to competitively inhibit estrogen binding to ER.[374-376] In addition, androstenediol, a weak androgen commonly found in human female plasma, competitively inhibits estrogen binding to ER at somewhat lower concentrations.[358] In rat uteri in vitro, extremely high concentrations of androgens (10^{-6} M) transfer ER to the nucleus and induce proteins that are normally induced only by estradiol. Androgen stimulation of induced protein can be blocked with antiestrogens but not with antiandrogens.[375] strongly supporting the thesis that androgens are affecting ER and not androgen receptor. Although androgens appear to be acting directly in in vitro systems, some controversy remains as to whether these androgen-mediated events occur in vivo.[376,377]

The possibility that androgen treatment might decrease ER in mammary tumors was suggested by Deshpande et al., [378] who reported that pretreatment with dromostanolone proprionate decreased the amount of injected [³H]estradiol present in human breast tumors compared with controls. A similar observation was made in rat mammary tumors. [379] We have now confirmed these earlier observations by showing a decrease in cytoplasmic ER in tumors during regression after androgen therapy.[380] From the above findings, it would be reasonable to speculate that androgens either deplete ER or render it inactive, so that andogenous estrogens could no longer stimulate tumor growth.

Clearly, androgen action on normal target tissues and androgen action on tumors may not share the same mechanism. If not, discovery of the actual mechanisms could lead to the design of more effective, nonviralizing androgen analogues for use in therapy, as well as to enhancing our understanding of endocrine control over mammary tumor growth.

7. Conclusions

Breast cancer is often hormone-responsive, since growth or regression of tumors can often be modulated by appropriate endocrine manipulations. Prolactin, estrogen, and progesterone appear to be the major hormones involved in regulation of breast tumor growth. Considerable insight into the mechanism of action of these hormones on stimulation of tumor growth has been provided by demonstration of specific receptors for each. The inference that each hormone acts independently through its receptor to control tumor growth is belied by current studies which show that certain hormones are capable of regulating the receptor sites, metabolism, or nuclear translocation of others. This may begin to explain the complex hormonal interactions and requirements of normal and neoplastic breast tissues. Considerable progress has thus been made in understanding the basis for success of various ablative therapies.

The pharmacologic actions of estrogens, androgens, and progestins in causing breast tumor regression is much less well understood. The role of hormone receptor sites has not been established in the mechanism of tumor regression caused by these pharmacological therapies. Nevertheless, when estrogen receptors are absent in a tumor, we can predict with accuracy that endocrine therapies will fail, whereas when they are present, the likelihood of a successful response to pharmacological or ablative therapy is high.

Receptor sites seem to be a common denominator and useful marker for hormone dependence or hormone responsiveness, irrespective of their actual role in the tumor regression process. Further investigations into the receptor functions should lead to new approaches in the endocrine management of patients with breast cancer.

8. References

1. G.T. Beatson, On the treatment of inoperable cases of carcinoma of the mamma: Suggestions for a new method of treatment with illustrative cases, *Lancet* 2, 104–107 (1896).
2. T.L. Dao, Ablation therapy for hormone-dependent tumors, *Annu. Rev. Med.* 23, 1–18 (1972).
3. B. Stoll, *Hormonal Management in Breast Cancer*, J.B. Lippincott, Philadelphia (1969).
4. J.F. Holland and E. Frei (eds.), *Cancer Medicine*, Lea and Febiger, Philadelphia (1973).
5. W.L. McGuire, G.C. Chamness, and M.E. Costlow, Progress in endocrinology and metabolism: "Hormone dependence in breast cancer," *Metabolism* 23, 75–100 (1974).
6. J. Meites, Relation of prolactin and estrogen to mammary tumorigenesis in the rat, *J. Natl. Cancer Inst.* 48, 1217–1224 (1972).
7. O.H. Pearson, R.M.L. Murray, G. Mozaffarian, and J. Pensky, in: *Prolactin and Carcinogenesis* (A.R. Boyns and K. Griffiths, eds.), pp. 154–157, Alpha Omega Alpha, Cardiff, Wales (1972).
8. F. Smithline, L. Sherman, and H.D. Kolodny, Prolactin and breast carcinoma, *N. Engl. J. Med.* 292, 783–792 (1975).
9. O.H. Pearson, O. Llerena, L. Llerena, A. Molina, and T.P. Butler, Prolactin dependent rat mammary cancer: A model for man? *Trans. Assoc. Am. Physicians* 82, 225–238 (1969).
10. H. Nagasawa and R. Yanai, Effects of prolactin or growth hormones on growth of carcinogen-induced mammary tumors of adreno-ovariectomized rats, *Int. J. Cancer* 6, 488–495 (1970).
11. A.E. Bogden, D.J. Taylor, E.Y.H Kuo, M.M. Mason, and A. Speropoulos, The effect of pherphenazine-induced serum prolactin response on estrogen-primed mammary tumor–host systems, 13762 and R-35 mammary adenocarcinomas, *Cancer Res.* 34, 3018–3025 (1974).
12. J. Meites, C.S. Nicholl, and P.K. Talwalker, in: *Advances in Neuroendocrinology* (A.V. Nalbandov, ed.), pp. 238–288, University of Illinois Press, Urbana (1963).
13. J.A. Clemens, C.W. Welsch, and J. Meites, Effects of hypothalamic lesions on incidence and growth of mammary tumors in carcinogen-treated rats, *Proc. Soc. Exp. Biol. Med.* 127, 969–972 (1968).
14. M.S. Klaiber, M. Gruenstein, D.R. Meranze, and M.B. Shimkin, Influence of hypothalamic lesions on the induction and growth of mammary cancers in Sprague-Dawley rats receiving 7,12-Dimethylbenz(a)anthracene, *Cancer Res.* 29, 999–1001 (1969).
15. H. Nagasawa and J. Meites, Effects of a hypothalamic estrogen implant on growth of carcinogen-induced mammary tumors in rats, *Cancer Res.* 30, 1327–1329 (1970).
16. J. Meites, K.H. Lu, W. Wuttke, H. Nagasawa, and S.K. Quadri, Recent studies on functions and control of prolactin secretion in rats, *Recent Prog. Horm. Res.* 28, 471–526 (1972).
17. T.P. Butler and O.H. Pearson, Regression of prolactin-dependent rat mammary carcinoma in response to antihormone treatment, *Cancer Res.* 31, 817–820 (1971).
18. W. Pierpaoli and E. Sorkin, Inhibition of growth of methycholanthrene-induced mammary carcinoma in rats by anti-adenohypophis serum, *Nature* 238, 58–59 (1972).

19. K.H. Lu, Y. Koch, and J. Meites, Direct inhibition by ergocornine of pituitary prolactin release, *Endocrinology* **89**, 229–233 (1971).

20. W. Wuttke, E.E. Cassell, and J. Meites, Effects of ergocornine on serum prolactin and LH, and on hypothalamic content of PIF and LRF, *Endocrinology* **88**, 737–741 (1971).

21. J.C. Heuson, C. Waelbroeck-Van Gaver, and N. Legros, Growth inhibition of rat mammary carcinoma and endocrine changes produced by 2-Br-α-ergocryptine, a suppressor of lactation and nidation, *Eur. J. Cancer* **6**, 353–356 (1970).

22. E.E. Cassell, J. Meites, and C.W. Welsch, Effects of ergocornine and ergocryptine on growth of 7,12-Dimethylbenzanthracene-induced mammary tumors in rats, *Cancer Res.* **31**, 1051–1053 (1971).

23. H. Stahelin, B. Burckhardt-Visher, and E. Fluckiger, Rat mammary cancer inhibition by a prolactin suppressor, 2-Bromo-α-Ergocryptine, *Experientia* **27**, 915–916 (1971).

24. S.K. Quadri and J. Meites, Regression of spontaneous mammary tumors in rats by ergot drugs, *Proc. Soc. Exp. Biol. Med.* **138**, 999–1001 (1971).

25. J.A. Clemens and C.J. Shaar, Inhibition by ergocornine of initiation and growth of 7,12-Dimethylbenzanthracene-induced mammary tumors in rats: Effect of tumor size, *Proc. Soc. Exp. Biol. Med.* **139**, 659–662 (1972).

26. C.W. Welsch, G. Iturri, and J. Meites, Comparative effects of hypophysectomy, ergocornine and ergocornine–reserpine treatments on rat mammary carcinoma, *Int. J. Cancer* **12**, 206–212 (1973).

27. S.K. Quadri, J.L. Clark, and J. Meites, Effects of LSD, pargyline and haloperidol on mammary tumor growth in rats, *Proc. Soc. Exp. Biol. Med.* **142**, 22–26 (1973).

28. S.K. Quadri, G.S. Kledzik, and J. Meites, Effects of L-Dopa and methyldopa on growth of mammary cancers in rats, *Proc. Soc. Exp. Biol. Med.* **142**, 759–761 (1973).

29. H.G. Floss, J.M. Cassady, and J.E. Robbers, Influence of ergot alkaloids on pituitary prolactin and prolactin-dependent processes, *J. Pharm. Sci.* **62**, 699–715 (1973).

30. S. Young, Induction of mammary carcinoma in hypophysectomized rats treated with 3-methylcholanthrene, oestradiol-17β, progesterone and growth hormone, *Nature* **190**, 356–357 (1961).

31. C.H. Li and W. Yang, The effect of bovine growth hormone on growth of mammary tumors in hypophysectomized rats, *Life Sci.* **15**, 761–764 (1975).

32. D. Sinha, D. Cooper, and T.L. Dao, The nature of estrogen and prolactin effect on mammary tumorigenesis, *Cancer Res.* **33**, 411–414 (1973).

33. T.L. Dao and H. Sunderland, Mammary carcinogenesis by 3-methylcholanthrene. 1. Hormonal aspects in tumor induction and growth, *J. Natl. Cancer Inst.* **23**, 567–586 (1959).

34. C. Huggins, R.C. Moon, and S. Morii, Extinction of experimental mammary cancer. I. Estradiol-17β and progesterone, *Proc. Natl. Acad. Sci. U.S.A.* **48**, 379–386 (1962).

35. G.M. McCormick and R.C. Moon, Effect of pregnancy and lactation on growth of mammary tumours induced by 7,12-Dimethylbenz(A)anthracene (DMBA), *Br. J. Cancer* **19**, 160–166 (1965).

36. H. Nagasawa and R. Yanai, Effect of human placental lactogen on growth of carcinogen-induced mammary tumors in rats, *Int. J. Cancer* **11**, 131–137 (1973).

37. G.M. McCormick and R.C. Moon, Hormones influencing postpartum growth of 7,12-Dimethylbenz(a)anthracene-induced rat mammary tumors, *Cancer Res.* **27**, 626–631 (1967).

38. G.M. McCormick, The effect of varying the length of the nursing period on the postpartum growth of chemically induced rat mammary tumors, *Cancer Res.* **32**, 1574–1576 (1972).

39. H. Tomogane, K. Ota, and A. Yokoyama, Suppression of progesterone secretion in lactating rats by administration of ergocornine and the effect of prolactin replacement, *J. Endocrinol.* **65**, 155–161 (1975).

40. W.R. Miller, Hyperprolactinemia and steroid metabolism by rat mammary adenocarcinomas, *Cancer Res.* **36**, 336–338 (1976).
41. R. Luft, H. Olivecrona, and B. Sjogren, Hypotysektomi pa narriska, *Nord. Med.* **47**, 351–354 (1952).
42. O.H. Pearson, C.D. West, V.P. Hollander, and N.E. Treves, Evaluation of endocrine therapy for advanced breast cancer, *J. Am. Med. Assoc.* **154**, 234–239 (1954).
43. O.H. Pearson, B.S. Ray, C. C. Harrold, C.D. West, M.D. Li, J.P. McClean, and M.B. Lipsett, Hypophysectomy in treatment of advanced cancer, *Trans. Assoc. Am. Physicians* **68**, 101–111 (1955).
44. O.H. Pearson and B.S. Ray, Results of hypophysectomy in the treatment of metastatic mammary carcinoma, *Cancer* **12**, 85–92 (1959).
45. M.B. Lipsett and D.M. Bergenstal, Lack of effect of human growth hormone and ovine prolactin on cancer in man, *Cancer Res.* **20**, 1172–1178 (1960).
46. W.B. Malarkey, L.S. Jacobs, and W.H. Daughaday, Levodopa suppression of prolactin in nonpeurperal galactorrhea, *N. Engl. J. Med.* **285**, 1160–1163 (1971).
47. D.L. Kleinberg, G.L. Noel, and A. Frantz, Chlorpromazine stimulation and L-Dopa suppression of plasma prolactin in man, *J. Clin. Endocrinol. Metab.* **33**, 873–876 (1971).
48. H.G. Friesen, H. Guyda, P. Hwang, J.E. Tyson, and A. Barbeau, Functional evaluation of prolactin secretion: A guide to therapy, *J. Clin. Invest.* **51**, 706–709 (1972).
49. R.P. Dickey and J.P. Minton, L-Dopa effect on prolactin, follicle-stimulating hormone, and luteinizing hormone in women with advanced breast cancer: A preliminary report, *Am. J. Obstet. Gynecol.* **114**, 267–269 (1972).
50. B.A. Stoll, Brain catecholamines in breast cancer: A hypothesis, *Lancet* **1**, 321 (1972).
51. R.M.L. Murray, G. Mozaffarian, and O.H. Pearson, in: *Prolactin and Carcinogenesis* (A.R. Boyns and K. Griffiths, eds.), pp. 158–161, Alpha Omega Alpha, Cardiff, Wales (1972).
52. A.G. Frantz, D.V. Habif, G.A. Hyman, and H.K. Suh, Remission of metastatic breast cancer after reduction of circulating prolactin in patients treated with L-Dopa, *Clin. Res.* **20**, 864 (1972).
53. A.G. Frantz, D.V. Habif, G.A. Hyman, H.K. Suh, J.F. Sassin, E.A. Zimmerman, G.L. Noel, and D.L. Kleinberg, in: *Human Prolactin* (J.L. Pasteels and C. Robyn, eds.), pp. 273–290, Excerpta Medica, Amsterdam (1973).
54. J.P. Minton, The response of breast cancer patients with bone pain to L-Dopa, *Cancer* **33**, 358–363 (1974).
55. E. del Pozo, R. Brun del Re, L. Varga, and H.G. Friesen, The inhibition of prolactin secretion in man by CB-154 (2-Br-α-ergocryptine), *J. Clin. Endocrinol. Metab.* **35**, 768–771 (1972).
56. L. Lemberger, R. Crabtree, J.A. Clemens, R.W. Dyke, and R.T. Woodburn, The inhibitory effect of an ergoline derivative (Lergotrile, Compound 83636) on prolactin secretion in man, *J. Clin. Endocrinol. Metab.* **39**, 579–584 (1974).
57. R.E. Cleary, R. Crabtree, and L. Lemberger, The effect of lergotrile on galactorrhea and gonadrotropin secretion, *J. Clin. Endocrinol. Metab.* **40**, 830–833 (1975).
58. J.E. Tyson, M. Khojandi, J. Huth, B. Smith, and P. Thomas, Inhibition of cyclic gonadotropin secretion by endogenous human prolactin, *Am. J. Obstet. Gynecol.* **121**, 375–379 (1975).
59. J.C. Heuson, A. Coume, and M. Staquet, Clinical trial of 2-Br-α-Ergocryptine (CB154) in advanced breast cancer, *Eur. J. Cancer* **8**, 155–156 (1972).
60. P.G. Guerzon and O.H. Pearson, Lergotrile Mesylate, a new prolactin inhibitor drug, *Clin. Res.* **22**, 632A (1974).
61. K.D. Schulz, P.-J. Czygan, E. del Pozo, and H.G. Friesen, in: *Human Prolactin* (J.L. Pasteels and C. Robyn, eds.), pp. 268–271, Excerpta Medica, Amsterdam (1973).

62. A.R. Boyns, E.N. Cole, K. Griffiths, M.M. Roberts, R. Buchan, R.G. Wilson, and A.P.M. Forrest, Plasma prolactin in breast cancer, *Eur. J. Cancer* **9**, 99–102 (1973).

63. R.G. Wilson, R. Buchan, M.M. Roberts, A.P.M. Forrest, A.R. Boyns, E.N. Cole, and K. Griffiths, Plasma prolactin and breast cancer, *Cancer* **33**, 1325–1327 (1974).

64. H.G. Kwa, M. De Jong-Bakker, E. Engelsman, and F.J. Cleton, Plasma prolactin in human breast cancer, *Lancet* **1**, 433–434 (1974).

65. S. Franks, D.N.L. Ralphs, V. Seagroatt, and H.S. Jacobs, Prolactin concentrations in patients with breast cancer, *Br. Med. J.* **4**, 320–321 (1974).

66. B.E. Henderson, V. Gerkins, I. Rosario, J. Casagrande, and M.C. Pike, Elevated serum levels of estrogen and prolactin in daughters of patients with breast cancer, *N. Engl. J. Med.* **293**, 790–795 (1975).

67. Boston Collaborative Drug Surveillance Program, Reserpine and breast cancer, *Lancet* **2**, 669–671 (1974).

68. B. Armstrong, N. Stevens, and R. Doll, Retrospective study of the association between use of rauwolfia derivatives and breast cancer in English women, *Lancet* **2**, 672–675 (1974).

69. O.P. Heinomen, S. Shapiro, L. Tuominen, and M.I. Turunen, Resperine use in relation to breast cancer, *Lancet* **2**, 675–677 (1974).

70. T.M. Mack, B.E. Henderson, V.R. Gerkins, M. Arthur, J. Baptista, and M.C. Pike, Reserpine and breast cancer in a retirement community, *N. Engl. J. Med.* **292**, 1366–1371 (1975).

71. W.M. O'Fallon, D.R. Labarthe, and L.T. Kurland, Rauwolfia derivatives and breast cancer, *Lancet* **2**, 292–296 (1975).

72. J.F. Sassin, A.G. Frantz, E.D. Weitzman, and S. Kapen, Human prolactin: 24 hour pattern with increased release during sleep, *Science* **177**, 1205–1207 (1972).

73. J.F. Sassin, A.G. Frantz, S. Kapen, and E.D. Weitzman, The nocturnal rise of human prolactin is dependent on sleep, *J. Clin. Endocrinol. Metab.* **37**, 436–440 (1973).

74. G. Ehni and N.E. Eckles, Interruption of the pituitary stalk in the patient with mammary cancer, *J. Neurosurg.* **16**, 628–652 (1959).

75. R.W. Turkington, L.E. Underwood, and J.J. Van Wyk, Elevated serum prolactin levels after pituitary-stalk section in man, *N. Engl. J. Med.* **285**, 707–710 (1971).

76. R.W. Turkington, G.C. Majumder, N. Kadohama, J.H. MacIndoe, and W.L. Frantz, Hormonal regulation of gene expression in mammary cells, *Recent Prog. Horm. Res.* **29**, 417–455 (1973).

77. G.N. Gill, Mechanism of ACTH action, *Metabolism* **21**, 571–588 (1972).

78. R.W. Turkington, Stimulation of RNA synthesis in isolated mammary cells by insulin and prolactin bound to sepharose, *Biochem. Biophys. Res. Commun.* **41**, 1362–1367 (1970).

79. M. Birkinshaw and I.R. Falconer, The localization of prolactin-labelled with radioactive iodine in rabbit mammary tissue, *J. Endocrinol.* **55**, 323–334 (1972).

80. H. Rajaniemi, A. Okasanen, and T. Vanha-Perttula, Distribution of ^{125}I-prolactin in mice and rats. Studies with whole-body and microautoradiography, *Horm. Res.* **5**, 6–20 (1974).

81. R.W. Turkington, Measurement of prolactin activity in human serum by the induction of specific milk proteins in mammary gland *in vitro, J. Clin. Endocrinol. Metab.* **33**, 210–216 (1971).

82. R.P.C. Shiu, P.A. Kelly, and H.G. Friesen, Radioreceptor assay for prolactin and other lactogenic hormones, *Science* **180**, 968–970 (1973).

83. W.L. Frantz, J.H. MacIndoe, and R.W. Turkington, Prolactin receptors: characteristics of the particulate fraction binding activity, *J. Endocrinol.* **60**, 485–497 (1974).

84. R.P.C. Shiu and H.G. Friesen, Properties of a prolactin receptor from the rabbit mammary gland, *Biochem. J.* **140**, 301–311 (1974).
85. B.I. Posner, P.A. Kelly, R.P.C. Shiu, and H.G. Friesen, Studies of insulin, growth hormone and prolactin binding: tissue distribution, species variation and characterization, *Endocrinology* **95**, 521–531 (1974).
86. M.E. Costlow, R.A. Buschow, N.J. Richert, and W.L. McGuire, Prolactin and estrogen binding in transplantable hormone-dependent and autonomous rat mammary carcinoma, *Cancer Res.* **35**, 970–974 (1975).
87. P.A. Kelly, C. Bradley, R.P.C. Shiu, J. Meites, and H.G. Friesen, Prolactin binding to rat mammary tumor tissue, *Proc. Soc. Exp. Biol. Med.* **146**, 816–819 (1974).
88. E.R. DeSombre, G. Kledzik, S. Marshall, and J. Meites, Estrogen and prolactin receptor concentration in rat mammary tumors and response to endocrine ablation, *Cancer Res.* **36**, 354–358 (1976).
89. R.W. Turkington, Prolactin receptors in mammary carcinoma cells, *Cancer Res.* **34**, 758–763 (1974).
90. M.E. Costlow, R.A. Buschow, and W.L. McGuire, Prolactin receptors in an estrogen receptor-deficient mammary carcinoma, *Science* **184**, 85–86 (1974).
91. H.H. Holcomb, M.E. Costlow, R.A. Buschow, and W.L. McGuire, Prolactin binding in rat mammary gland during pregnancy and lactation, *Biochim. Biophys. Acta* **428**, 104–112 (1976).
92. M.E. Costlow, R.A. Buschow, and W.L. McGuire, Prolactin receptors and androgen induced regression of DMBA-induced mammary carcinoma, *Cancer Res.* **36**, 3324–3329 (1976).
93. I.M. Holdaway and H.G. Friesen, Correlation between hormone binding and growth response of rat mammary tumor, *Cancer Res.* **36**, 1562–1567 (1976).
94. G.H. Sasaki and B.S. Leung, Prolactin stimulation of estrogen receptor *in vitro* in 7,12-Dimethylbenz(A)anthracene-induced mammary tumor, *Res. Commun. Chem. Pathol. Pharmacol.* **8**, 409–412 (1974).
95. F. Vignon and H. Rochefort, Régulation des "réceptors" des oestrogines dans les tumeurs mammaires: effet de la prolactine *in vivo*, *C. R. Acad. Sci.* **278**, 103–106 (1974).
96. F. Vignon and H. Rochefort, Regulation of estrogen receptors in ovarian-dependent rat mammary tumors. I. Effects of castration and prolactin, *Endocrinology* **98**, 722–729 (1976).
97. E.J. Diamond, S. Koprak, S.K. Shen, and V.P. Hollander, The conversion of an ovariectomy-nonresponsive to an ovariectomy-responsive mammary tumor strain, *Cancer Res.* **36**, 77–80 (1976).
98. B.I. Posner, P.A. Kelly, and H.G. Friesen, Induction of a lactogenic receptor in rat liver: Influence of estrogen and the pituitary, *Proc. Natl. Acad. Sci. U.S.A.* **71**, 2407–2410 (1974).
99. B.I. Posner, P.A. Kelly, and H.G. Friesen, Prolactin receptors in rat liver: Possible induction by prolactin, *Science* **188**, 57–59 (1975).
100. M.E. Costlow, R.A. Buschow, and W.L. McGuire, Prolactin stimulation of prolactin receptors in rat liver, *Life. Sci.* **17**, 1457–1466 (1975).
101. M. Gelato, S. Marshall, M. Boudreau, J. Bruni, and G.A. Campbell, Effects of thyroid and ovaries on prolactin binding in rat liver, *Endocrinology* **96**, 1292–1296 (1975).
102. R. Hilf, I. Michel, and C. Bell, Biochemical and morphological responses of normal and neoplastic mammary tissue to hormonal treatment, *Recent Prog. Horm. Res.* **23**, 229–295 (1967).
103. W.L. McGuire, Hormonal stimulation of lactose synthetase in mammary carcinoma, *Science* **165**, 1013–1014 (1969).

104. N.J. Nardacci and W.L. McGuire, A specific marker for prolactin responsiveness in experimental breast cancer: Lactalbumin mRNA, *Clin. Res.* **24**, 462A (1976).
105. W.L. McGuire, J.A. Julian, and G.C. Chamness, A dissociation between ovarian dependent growth and estrogen sensitivity in mammary carcinoma, *Endocrinology* **89**, 969–973 (1971).
106. W.L. McGuire, K. Huff, A.W. Jennings, and G.C. Chamness, Mammary carcinoma: A specific biochemical defect in autonomous tumors, *Science* **175**, 335–336 (1972).
107. I. Schorr, P. Rathnam, B.B. Saxena, and R.L. Ney, Multiple specific hormone receptors in the adenylate cyclase of an adrenocortical carcinoma, *J. Biol. Chem.* **246**, 5806–5811 (1971).
108. W.R. Lyons, C.H. Li, and R.E. Johnson, The hormonal control of mammary growth and lactation, *Recent Prog. Horm. Res.* **14**, 219–254 (1958).
109. K. Ahren and D. Jacobsohn, Mammary gland growth in hypophysectomized rats injected with ovarian hormones and insulin, *Acta Physiol. Scand.* **37**, 190–203 (1956).
110. A. Norgren, Action of different doses of oestrone on mammary gland of hypophysectomized castrated rabbits, *Acta Univ. Lund.* **1**, 1–24 (1967).
111. H. Nagasawa and R. Yanai, Increased mammary gland response to pituitary mammotropic hormones by estrogen in rats, *Endocrinol. Jpn.* **18**, 53–56 (1971).
112. J. Meites and C.S. Nicoll, Adenohypophysis: Prolactin, *Annu. Rev. Physiol.* **28**, 57–88 (1966).
113. A. Sterental, J.M. Dominguez, C. Weissman, and O.H. Pearson, Pituitary role in the estrogen dependency of experimental mammary cancer, *Cancer Res.* **23**, 481–484 (1963).
114. C.J. Bradley, G.S. Kledzik, and J. Meites, Prolactin and estrogen dependency of rat mammary cancers at early and late stages of development, *Cancer Res.* **36**, 319–324 (1976).
115. S.-I. Murota and V.P. Hollander, Role of ovarian hormones in the growth of transplantable mammary carcinoma, *Endocrinology* **89**, 560–564 (1971).
116. B.V. Caldwell, S.A. Tillson, H. Esber, and I.H. Thorneycroft, Survival of tumours after immunization against oestrogens, *Nature* **231**, 118–119 (1971).
117. O.H. Pearson and H. Nasr, Hormonal steroids, *Excerpta Med. Int. Congr. Ser.* **219**, 602 (1970).
118. H. Nagasawa and R. Yanai, Reduction of pituitary isograft of inhibitory effect of large dose of estrogen on incidence of mammary tumors induced by carcinogen in ovariectomized rats, *Int. J. Cancer* **8**, 463–467 (1971).
119. J. Meites, E.E. Cassell, and J.H. Clark, Estrogen inhibition of mammary tumor growth in rats; counteraction by prolactin, *Proc. Soc. Exp. Biol. Med.* **137**, 1225–1227 (1971).
120. R.F. Glascock and W.G. Hoekstra, Selective accumulation of tritium-labelled hexoestrol by the reproductive organs of immature female goats and sheep, *Biochem. J.* **72**, 673–682 (1959).
121. E.V. Jensen and H.I. Jacobson, in: *Biological Activities of Steroids in Relation to Cancer* (G. Pincus and E.P. Vollmer, eds.), pp. 161–178, Academic Press, New York (1960).
122. P.J. Folca, R.F. Glascock, and W.T. Irvine, Studies with tritium-labelled hexoestrol in advanced breast cancer, *Lancet* **2**, 796–802 (1961).
123. W.H. Pearlman, R. De Hertogh, K.R. Laumas, and M.R.S. Pearlman, Metabolism and tissue uptake of estrogen in women with advanced carcinoma of the breast, *J. Clin. Endocrinol. Metab.* **29**, 707–720 (1969).
124. F.G. Ellis, T.V. Berne, N. Deshpande, F.O. Belzer, and R.D. Bulbrook, The uptake of tritiated steroids by human breast carcinoma, *Surg. Gynecol. Obstet.* **128**, 975–984 (1969).

125. F. James, V.H.T. James, A.E. Carter, and W.T. Irvine, A comparison of *in vivo* and *in vitro* uptake of estradiol by human breast tumors and the relationship of steroid excretion, *Cancer Res.* **31** 1268–1272 (1971).

126. H. Braunsberg, V.H.T. James, W.T. Irvine, C.W. Jamieson, F. James, R.A. Sellwood, A.E. Carter, and M. Hulbert, Prognostic significance of oestrogen uptake by human breast cancer tissue, *Lancet* **1**, 163–165 (1973).

127. R.J.B. King, D.M. Cowan, and D.R. Inman, The uptake of [6,7-³H]oestradiol by dimethylbenzanthracene-induced rat mammary tumours, *J. Endocrinol.* **32**, 83–90 (1965).

128. R.J.B. King, J. Gordon, D.M. Cowan, and D.R. Inman, The intranuclear localization of [6,7-³H]oestradiol-17β in dimethylbenzanthracene-induced rat mammary adenocarcinoma and other tissues, *J. Endocrinol.* **36**, 139–150 (1966).

129. B.G. Mobbs, The uptake of tritiated oestradiol by dimethylbenzanthracene-induced mammary tumours of the rat, *J. Endocrinol.* **36**, 409–414 (1966).

130. S. Sander and A. Attramadal, The *in vivo* uptake of oestradiol-17β by hormone responsive and unresponsive breast tumors of the rat, *Acta Pathol. Microbiol. Scand.* **74**, 169–178 (1968).

131. L. Terenius, Parallelism between oestrogen binding capacity and hormone responsiveness of mammary tumours in GR/A mice, *Eur. J. Cancer* **8**, 55–58 (1972).

132. B.G. Mobbs, Uptake of [³H]oestradiol by dimethylbenzanthracene-induced rat mammary tumours regressing spontaneously or after ovariectomy, *J. Endocrinol.* **44**, 463–464 (1969).

133. E.V. Jensen, E.R. DeSombre, and P.W. Jungblut, in: *Endogenous Factors Influencing Host–Tumor Balance* (R.W. Wissler, T.L. Dao, and S. Wood, Jr., eds.), pp. 15–30, University of Chicago Press, Chicago (1967).

134. L. Terenius, Selective retention of estrogen isomers in estrogen dependent breast tumors of rats demonstrated by *in vitro* methods, *Cancer Res.* **28**, 328–337 (1968).

135. E.V. Jensen and E.R. DeSombre, Mechanism of action of the female sex hormones, *Annu. Rev. Biochem.* **41**, 203–230 (1972).

136. J. Gorski, D.O. Toft, G. Shyamala, D. Smith, and A. Notides, Hormone receptors: Studies on the interaction of estrogen with the uterus, *Recent Prog. Horm. Res.* **24** 45–80 (1968).

137. G.C. Mueller, B. Vonderhaar, U.H. Kim, and M.L. Mahieu, Estrogen action: An inroad to cell biology, *Recent Prog. Horm. Res.* **28**, 1–49 (1972).

138. F. Bresciani, G.A. Puca, E. Nola, M. Salvatore, and I. Ardovino, Meccanismo dell'azione estrogena e transformazione neoplastica, *Atti Soc. Ital. Patol.* **11**, 203–224 (1969).

139. W.L. McGuire and J.A. Julian, Comparison of macromolecular binding of estradiol in hormone dependent and hormone independent rat mammary carcinoma, *Cancer Res.* **31**, 1440–1445 (1971).

140. W.L. McGuire, P.P. Carbone, M.E. Sears, and G.C. Escher, in: *Estrogen Receptors in Human Breast Cancer* (W.L. McGuire, P.P. Carbone, and E.P. Vollmer, eds.), pp. 1–7, Raven Press, New York (1975).

141. S.G. Korenman, Estrogen receptor assay in human breast cancer, *J. Natl. Cancer Inst.* **55**, 543–545 (1975).

142. G.C. Chamness, K. Huff, and W.L. McGuire, Protamine-precipitated estrogen receptor: A solid-phase ligand exchange assay, *Steroids* **25**, 627–635 (1975).

143. D.T. Zava, N.Y. Harrington, and W.L. McGuire, A nuclear exchange assay for estradiol receptor, *Biochemistry* **15**, 4292–4297 (1976).

144. B.S. Leung and G.H. Sasaki, On the mechanism of prolactin and estrogen action in 7,12-Dimethylbenz(A)anthracene-induced mammary carcinoma in the rat. II. *In vivo* tumor responses and estrogen receptor, *Endocrinology* **97**, 564–572 (1975).

145. Y. Nomura, Y. Abe, and K. Inokuchi, Specific estrogen receptor and its relation to response to oophorectomy in rat mammary cancer induced by 7,12-Dimethylbenz(a)anthracene, *Gann* **65**, 523–528 (1974).
146. G. Shyamala, Estradiol receptors in mouse mammary tumors—absence of the transfer of bound estradiol from the cytoplasm to the nucleus, *Biochem. Biophys. Res. Commun.* **46**, 1623–1630 (1972).
147. F. Vignon and H. Rochefort, Estrogen receptor studies in experimental tumors, in: *Proc. 10th Meeting on Mammary Cancer*, Kobe, Japan, p. 42 (1976).
148. W.L. McGuire, K. Huff, and G.C. Chamness, Temperature dependent binding of estrogen receptor to chromatin, *Biochemistry* **11**, 4562–4565 (1972).
149. W.L. McGuire and M. De La Garza, Similarity of the estrogen receptor in human and rat mammary carcinoma, *J. Clin. Endocrinol. Metab.* **36**, 548–552 (1973).
150. W.L. McGuire, Estrogen receptors in human breast cancer, *J. Clin. Invest.* **52**, 73–77 (1973).
151. W.L. McGuire and M. De La Garza, Improved sensitivity in the measurement of estrogen receptor in human breast cancer, *J. Clin. Endocrinol. Metab.* **37**, 986–989 (1973).
152. W.L. McGuire, O.H. Pearson, and A. Segaloff, in: *Estrogen Receptors in Human Breast Cancer* (W.L. McGuire, P.P. Carbone, and E.P. Vollmer, eds.), pp. 17–30, Raven Press, New York (1975).
153. P.P. Rosen, C.J. Mendendez-Bolet, J.S. Nisselbaum, J.A. Urban, V. Mike, A. Fracchia, and M.K. Schwartz, Pathological review of breast lesions analyzed for estrogen receptor protein, *Cancer Res.* **35**, 3187–3194 (1975).
154. P. Feherty, G. Farrer-Brown, and A.E. Kellie, Oestradiol receptors in carcinoma and benign disease of the breast: an *in vitro* assay, *Br. J. Cancer* **25**, 697–710 (1971).
155. S.G. Korenman and B.A. Dukes, Specific estrogen binding by the cytoplasm of human breast carcinoma, *J. Clin. Endocrinol. Metab.* **30**, 639–645 (1970).
156. R. Hahnel, E. Twaddle, and A.B. Vivian, Estrogen receptors in human breast cancer. II. *In vitro* binding of estradiol by benign and malignant tumors, *Steroids* **18**, 681–708 (1971).
157. G.A. Puca and F. Bresciani, Interactions of 6,7-^{3}H-17β-estradiol with mammary gland and other organs of the C3H mouse *in vivo*, *Endocrinology* **85**, 1–10 (1969).
158. J.L. Wittliff, D.G. Gardner, W.L. Battema, and P.J. Gilbert, Specific estrogen-receptors in the neoplastic and lactating mammary gland of the rat, *Biochem. Biophys. Res. Commun.* **48**, 119–125 (1972).
159. G. Shyamala and S. Nandi, Interactions of 6,7-^{3}H-17β-estradiol with the mouse lactating mammary tissue *in vivo* and *in vitro*, *Endocrinology* **91**, 861–867 (1972).
160. A.J.W. Hsueh, E.J. Peck, Jr., and J.H. Clark, Oestrogen receptors in the mammary gland of the lactating rat, *J. Endocrinol.* **58**, 503–511 (1973).
161. J.A. Katzenellenbogen, H.J. Johnson, and K.E. Carlson, Studies on the uterine, cytoplasmic estrogen binding protein. Thermostability and ligand dissociation rate. An assay of empty and filled sites by exchange, *Biochemistry* **12**, 4092–4099 (1973).
162. H. Truong, C. Geynet, C. Millet, O. Soulignac, R. Boucourt, M. Vignau, V. Torelli, and E.E. Baulieu, Purification of estradiol receptor by affinity chromatography. Representative experiments, *FEBS Lett.* **35**, 289–294 (1973).
163. J.L. Daehnfeldt, Endogenously blocked high affinity estradiol receptors in the immature and mature rat uterus, *Proc. Soc. Exp. Biol. Med.* **146**, 159–162 (1974).
164. K.B. Horwitz, M.E. Costlow, and W.L. McGuire, MCF-7: A human breast cancer cell line with estrogen, androgen, progesterone, and glucocorticoid receptors, *Steroids* **26**, 785–795 (1975).
165. K.B. Horwitz, W.L. McGuire, O.H. Pearson, and A. Segaloff, Predicting response to endocrine therapy in human breast cancer: A hypothesis, *Science* **189**, 726–727 (1975).

166. R.E. Buller, W.T. Schrader, and B.W. O'Malley, Progesterone-binding components of chick oviduct, *J. Biol. Chem.* **250**, 809–818 (1975).
167. G.C. Chamness, A.W. Jennings, and W.L. McGuire, Oestrogen receptor binding is not restricted to target nuclei, *Nature* **241**, 458–460 (1973).
168. G.C. Chamness, A.W. Jennings, and W.L. McGuire, Estrogen receptor binding to isolated nuclei. A nonsaturable process, *Biochemistry* **13**, 327–331 (1974).
169. R.E. Shepherd, K. Huff, and W.L. McGuire, Non-interaction between *in vivo* and cell free nuclear binding of estrogen receptor, *Endocr. Res. Commun.* **1**, 73–85 (1974).
170. J.H. Clark and E.J. Peck, Nuclear retention of receptor–oestrogen complex and nuclear acceptor sites, *Nature* **260**, 635–637 (1976).
171. D.T. Zava, G.C. Chamness, K.B. Horwitz, and W.L. McGuire, Human breast cancer: Biologically active estrogen receptor in the absence of estrogen? *Science* (1977), in press.
172. K.D. Schulz, B. Haselmeier, and F. Holzel, The influence of Clomid and its isomers upon dimethylbenzanthracene-induced rat mammary tumours, *Acta Endocrinol. Suppl.* **138**, 236 (1969).
173. L. Terenius, Anti-oestrogens and breast cancer, *Eur. J. Cancer* **7**, 57–64 (1971).
174. E. DeSombre and L.Y. Arbogast, Effect of the antiestrogen CI 628 on the growth of rat mammary tumors, *Cancer Res.* **34**, 1971–1976 (1974).
175. V.C. Jordan and S. Koerner, Tamoxifen as an anti-tumour agent: role of oestradiol and prolactin, *J. Endocrinol.* **68**, 305–311 (1976).
176. G.H. Gallez, J.C. Heuson, and C.H. Waelbroeck, Growth-stimulating effect of nafoxidine on rat mammary tumor after ovariectomy, *Eur. J. Cancer* **9**, 699–700 (1973).
177. J.C. Heuson, C. Waelbroeck, N. Legros, G. Gallez, C. Robyn, and M. L'Hermite, Inhibition of DMBA-induced mammary carcinogenesis in the rat by 2-Br-α-ergocryptine (CB154), an inhibitor of prolactin secretion, and by nafoxidine (U-11,100A) an estrogen antagonist, *Gynecol. Invest.* **2**, 130–137 (1972).
178. V.C. Jordan and T. Jaspan, Tamoxifen as an anti-tumour agent: oestrogen binding as a predictive test for tumour response, *J. Endocrinol.* **68**, 453–460 (1976).
179. M.J. O'Halloran and P.G. Maddock, ICI 46,474 in breast cancer, *J. Ir. Med. Assoc.* **67**, 38–39 (1974).
180. M.P. Cole, C.T.A. Jones, and I.D.H. Todd, A new antiestrogenic agent in late breast cancer. An early clinical appraisal of ICI 46,474, *Br. J. Cancer* **25**, 270–275 (1971).
181. H.W.C. Ward, Antioestrogen therapy for breast cancer: A trial of tamoxifen at 2 dose levels, *Br. Med. J.* **1**, 13–14 (1973).
182. J.C. Heuson, A. Coume, and M. Staquet (For the E.O.R.T.C. Breast Cancer Group), Clinical trial of nafoxidine, an oestrogen antagonist in advanced breast cancer, *Eur. J. Cancer* **8**, 387–389 (1972).
183. H.J.G. Bloom and E. Boesen, Antioestrogens in treatment of breast cancer: Value of nafoxidine in 52 advanced cases, *Br. Med. J.* **2**, 7–10 (1974).
184. J.C. Heuson, E. Engelsman, J. Blonk-vander Wijst, H. Maass, A. Drochmans, J. Michel, H. Nowakowski, and A. Gorins, Comparative trial of nafoxidine and ethinyloestradiol in advanced breast cancer: An E.O.R.T.C. study, *Br. Med. J.* **2**, 711–713 (1975).
185. E. Hecker, I. Vegh, C.M. Levy, C.A. Magin, J.C. Martinez, J. Loureino, and R.E. Garola, Clinical trial of clomiphene in advanced breast cancer, *Eur. J. Cancer* **10**, 747–749 (1974).
186. L. Terenius, Structure–activity relationships of anti-oestrogens with regard to interaction with 17β-oestradiol in the mouse uterus and vagina, *Acta Endocrinol.* **66**, 431–447 (1971).
187. H. Rochefort, F. Lignon, and F. Capony, Effect of antiestrogens on uterine estradiol receptors, *Gynecol. Invest.* **3**, 43–62 (1972).

188. J.H. Clark, J.N. Anderson, and E.J. Peck, Jr., Estrogen receptor–antiestrogen complex: atypical binding by uterine nuclei and effects on uterine growth, *Steroids* **22**, 707–718 (1973).

189. B.S. Katzenellenbogen and E.R. Ferguson, Antiestrogen action in the uterus: biological ineffectiveness of nuclear bound estradiol after antiestrogen, *Endocrinology* **97**, 1–12 (1975).

190. J.H. Clark, E.J. Peck, Jr., and J.N. Anderson, Oestrogen receptors and antagonism of steroid hormone action, *Nature* **251**, 446–448 (1974).

191. V.C. Jordan and S. Koerner, Tamoxifen (ICI 46,474) and the human carcinoma 8 S oestrogen receptor, *Eur. J. Cancer* **11**, 205–206 (1975).

192. R. Garola, C.M. Levy, I. Vegh, C. Magin, J.C. Martinez, and E. Hecker, *In vivo* blockade of the estradiol-binding-protein (EBP) by clomiphene citrate in human breast cancer, *Oncology* **30**, 105–112 (1974).

193. M.E. Lippman and G. Bolan, Oestrogen-responsive human breast cancer in long term tissue culture, *Nature* **256**, 592–593 (1975).

194. V.C. Jordan, S. Koerner, and C. Robison, Inhibition of oestrogen-stimulated prolactin release by anti-oestrogens, *J. Endocrinol.* **65**, 151–152 (1975).

195. B.S. Leung, G.H. Sasaki, and J. Leung, Estrogen–prolactin dependency in 7,12-dimethylbenz(a)anthracene-induced tumors, *Cancer Res.* **35**, 621–627 (1975).

196. P. Cole and B. MacMahon, Oestrogen fractions during early reproductive life in the etiology of breast cancer, *Lancet* **1**, 604–606 (1969).

197. B. MacMahon, P. Cole, and J. Brown, Etiology of human breast cancer: A review, *J. Natl. Cancer Inst.* **50**, 21–42 (1973).

198. L.E. Dickinson, B. MacMahon, P. Cole, and J.B. Brown, Estrogen profiles of oriental and caucasian women in Hawaii, *N. Engl. J. Med.* **291**, 1211–1213 (1974).

199. H.M. Lemon, Endocrine influences on human mammary cancer formation. A critique, *Cancer* **23**, 781–790 (1969).

200. H.M. Lemon, Abnormal estrogen metabolism and tissue estrogen receptor proteins in breast cancer, *Cancer* **25**, 423–435 (1970).

201. H.M. Lemon, D.M. Miller, and J.F. Foley, Competition between steroids for hormonal receptor, *Natl. Cancer Inst. Monogr.—Prediction of Response in Cancer Therapy* **34**, 77–83 (1971).

202. H.M. Lemon, Estriol prevention of mammary carcinoma induced by 7,12-dimethylbenzanthracene and procarlazine, *Cancer Res.* **35**, 1341–1353 (1975).

203. S.G. Korenman, Comparative binding affinity of estrogens and its relation to estrogenic potency, *Steroids* **13**, 163–178 (1969).

204. D.L. Loriaux, H.J. Ruder, D.R. Knab, and M.B. Lipsett, Estrone sulfate, estrone, estradiol and estriol plasma levels in human pregnancy, *J. Clin. Endocrinol. Metab.* **35**, 887–891 (1972).

205. M.B. Lipsett, Oestrogen profiles and breast cancer, *Lancet* **2**, 1378 (1971).

206. T.S. Ruh, B.S. Katzenellenbogen, J.A. Katzenellenbogen, and J. Gorski, Estrone interaction with the rat uterus: *in vitro* response and nuclear uptake, *Endocrinology* **92**, 125–134 (1973).

207. G. Rudali, F. Apiou, and B. Muel, Mammary cancer produced in mice with estriol, *Eur. J. Cancer* **11**, 39–41 (1975).

208. B.M. Sherman and S.G. Korenman, Inadequate corpus luteum function: A pathophysiological interpretation of human breast cancer epidemiology, *Cancer* **33**, 1306–1312 (1974).

209. J.J. Barlow, K. Emerson, Jr., and B.N. Saxena, Estradiol production after ovariectomy for carcinoma of the breast, *N. Engl. J. Med.* **280**, 633–637 (1969).

210. C. Longcope, Metabolic clearance and blood production rates of estrogens in postmenopausal women, *Am. J. Obstet. Gynecol.* **111**, 778–781 (1971).

211. M.A. Kirschner and J.P. Taylor, Urinary estrogen production rates in normal and endocrine-ablated subjects, *J. Clin. Endocrinol. Metab.* **35,** 513–521 (1972).
212. J.M. Grodin, P.K. Siiteri, and P.C. MacDonald, Source of estrogen production in postmenopausal women, *J. Clin. Endocrinol. Metab.* **36,** 207–214 (1973).
213. H.L. Judd, G.E. Judd, W.E. Lucas, and S.S.C. Yen, Endocrine function of the post-menopausal ovary: Concentration of androgens and estrogens in ovarian and peripheral vein blood, *J. Clin. Endocrinol. Metab.* **39,** 1020–1024 (1974).
214. A. Lipton and R.J. Santen, Medical andrenalectomy using aminoglutethimide and dexamethasone in advanced breast cancer, *Cancer* **33,** 503–512 (1974).
215. R.N. Dexter, L.M. Fishman, R.L. Ney, and G.W. Liddle, Inhibition of adrenal cor-ticosteroid synthesis by aminoglutethimide: Studies of the mechanism of action, *J. Clin. Endocrinol. Metab.* **27,** 473–480 (1967).
216. R.R. Cash, J. Brough, M.N.P. Cohen, and P.S. Satoh, Aminoglutethimide (Elipten–Ciba) as an inhibition of adrenal steroidogenesis: mechanism of action and therapeu-tic trial, *J. Clin. Endocrinol. Metab.* **27,** 1239–1248 (1967).
217. T. Hall, J.J. Barlow, C.T. Griffiths, and Z. Saba, Treatment of metastatic breast cancer with aminoglutethimide, *Clin. Res.* **17,** 402 (1969).
218. C.T. Griffiths, T.C. Hall, Z. Saba, J.J. Barlow, and H.B. Nevinny, Preliminary trial of aminoglutethimide in breast cancer, *Cancer* **32,** 32–37 (1973).
219. R.J. Santen, A. Lipton, and J. Kendall, Successful medical adrenalectomy with aminoglutethimide: Role of altered drug metabolism, *J. Am. Med. Assoc.* **230,** 1661–1665 (1974).
220. W.E. Poel, Progesterone enhancement of mammary tumor development as a model of co-carcinogenesis, *Br. J. Cancer* **22,** 867–873 (1968).
221. C. Huggins and N.C. Yang, Induction and extinction of mammary cancer, *Science* **137,** 257–262 (1962).
222. C. Huggins, Two principles in endocrine therapy of cancers: Hormone deprival and hormone interference, *Cancer Res.* **25,** 1163–1175 (1965).
223. G.M. McCormick and R.C. Moon, Effect of increasing doses of estrogen and proges-terone on mammary carcinogenesis in the rat, *Eur. J. Cancer* **9,** 483–486 (1973).
224. F.M. Muggia, P.A. Casilleth, M. Ochoa, F.A. Flatow, A. Gellhorn, and G.A. Hyman, Treatment of breast cancer with medroxyprogesterone, *Ann. Int. Med.* **68,** 328–337 (1968).
225. B.A. Stoll, Vaginal cytologyas, an aid to hormone therapy in postmenopausal cancer of the breast, *Cancer* **20,** 1807–1813 (1967).
226. Council on Drugs, Androgens and estrogens in the treatment of disseminated mam-mary carcinoma, *J. Am. Med. Assoc.* **172,** 1271–1283 (1960).
227. L.G. Growley and I. MacDonald, Delalutin and estrogens for the treatment of ad-vanced mammary carcinoma in the postmenopausal women, *Cancer* **18,** 436–446 (1965).
228. B.A. Stoll, Progestin therapy of breast cancer: Comparison of agents, *Br. Med. J.* **3,** 338–341 (1967).
229. B.A. Stoll, Effect of tyndiol, an oral contraceptive, on breast cancer, *Br. Med. J.* **1,** 150–153 (1967).
230. L. Sadoff and W. Lusk, The effect of large doses of medroxyprogesterone acetate (MPA) on urinary estrogen levels and serum levels of cortisol, T⁴, LH, and testos-terone in patients with advanced cancer, *Obstet. Gynecol.* **43,** 262–266 (1974).
231. R.L. Landau, E.N. Ehrlich, and C. Huggins, Estradiol benzoate and progesterone in advanced human breast cancer, *J. Am. Med. Assoc.* **182,** 632–636 (1962).
232. B.J. Kennedy, Hormone therapy for advanced breast cancer, *Cancer* **18,** 1551–1557 (1965).

233. B.J. Kennedy and L. French, Hypophysectomy in advanced breast cancer, *Am. J. Surg.* **110**, 411–414 (1965).

234. M.J. Bryson and M.L. Sweat, Metabolism of progesterone and human myometrium, *Endocrinology* **84**, 1071–1075 (1969).

235. D.T. Armstrong and E.R. King, Uterine progesterone metabolism and progestational response: effects of estrogen and prolactin, *Endocrinology* **89**, 191–197 (1971).

236. I. Hashimoto, D.M. Hendricks, L.L. Anderson, and R.M. Melampy, Progesterone and pregn-4-en-20α-ol-3-one and ovarian venous blood during various reproductive states in the rat, *Endocrinology* **82**, 333–341 (1968).

237. D. Egert and H. Maass, Progesterone in the uterus. III. On the question of progesterone metabolism in the uterus of pregnant rats, *Acta Endocrinol.* **77**, 160–170 (1974).

238. W.G. Wiest, in: *The Sex Steroids* (K.W. McKerns, ed.), pp. 295–313, Plenum Press, New York (1971).

239. J.A. Collins and D.M. Jewkes, Progesterone metabolism by proliferative and secretory human endometrium, *Am. J. Obstet. Gynecol.* **118**, 179–185 (1974).

240. W.G. Wiest, *In vitro* metabolism of progesterone and 20-α-hydroxypregn-4-en-3-one by tissues of the female rat, *Endocrinology* **73**, 310–316 (1963).

241. D.E.M. Lawson and W.H. Pearlman, The metabolism *in vivo* of progesterone-7-³H; its localization in the mammary gland, uterus, and other tissues of the pregnant rat, *J. Biol. Chem.* **239**, 3226–3232 (1964).

242. R.T. Chatterton, in: *The Sex Steroids* (K.W. McKerns, ed.), pp. 345–382, Plenum Press, New York (1971).

243. K.C. Podratz, T.W. Munns, and P.A. Katzman, Metabolism of progesterone and mouse vaginal tissue, *Steroids* **24**, 775–792 (1974).

244. T. Tabei, H. Haga, W.L. Heinrichs, and W.L. Herrmann, Metabolism of progesterone by rat brain, pituitary gland and other tissues, *Steroids* **23**, 651–666 (1974).

245. B.W. O'Malley, W.L. McGuire, P.O. Kohler, and S.G. Korenman, Studies on the mechanism of steroid hormone regulation of synthesis of specific hormones, *Recent Prog. Horm. Res.* **25**, 105–160 (1969).

246. M.D. Morgan and J.D. Wilson, Intranuclear metabolism of progesterone-1,2-³H in the hen oviduct, *J. Biol. Chem.* **245**, 3781–3789 (1970).

247. N. Deshpande, Hormonal imbalance in breast cancer, *J. Steroid Biochem.* **6**, 735–741 (1975).

248. N. Bruchovsky and J.D. Wilson, The conversion of testosterone to 5α-androgen-17β-ol-3-one by rat prostate *in vivo* and *in vitro*, *J. Biol. Chem.* **243**, 2012–2021 (1968).

249. J.D. Wilson, Recent studies on the mechanism of action of testosterone, *N. Engl. J. Med.* **287**, 1284–1291 (1972).

250. R.T. Chatterton, Jr., A.J. Chatteron, and L. Hellman, Metabolism of progesterone by the rabbit mammary gland, *Endocrinology* **85**, 16–24 (1969).

251. J. Saffran, B.K. Loeser, B.M. Haas, and H.E. Stavely, Metabolism of progesterone in rat uterus, *Steroids* **23**, 117–131 (1974).

252. W.W. Leavitt and C.J. Grossman, Characterization of binding components for progesterone and 5α-pregnane-3,20-dione in the hamster uterus, *Proc. Natl. Acad. Sci. U.S.A.* **71**, 4341–4345 (1974).

253. J.C. Coffey, *In vitro* progesterone in rat submaxillary gland; the formation of 20α-hydroxy-4-pregnen-3-one and other substances, *Steroids* **22**, 561–566 (1973).

254. C.A. Strott, Metabolism of progesterone in the chick oviduct: relation to the progesterone receptor and biological activity, *Endocrinology* **95**, 826–837 (1974).

255. B.W. O'Malley and W.T. Schrader, Progesterone receptor components: identification of subunits binding to the target-cell genome, *J. Steroid Biochem.* **3**, 617–629 (1972).

256. L.E. Faber, M.L. Sandmann, and H.E. Stavely, Progesterone binding in uterine cytosols of the guinea pig, *J. Biol. Chem.* **247**, 8000–8004 (1972).

257. E. Milgrom, L. Thi, M. Atger, and E.-E. Baulieu, Mechanisms of regulating the concentration and the conformation of progesterone receptor(s) in the uterus, *J. Biol. Chem.* **248**, 6366–6374 (1973).

258. M. Atger, E.-E. Baulieu, and E. Milgrom, An investigation of progesterone receptors in guinea pig vagina, uterine cervix, mammary glands, pituitary, and hypothalamus, *Endocrinology* **94**, 161–167 (1974).

259. K. Kontula, O. Jaane, E. Rajakoski, E. Tanhuapaa, and R. Vihko, Ligand specificity of progesterone binding proteins in guinea pig and sheep, *J. Steroid Biochem.* **5**, 39–44 (1974).

260. M.L. Freifeld, P.D. Feil, and C.W. Bardin, The *in vivo* regulation of the progesterone "receptor" in guinea pig uterus: Dependence on estrogen and progesterone, *Steroids* **23**, 93–103 (1974).

261. D. Philibert and J.-P. Raynaud, Progesterone binding in the immature rabbit and guinea pig, *Endocrinology* **94**, 627–632 (1974).

262. P.D. Feil and C.W. Bardin, Cytoplasmic and nuclear progesterone receptor in the guinea pig uterus, *Endocrinology* **97**, 1398–1407 (1975).

263. W.W. Leavitt, D.O. Toft, C.A. Strott, and B.W. O'Malley, A specific progesterone receptor in the hamster uterus: Physiologic properties and regulation during the estrous cycle, *Endocrinology* **94**, 1041–1053 (1974).

264. L.E. Faber, M.L. Sandmann, and H.E. Stavely, Progesterone binding proteins of the rat and rabbit uterus, *J. Biol. Chem.* **247**, 5648–5649 (1972).

265. L. Faber, M.L. Sandmann, and H. Stavely, Progesterone and corticosterone binding in rabbit uterine cytosols, *Endocrinology* **93**, 74–80 (1973).

266. J. Davies, J.R.G. Challis, and K.J. Ryan, Progesterone receptors and the myometrium of pregnant rabbits, *Endocrinology* **95**, 164–173 (1974).

267. P.D. Feil, S.R. Glasser, D.O. Toft, and B.W. O'Malley, Progesterone binding in the mouse and rat uterus, *Endocrinology* **91**, 738–746 (1972).

268. D. Philibert and J.-P. Raynaud, Progesterone binding in the immature mouse and rat uterus, *Steroids* **22**, 89–99 (1973).

269. J. Saffran, B.K. Loeser, B. Haas, and H.E. Stavely, Binding of progesterone by rat uterus *in vitro*, *Biochem. Biophys. Res. Commun.* **53**, 202–209 (1973).

270. A.J.W. Hsueh, E.J. Peck, Jr., and J.H. Clark, Receptor progesterone complex in the nuclear fraction of the rat uterus demonstrated by tritiated progesterone exchange, *Steroids* **24**, 599–611 (1974).

271. K. Kontula, O. Janne, T. Luukkainen, and R. Vihko, Progesterone binding protein in human myometrium. Ligand specificity and some physiochemical characteristics, *Biochim. Biophys. Acta* **328**, 145–153 (1973).

272. H.E. Smith, R.G. Smith, D.O. Toft, J.R. Neergaard, E. Burrows, and B.W. O'Malley, Binding of steroids to progesterone receptor proteins in chick oviduct and human uterus, *J. Biol. Chem.* **249**, 5924–5932 (1974).

273. P.C.M. Young and R.E. Cleary, Characterization and properties of progesterone binding components in human endometrium, *J. Clin. Endocrinol. Metab.* **39**, 425–439 (1974).

274. K. Pollow, H. Lubbert, E. Boquoi, G. Kruezer, and B. Pollow, Characterization and comparison of receptors for 17β-estradiol and progesterone in human proliferative endometrium and endometrial carcinoma, *Endocrinology* **96**, 319–328 (1974).

275. M. Haukkamaa and T. Luukkainen, The cytoplasmic progesterone receptor of human endometrium during the menstrual cycle, *J. Steroid Biochem.* **5**, 447–452 (1974).

276. K. Kontula, O. Janne, T. Luukkainen, and R. Vihko, Progesterone binding protein in

human myometrium. Influence of metal ions on binding, *J. Clin. Endocrinol. Metab.* **38**, 500–503 (1974).

277. R.G. Smith, C.A. Iramain, V.C. Buttram, Jr., and B.W. O'Malley, Purification of human uterine progesterone receptor, *Nature* **253**, 271–272 (1975).

278. M.R. Sherman, P.L. Corvol, and B.W. O'Malley, Progesterone binding components of chick oviduct. I. Preliminary characterization of cytoplasmic components, *J. Biol. Chem.* **245**, 6085–6096 (1970).

279. D.O. Toft and B.W. O'Malley, Target tissue receptors for progesterone: the influence of estrogen, *Endocrinology* **90**, 1041–1045 (1972).

280. W.T. Schrader, D.O. Toft, and B.W. O'Malley, Progesterone-binding protein of chick oviduct, *J. Biol. Chem.* **247**, 2401–2407 (1972).

281. N. Deshpande, R.D. Bulbrook, and F.O. Belzer, An apparent selective accumulation of progesterone by the human breast, *Excerpta Med. Int. Congr. Ser.* **132**, 750–753 (1966).

282. L. Terenius, Estrogen and progestin binders in human and rat mammary carcinoma, *Eur. J. Cancer* **9**, 291–294 (1973).

283. G. Shyamala, Specific cytoplasmic glucocorticoid hormone receptors in lactating mammary glands, *Biochemistry* **12**, 3085–3090 (1973).

284. D.G. Gardner and J.L. Wittliff, Characterization of a distinct glucocorticoid-binding protein in the lactating mammary gland of the rat, *Biochim. Biophys. Acta* **320**, 617–627 (1973).

285. K.B. Horwitz, Progesterone receptors and hormone dependent breast cancer, Doctoral dissertation, University of Texas Southwestern Medical School at Dallas, pp. 80–85 (1975).

286. A.J.W. Hsueh, E.J. Peck, Jr., and J.H. Clark, Progesterone antagonism of estrogen receptor and estradiol-induced uterine growth, *Nature* **254**, 337–338 (1975).

287. D.W. Bullock and G.F. Wellen, Regulation of a specific uterine protein by estradiol and progesterone in ovariectomized rabbits, *Proc. Soc. Exp. Biol. Med.* **146**, 294–298 (1974).

288. E.M. Armstrong and I.A.R. More, Ultrastructural demonstration of the mode of action of an antioestrogen (Tamoxifen), *Cytobios* **11**, 13–16 (1974).

289. J.C. Heuson, C. Waelbroeck, N. Legros, G. Gallez, C. Robyn, and M. L'Hermite, Inhibition of DMBA-induced mammary carcinogenesis in the rat by 2-Br-α-Ergocryptine (CB-154), an inhibitor of prolactin secretion, and by Nafoxidine (U-11,100A), an estrogen antagonist, *Gynecol. Invest.* **2**, 130–137 (1971/1972).

290. A.J.W. Hsueh, E.J. Peck, Jr., and J.H. Clark, Control of uterine estrogen receptor levels by progesterone, *Endocrinology* **98**, 438–444 (1976).

291. M.L. Voorhess, Masculinization of the female fetus associated with Noerthindrone–Mestranol therapy during pregnancy, *J. Pediatr.* **71**, 128–131 (1967).

292. G.K. Suchowsky and K. Junkmann, A study of the virilizing effect of progesterone on the female rat fetus, *Endocrinology* **68**, 341–349 (1961).

293. I. Mowszowicz, D. Bieber, K. Chung, L.P. Bullock, and C.W. Bardin, Syandrogenic and antiandrogenic effect of progestins: Comparison with nonprogestational antiandrogens, *Endocrinology* **95**, 1589–1599 (1974).

294. M.S. Fahim and D.G. Hall, Effect of ovarian steroids on hepatic metabolism. I. Progesterone, *Am. J. Obstet. Gynecol.* **106**, 183–186 (1970).

295. L.P. Bullock, P.L. Barthe, I. Mowszowicz, D.N. Orth, and C.W. Bardin, The effect of progestins on submaxillary gland epidermal growth factor: demonstration of androgenic, syandrogenic and antiandrogenic actions, *Endocrinology* **97**, 189–195 (1975).

296. E. Naqvi, M.X. Zarrow, and V.H. Dennberg, Inhibition of androgen-induced precocious puberty by progesterone, *Endocrinology* **84**, 669–670 (1969).

297. K. Kratchwil, *In vitro* analysis of the hormonal basis for the sexual dimorphism in the

embryonic development of the mouse mammary gland, *J. Embryol. Exp. Morphol.* **25,** 141–153 (1971).

298. G.G. Rousseau, J.D. Baxter, and G.M. Tomkins, Glucocorticoid receptors: relations between steroid binding and biological effects, *J. Mol. Biol.* **67,** 99–115 (1972).

299. D.G. Gardner and J.L. Wittliff, Demonstration of a glucocorticoid hormone-receptor complex in the cytoplasm of a hormone-responsive tumour, *Br. J. Cancer* **27,** 441–444 (1973).

300. G. Shyamala, Glucocorticoid receptors in mouse mammary tumors, *J. Biol. Chem.* **249,** 2160–2163 (1974).

301. K.B. Horwitz and W.L. McGuire, Specific progesterone receptors in human breast cancer, *Steroids* **25,** 497–505 (1975).

302. W.W. Thatcher and H.A. Tucker, Adrenal function during prolonged lactation, *Proc. Soc. Exp. Biol. Med.* **134,** 915–918 (1970).

303. W.W. Thatcher and H.A. Tucker, Lactational performance of rats injected with oxytocin cortisol-21-acetate, prolactin and growth hormone during prolonged lactation, *Endocrinology* **86,** 237–240 (1970).

304. T. Oka and Y.J. Topper, Hormone-dependent accumulation of rough endoplasmic reticulum in mouse mammary epithelial cells *in vitro, J. Biol. Chem.* **246,** 7701–7707 (1971).

305. O. Takumi and J.W. Perry, Spermidine as a possible mediator of glucocorticoid effect on milk protein synthesis in mouse mammary epithelium *in vitro, J. Biol. Chem.* **249,** 7647–7652 (1974).

306. R.J.B. King and W.I.P. Mainwaring, *Steroid–Cell Interactions,* University Park Press, Baltimore (1974).

307. J.D. Baxter, G.G. Rousseau, M.C. Benson, R.L. Garcea, J. Ito, and G.M. Tomkins, Role of DNA and specific cytoplasmic receptors in glucocorticoid action, *Proc. Natl. Acad. Sci. U.S.A.* **69,** 1892–1896 (1972).

308. G.G. Rousseau, S.J. Higgins, J.D. Baxter, and G.M. Tomkins, Nuclear acceptor sites for glucocorticoid receptors, *J. Steroid Biochem.* **5,** 935–939 (1974).

309. N. Defer, B. Dastugue, and J. Kruh, Rat liver chromatin non-histone proteins and glucocorticoid binding, *Biochimie* **56,** 1549–1557 (1974).

310. G.G. Rousseau, Interaction of steroids with hepatoma cells: molecular mechanisms of glucocorticoid hormone action, *J. Steroid Biochem.* **6,** 75–89 (1975).

311. A. Munck and C. Wira, in: *Advances in the Biosciences 7* (G. Raspe, ed.), pp. 301–330, Pergamon Vieweg, Oxford (1970).

312. N. Hollander and Y.W. Chiu, *In vitro* binding of cortisol-1-2-³H by a substance in the supernatant faction of P1798 mouse lymphosarcoma, *Biochem. Biophys. Res. Commun.* **25,** 291–297 (1966).

313. J.D. Baxter, A.W. Harris, G.M. Tomkins, and M. Cohn, Glucocorticoid receptors in lymphoma cells in culture: relationship to glucocorticoid killing activity, *Science* **171,** 189–191 (1971).

314. M. Lippman, R. Halterman, S. Perry, B. Leventhal, and E.B. Thompson, Glucocorticoid binding proteins in human leukaemic lymphoblasts, *Nature* **242,** 157–158 (1973).

315. C.H. Sibley and G.M. Tomkins, Mechanisms of steroid resistance, *Cell* **2,** 221–227 (1974).

316. U. Gehring and G.M. Tomkins, A new mechanism for steroid unresponsiveness: loss of nuclear binding activity of a steroid hormone receptor, *Cell* **2,** 301–306 (1974).

317. K.R. Yamamoto, M.R. Stampfer, and G.M. Tompkins, Receptors from glucocorticoid-sensitive lymphoma cells and two classes of insensitive clones: physical and DNA-binding properties, *Proc. Natl. Acad. Sci. U.S.A.* **71,** 3901–3905 (1974).

318. L.L. Sparks, T.A. Daane, T. Hayashida, R.D. Cole, W.R. Lyons, and C.H. Li, The

effects of pituitary and adrenal hormones on the growth of a transplanted mammary adenocarcinoma in C3H mice, *Cancer* **8**, 271–284 (1955).

319. R. Hilf, I. Michel, C. Bell, J.J. Freeman, and A. Borman, Biochemical and morphologic properties of a new lactating mammary tumor line in the rat, *Cancer Res.* **25**, 286–299 (1965).

320. L. Kornel, On the effects and the mechanism of corticosteroids in normal and neoplastic target tissue: Findings and hypotheses, *Acta Endocrinol.* **74**, 1–45 (1973).

321. C.M. McGrath, Replication of mammary tumor virus in tumor cell cultures: Dependence on hormone-induced cellular organization, *J. Natl. Cancer Inst.* **47**, 455–467 (1971).

322. H.A. Young, E.M. Scolnick, and W.P. Parks, Glucocorticoid–receptor interactions and induction of murine mammary tumor virus, *J. Biol. Chem.* **250**, 3337–3343 (1975).

323. A. Pihl, S. Sander, I. Brennhoud, and S. Olsens, in: *Estrogen Receptors in Human Breast Cancer* (W.L. McGuire, P.P. Carbone, and E.P. Vollmer, eds.), pp. 193–203, Raven Press, New York (1975).

324. M.B. Lipsett, Why corticoids are effective against a wide variety of cancers, *Ann. N. Y. Acad. Sci.* **230**, 489–490 (1974).

325. H.A. Tucker, B.L. Larson, and J. Gorski, Cortisol binding in cultured bovine mammary cells, *Endocrinology* **89**, 152–160 (1971).

326. R.W. Turnell, P.C. Beers, and J.L. Wittliff, Glucocorticoid-binding macromolecules in the lactating mammary gland of the vole, *Endocrinology* **95**, 1770–1773 (1974).

327. J.E. Goral and J.L. Wittliff, Comparison of glucocorticoid-binding proteins in normal and neoplastic mammary tissues of the rat, *Biochemistry* **14**, 2944–2952 (1975).

328. G. Shyamala, Glucocorticoid receptors in mouse mammary tumors: Specific binding to nuclear components, *Biochemistry* **14**, 437–444 (1975).

329. E.E. Baulieu, The action of hormone metabolites: A new concept in endocrinology, *Ann. Clin. Res.* **2**, 246–250 (1970).

330. L.P. Bullock and C.W. Bardin, Androgen receptors in mouse kidney: A study of male, female and androgen-insensitive (*tfm/y*) mice, *Endocrinology* **94**, 746–756 (1974).

331. L.P. Bullock and C.W. Bardin, *In vivo* androgen retention in mouse kidney, *Steroids* **25**, 107–119 (1975).

332. U. Gehring, G.M. Tomkins, and S. Ohno, Effect of androgen insensitivity mutation on a cytoplasmic receptor for dihydrotestosterone, *Nature* **232**, 106–107 (1971).

333. B. Attardi and S. Ohno, Cytosol androgen receptor from kidney of normal and testicular feminized (Tfm) mice, *Cell* **2**, 205–212 (1974).

334. L.P. Bullock and C.W. Bardin, Androgen receptors in testicular feminization, *J. Clin. Endocrinol. Metab.* **35**, 935–937 (1972).

335. L.P. Bullock and C.W. Bardin, *In vivo* and *in vitro* testosterone metabolism by the androgen insensitive rat, *J. Steroid Biochem.* **4**, 139–151 (1973).

336. J. Imperato-McGinley, L. Guerrero, T. Gautier, and R.E. Peterson, Steroid 5α-reductase deficiency in man: An inherited form of male pseudohermaphroditism, *Science* **186**, 1213–1215 (1974).

337. W. Mainwaring and F.R. Mangan, A study of the androgen receptors in a variety of androgen-sensitive tissues, *J. Endocrinol.* **59**, 121–139 (1973).

338. S.A. Shain and L.R. Axelrod, Reduced high affinity 5-α-dihydrotestosterone receptor capacity in the ventral prostate of the aging rat, *Steroids* **21**, 801–812 (1973).

339. I. Jung and E.E. Baulieu, Neo-nuclear androgen receptor in rat ventral prostate, *Biochimie* **53**, 807–817 (1971).

340. J.N. Sullivan and C.A. Strott, Evidence for an androgen-independent mechanism regulating the levels of receptor in target tissue, *J. Biol. Chem.* **248**, 3202–3208 (1973).

341. N. Bruchovsky and S. Craven, Prostatic involution: Effect on androgen-receptors and intracellular androgen transport, *Biochem. Biophys. Res. Commun.* **62**, 837–843 (1975).

342. S. Liao, D.K. Howell, and T.-M. Chang, Action of a nonsteroidal antiandrogen, flutamide, on the receptor binding and nuclear retention of 5-α-dihydrotestosterone in rat ventral prostate, *Endocrinology* **94**, 1205–1209 (1974).

343. E.A. Peets, M.F. Henson, and R. Neri, On the mechanism of the antiandrogenic action of flutamide (α,α,α-Trifluoro-2-methyl-4'-nitro-*m*-propionotoluidide) in the rat, *Endocrinology* **94**, 532–540 (1974).

344. L. Terenius, Affinities of progestogen and estrogen receptors in rabbit uterus for synthetic progestens, *Steroids* **23**, 909–919 (1974).

345. C. Huggins, L.C. Grand, and F.P. Brillantes, Mammary cancer induced by a single feeding of polynuclear hydrocarbons, and its suppression, *Nature* **189**, 204–207 (1961).

346. J. Furth, Vistas in the etiology and pathogenesis of tumors, *Fed. Proc. Fed. Am. Soc. Exp. Biol.* **20**, 865–873 (1961).

347. E. Heise and M. Gorlich, Growth and therapy of mammary tumors induced by 7,12-Dimethylbenzanthracene in rats, *Br. J. Cancer* **20**, 539–545 (1966).

348. Cooperative Breast Cancer Group, Testosterone propionate therapy in breast cancer, *J. Am. Med. Assoc.* **188**, 1069–1072 (1964).

349. I.S. Goldenberg, N. Waters, R.S. Ravdin, F.J. Ansfield, and A. Segaloff, Androgenic therapy for advanced breast cancer in women, *J. Am. Med. Assoc.* **223**, 1267–1268 (1973).

350. H. Volk, R.J. Deupree, I.S. Goldenberg, R.C. Wilde, R.A. Carabasi, and G.C. Escher, A dose response evaluation of Delta-1-testololactone in advanced breast cancer, *Cancer* **33**, 9–13 (1974).

351. W.L. McGuire, Current status of estrogen receptors in human breast cancer, *Cancer* **36**, 638–644 (1975).

352. M. Lyon and P.H. Glenister, Evidence from *Tfm/0* that androgen is inessential for reproduction in female mice, *Nature* **247**, 366–367 (1974).

353. S. Ohno, L. Christian, and B. Attardi, Role of testosterone in normal female function, *Nature (London) New Biol.* **243** 119–120 (1973).

354. W. Elger and F. Neumann, The role of androgens in differentiation of the mammary gland in male mouse fetuses, *Proc. Soc. Exp. Biol. Med.* **123**, 637–640 (1966).

355. F. Neumann and W. Elger, The effect of the anti-androgen 1,2α-methylene-6-chloro-Δ4,6-pregradiene-17α-OL-3,20-dione-17α-acetate (cyproterone acetate) on the development of the mammary glands of male foetal rats, *J. Endocrinol.* **36**, 347–353 (1966).

356. R.K. Wagner, L. Gorlich, and P.W. Jungblut, Dihydrotestosterone receptor in human mammary cancer, *Acta Endocrinol.* **173**, 65 (1973).

357. J.P. Persijn, C.B. Korsten, and E. Engelsman, Oestrogen and androgen receptors in breast cancer and response to endocrine therapy, *Br. Med. J.* **4**, 503 (1975).

358. J. Poortman, J.A.C. Pregnen, F. Schwarz, and J.H.H. Thijssen, Interaction of Δ⁵-androstene-3β-17β-diol with estradiol and dihydrotestosterone receptors in human myometrial and mammary cancer tissue, *J. Clin. Endocrinol. Metab.* **40**, 373–379 (1975).

359. M.E. Lippman, G. Bolan and K. Huff, Human breast cancer responsive to androgen in long term tissue culture, *Nature* **258**, 339–341 (1975).

360. W.R. Miller, D. McDonald, A.P.M. Forrest, and A.A. Shivas, Metabolism of androgens by human breast tissue, *Lancet* **1**, 912–913 (1973).

361. L. Raith, A. Wirtz, M. Wiedemann, and H.J. Karl, Metabolism of testosterone and androstendione in human breast carcinoma and its relation to sexual hormone receptors, *Acta Endocrinol.* **177**, 28–29 (1973).

362. J.S. Jenkins and S. Ash, Metabolism of testosterone by human breast tumors, *Lancet* **2**, 513–514 (1972).
363. L.I. Rose, R.H. Underwood, M.T. Dunning, G. Williams, and G.S. Pinkus, Testosterone metabolism in benign and malignant breast lesions, *Cancer* **36**, 399–403 (1975).
364. N. Bruchovsky and J.W. Meakin, The metabolism and binding of testosterone in androgen-dependent and autonomous transplantable mouse mammary tumors, *Cancer Res.* **33**, 1689–1695 (1973).
365. K. Yamaguchi, H. Kasai, T. Minesita, K. Kotoh, and K. Matsumoto, 5α-Reduction and binding of testosterone in androgen-dependent and independent mouse mammary tumors, *Endocrinology* **95**, 1424–1430 (1974).
366. N. Bruchovsky, D.J.A. Sutherland, J.W. Meakin, and T. Minesita, Androgen receptors: relationship to growth response and to intracellular androgen transport in nine variant lines of the Shionogi mouse mammary tumor, *Biochim. Biophys. Acta* **381**, 61–71 (1975).
367. J.A. Smith and R.J.B. King, Effects of steroids on growth of an androgen-dependent mouse mammary carcinoma in cell culture, *Exp. Cell Res.* **73**, 351–359 (1972).
368. D.J.A. Sutherland, E.C. Robins, and J.W. Meakin, Effects of androgens on Shionogi carcinoma 115 cells *in vitro*, *J. Natl. Cancer Inst.* **52**, 37–48 (1974).
369. J. Gordon, J.A. Smith, and R.J.B. King, Metabolism and binding of androgens by mouse mammary tumour cells in culture, *Mol. Cell. Endocrinol.* **1**, 259–270 (1974).
370. S.K. Quadri, G.S. Kledzik, and J. Meites, Counteraction by prolactin of androgen-induced inhibition of mammary tumor growth in rats, *J. Natl. Cancer Inst.* **52**, 875–878 (1974).
371. P.S. Kalra, C.P. Fawcett, L. Krulich, and S.M. McCann, The effects of gonadal steroids on plasma gonadotropins and prolactin in the rat, *Endocrinology* **92**, 1256–1268 (1973).
372. Y.J. Abul-Hajj, Metabolism of dehydroepiandrosterone by hormone dependent and hormone independent human breast carcinoma, *Steroids* **26**, 488–500 (1975).
373. A. Nimrod and K.J. Ryan, Aromatization of androgens by human abdominal and breast fat tissue, *J. Clin. Endocrinol. Metab.* **40**, 367–372 (1975).
374. H. Rochefort, F. Lignon, and F. Capony, Formation of estrogen nuclear receptor in uterus: Effect of androgens, estrone and nafoxidine, *Biochem. Biophys. Res. Commun.* **47**, 662–676 (1972).
375. T.S. Ruh and M.F. Ruh, Androgen induction of a specific uterine protein, *Endocrinology* **97**, 1144–1150 (1975).
376. W.N. Schmidt, M.A. Sadler, and B.S. Katzenellenbogen, Androgen–uterine interaction: Nuclear translocation of the estrogen receptor and induction of the synthesis of the uterine-induced protein (IP) by high concentrations of androgens *in vitro* but not *in vivo*, *Endocrinology* **98**, 702–716 (1976).
377. H. Rochefort, in: *Research on Steroids* Pergamon Vieweg, Oxford (1976), in press.
378. N. Deshpande, V. Jensen, R.D. Bulbrook, T. Berne, and F. Ellis, Accumulation of tritiated oestradiol by human breast tissue, *Steroids* **10**, 219–232 (1967).
379. B.G. Mobbs, The effect of testosterone treatment on the uptake of ³H-oestradiol-17β by dimethylbenzanthracene-induced rat mammary tumors, *J. Endocrinol.* **48**, 293–294 (1970).
380. D.T. Zava and W.L. McGuire, Androgen induced depletion of estrogen receptor in rat mammary tumors, *Cancer Res.* (1977), in press.

6

The Changing Role of Radiation Therapy in Breast Cancer

A STUDY IN THERAPEUTIC CONTROVERSY

HENRY M. KEYS AND PHILIP RUBIN

1. Introduction

Change in therapy has become the standard approach for the management of breast cancer in this multidisciplinary era. The role of radiation therapy is changing, as is the role of surgery. Radical mastectomy is no longer generally acceptable as the treatment of choice by surgeons, and routine postoperative radiation therapy is in dispute among radiation oncologists. With newer methods of detection and advances in adjuvant chemotherapy programs, a new literature is emerging and new approaches offering better survival results and better cosmesis are promised. Individualization, rather than standardization, marks the therapeutic effort in most cancer centers.

Virtually all forms of treatment and, in particular, radiation therapy, are controversial in breast cancer care. The most dramatic impact during this past year upon the role of radiation therapy in breast cancer has been the success achieved in adjuvant chemotherapy programs. The axiom of the need for five-year and ten-year survival results to be certain of gains in this disease has been supplanted by computerized and projected relapse-free survival curves with median follow-up times of one to two years. National Cooperative Group studies and foreign controlled

HENRY M. KEYS AND PHILIP RUBIN · Division of Radiation Oncology, Strong Memorial Hospital, Rochester, New York. This paper was supported in part by the Clinical Radiation Research Center Grant No. CA-11051-08.

trials have replaced the large series of major cancer institutions and universities. Enthusiasm for early results needs to be tempered by time, and the broader participation in protocols by clinicians needs to be more widely accepted.

Central to all studies is the comparability of patients. Randomization is only one aspect in clinical studies where patient selection can modify outcome. Proper and agreed-upon staging and classification of breast cancer patients are essential for comparison of end results. There is a need to develop a therapeutic index which reports survival in terms of not only relapse-free rates, but also complication-free survival. Combinations of treatment modalities currently are prescribed for all stages, but such treatment still needs to be graduated and optimized for the different stages of advancement upon presentation. The best combination of treatment offers not only the promise of the best survival, but also less toxicity.

The controversies surrounding the use of radiation therapy in breast cancer are the format of presentation in this chapter. This will be done by examining a controversial issue for each stage of advancement of breast cancer. This format will allow for the examination of conservatism versus radicalism in treatment, optimum combination of treatment, immunosuppression by radiation, indications for definitive postoperative and preoperative radiation therapy, best and current results of radiation therapy, and recommendations as to which radiation techniques to use with illustrative cases.

2. Stage I

2.1. The Controversy

Statement of Controversy: Can excisional biopsy (tylectomy) and radiation be as effective as radical mastectomy in early breast cancer? Is radiation carcinogenic and capable of inducing second primaries?

There are many data in the literature indicating that the results with tylectomy or lumpectomy are comparable to radical mastectomy.[1–11] However, there have been no randomized prospective trials to attempt to answer this question. Over the years, selected groups of patients have been treated for localized Stage I breast cancer using this more conservative approach of excising the lump or mass and irradiation. Table I summarizes the results of several series. Although a number of early papers emphasized the good survival (comparable to radical mastectomy series) obtained by their patients, it is now generally recognized that survival reflects the presence or absence of systemic metastatic dis-

Table I

Results of Tylectomy and Radiation Therapy for Early Breast Cancer

Author, year	No. of patients	Survival	Relapse-free survival	Recurrence[a]	Dose (rads)	Comment
Atkins et al., 1972[2]	St. I: 112 St. II: 70	78% } 5 yr 56%		13% 43%	2500 → 3800 2500 → 3800	Very low doses
Farrow et al., 1971[2]	St. I: 28 St. II: 49			50% 68%	3000 → 9000	55% had less than 6000 rads
Rissanen, 1969[3]	St. I: 415	79% 5 yr 71% 10 yr		25%	2500 → 3500	Low doses
Peters, 1970[4]	St. I: 66		62.1%	10.8% T, 4.6% N	4500	Intermediate dose
Proznitz et al., 1975[5]	St. I: 13 St. II: 19		{ 94%	3%T	6000+	Boosting implant often done
Wise et al., 1971[11]	St. I: 49 St. II: 47	95% 5 yr[b] 71% 5 yr[b]		9.4% T	6100 average	All external treatment
Fletcher, 1972[6]	St. I: 69 St. II: 13		87% 78%	3%	5000	All external treatment
Hellman, 1976[7]	St. I } St. II } 60	90% 4 yr 60% 4 yr	95% 75%	0 0	5000 → 7000 5000 → 8000 5000 → 8000	Most had interstitial boost

[a]Local = T; regional = N.
[b]Predicted "ultimate survival" (Boag–Warner method).

ease at the time of diagnosis, and as such is not significantly affected by local forms of treatment, such as radiation therapy and surgery.

Local and regional recurrence (or its prevention) is a more appropriate indication of the effectiveness of locoregional treatment methods, i.e., radiation therapy and/or surgery. The more recent reports reflect that realization and analyze their patients for the ability of the treatment provided to control disease in the area to which it is applied as well as to produce survival rates. The argument for radical surgery in localized breast cancer is that superior local control is obtained by this technique. Indeed, local–regional recurrences are uncommon after radical mastectomy in Stage I breast cancer. By contrast, there exist series of patients treated with radiation therapy only after biopsy or excision in which the local–regional recurrence rate is reported to be moderately or extraordinarily high, suggesting that surgical local control is better. The experiences most often cited in this context (the first three in Table I) are those of Atkins et. al.,[1] Farrow et al.,[2] and Rissanen.[3]

The first report is the London Guys Hospital trial reported by Atkins et al.[1] This was a well-controlled prospective trial, with patients having Stage I or II carcinoma of the breast randomly assigned to either radical mastectomy, thio-TEPA, and postoperative irradiation versus wide local excision, thio-TEPA, and radiation therapy. Overall, there was no difference in survival between the two treatment regimes. However, when Stage I and II are studied separately, a significant survival advantage is seen in the Stage II patients who had radical mastectomy—when the small number of patients available for ten-year follow-up are compared, but not when the larger five-year follow-up is tallied. The survival in Stage I patients was identical for the two treatment arms. Local recurrences were more common in the local-excision groups, both Stage I (15% versus 4%) and Stage II (43% versus 11%). After radical mastectomy, 12 of 13 local recurrences were in the chestwall skin, and the incidence of cutaneous recurrence was about the same in the excision group. The most common recurrent site in the latter group was the axilla, which accounted for almost one-half the recurrences in both Stages I and II.

The preceding analysis excludes the most important fact about this study, the low radiation dose utilized. The radiation dose employed was 2500–2700 rads in 12 days to the supraclavicular and axillary areas and 3800 rads in three weeks to the breast. These doses are inadequately low by current standards,[12] so that the high local and, especially, regional (axillary) rates of reappearance of disease are to be expected. The 25% local recurrence rate reported by Rissanen in a large series (415) of Stage I patients[3] is similarly expected for the same reason.

The third paper reporting a high recurrence rate is that of Farrow *et al.*[2] This seemingly randomized study, because of the number chosen of each series, accumulated 77 patients for each of three different treatments, in a retrospective review. For comparison, one group was treated with radiation after various forms of biopsy or local excision and a matched cohort of patients were picked from several thousand treated by radical mastectomy alone or with postoperative irradiation. While the clinical characteristics of the three groups were essentially identical, the recurrence rates certainly were not, and the degree of axillary node involvement was not. Not enough information is given to assess the adequacy of the irradiation techniques, but in terms of dose, 55% of the patients had less than 6000 rads, and both local control and survival appeared better above that level. Most of the patients had sizable remaining tumor after aspiration or incisional biopsy (average 5.1 cm), as well as axillary adenopathy in 49 of 77 patients. Doses of 3000 to 6000 rads would not be expected to control such disease. The fact that these patients were treated in three different hospitals, over many years, by a variety of physicians using many techniques, also undoubtedly added to the overall poor results, and discards this as a meaningful study or experience.

The other side of the controversy rests on the evidence reported by several authors that limited surgery and radiation for localized Stage I cancer can be effective with good cosmetic result, low risk of local recurrence, and at no significant survival disadvantage. In other words, the treatment by radiation therapy after minimal surgery is a reasonable alternative. Series 4–8 in Table I summarize these studies.

Peters[4] found a group of 66 patients treated by excisional biopsy and irradiation in a larger review of breast cancer treatment for localized stages at the Princess Margaret Hospital. After segmental resection, 4500 rads (usually) was given in four weeks to the breast and surrounding nodal areas. This resulted in only 10.8% local and 4.6% regional recurrence. The basis for selection is not detailed, but most likely involved refusal of surgery or medical contraindication to more extensive surgery. Similarly, 96 Stage I and Stage II mammary cancer patients were treated by simple excision and radiation therapy to an average dose of 6100 rads in nine weeks, and the results were reported by Wise *et al.*[11] Survival was good (five-year survival: Stage I = 95%, Stage II = 71%), and only nine patients (9.4%) suffered local recurrences.

The best results, however, are reported in the most recent series (Prosnitz *et al.*,[5] Fletcher,[6] and Hellman[7,8]). After excision (or, in some cases, biopsy) in selected Stage I patients, carefully individualized irradiation was delivered to the breast and surrounding lymph node areas. Doses of 5000 rads to areas without clinical evidence of disease were supplemented by external beam boosting arrangements (Fletcher) or interstitial techniques to raise the dose in high-risk areas to 6500 to 8000 rads (Hellman). The local recurrence rates of 0–3% and relapse-free survival at four years of 87–95% attest to the effectiveness of this approach.

In the foregoing discussion, both Stage I and Stage II patients were about equal in numbers and included in most of the papers cited. Thus, even in patients with axillary metastases, a conservative approach coupled with aggressive local and regional radiation can give very high local control rates and relapse-free survival (75–78% for four years). There is little doubt, however, that this approach is highly effective in T_1 and T_2, N_0, M_0 Stage I patients.

One difficulty encountered with the irradiated breast is that it is not easy to assess in follow-up examinations. Fibrofatty atrophy, skin and subcutaneous thickening, and preexisting fibrocystic disease make interpretation of palpatory findings a challenge, especially for the inexperienced examiner. Our own experience corroborates that of Wise et al.,[11] who noted that several apparent recurrences were, in fact, benign when biopsied.

Mammography may be helpful, especially in following the regression of mammographically visible lesions. However, serial studies (rather than single observations) are essential, and the dynamic alterations with time, which result from irradiation, may confuse the picture somewhat. Table II, from Bloomer et al.,[13] outlines the sequential changes expected after irradiation.

The carcinogenic effect of radiation should be mentioned here, as its potential detrimental effect could be a concern in those patients with a

Table II
Expected Mammographic Changes Following Definitive Breast Irradiation[a]

Mammographic finding	<6 months	>6 months
Size of mass	Decreased	Absent
Skin thickening	Variable	Present
Peau d'orange	Decreased	Increased
Inflammatory carcinoma	Increased	Increased
Prominent draining veins	Decreased	Decreased
Subcutaneous fibrosis	Progressive increase	Progressive increase
Size of breast	Progressive retraction (dose-dependent)	Progressive retraction (dose-dependent)
Calcifications	No significant change	No significant change

[a]From Bloomer et al. [13]

relatively good prognosis. The BEIR (Biological Effects of Ionizing Radiations) Report of 1972[14] discusses in detail the life-shortening effect of low-dose irradiation and carefully analyzes the impact of various doses of such irradiation on present and future generations. This sobering document is well worth reading, but it is important to recognize that low-dose whole-population data cannot be extrapolated to higher doses. In fact, second neoplasms can occur after radiation therapy, but do so only rarely, and then more often after low to intermediate doses. As a practical concern, the likelihood of cancer induction after radiation therapy of localized breast cancer is very small.[15]

2.2. Indications for Treatment

Conservative surgical excision of the mass or lump and radiation therapy are a reasonable alternative to radical mastectomy for early breast cancer. Women with slightly larger lesions in the central or medial portions of small breasts may have so little breast left that the cosmetic effect is poor. Also, some patients with extremely large breasts may be tecnically difficult to irradiate uniformly. However, for the majority of patients with clinical Stage I breast cancer, there is an alternative to radical mastectomy which has given equally good results to the more traditional approach. To assure that the patient has a choice of treatment, excisional biopsy and subsequent discussion with the patient are required, rather than frozen biopsy and immediate mastectomy while the patient is anesthesized if the biopsy is positive.

Should surgical "staging" of the axilla be part of such a program? There is some enthusiasm for limited axillary exploration to establish the status of axillary nodes for prognostic purposes, and to "debulk" the positive nodal disease encountered. There is a logic to this approach, particularly to detect those high-risk patients with multiple nodes involved for systemic adjuvant chemotherapy. However, the probability of finding nodal metastases is approximately one out of three,[11] and the radiation doses employed would be expected to control greater than 90% of the occult nodal disease present.[12] We currently favor axillary staging procedures which aid in treatment decisions for patients and which can provide useful information for both the choice of adjuvant chemotherapy and future analysis of the result of treatment.

Which form of biopsy is best: excisional, incisional, or aspiration? We advocate excisional biopsy, wedge resection, or tylectomy whenever possible, although generous margins around tumors are not essential. It is technically easier and biologically better to treat patients who have no gross residual tumor, whereas higher doses must be employed to achieve the same high local control rate if the mass was not removed.

The radiobiological arguments are identical for radiation control of local chest-wall recurrence with or without mastectomy.

2.3. Technique of Treatment

Each patient should have an individualized treatment plan designed to deliver the desired doses where prescribed and to spare normal uninvolved tissue to the greatest degree possible. All treatment should be given with modern megavoltage equipment.

The aim of treatment is to eradicate any residual tumor in the breast as well as the axillary, supraclavicular, and internal mammary lymph nodes. Doses of 4500 rads in four weeks or 5000 rads in five weeks are recommended for occult metastatic deposits in lymph node areas. After apparently complete excision of the primary breast cancer, 5000 rads

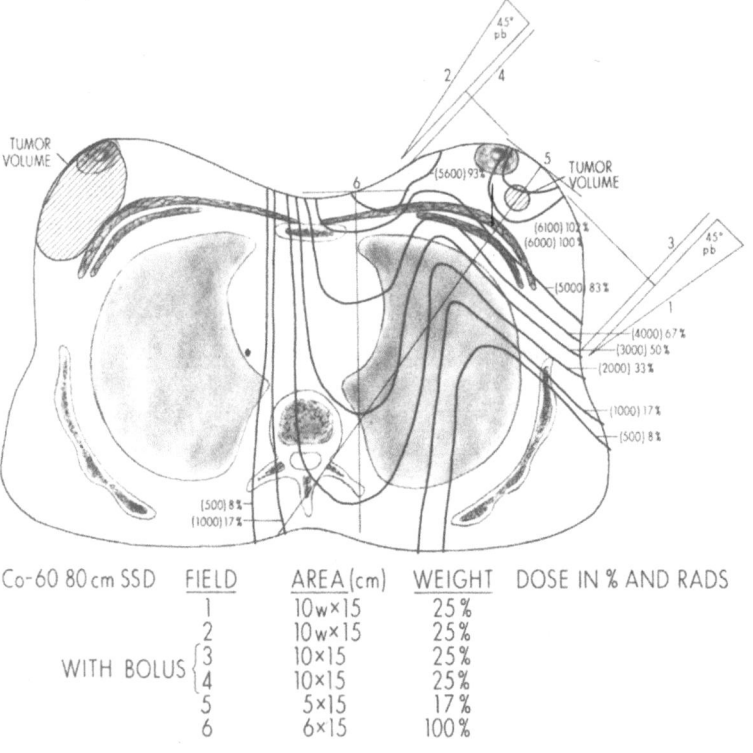

Co-60 80 cm SSD	FIELD	AREA (cm)	WEIGHT	DOSE IN % AND RADS
	1	10 w×15	25%	
	2	10 w×15	25%	
WITH BOLUS {	3	10×15	25%	
	4	10×15	25%	
	5	5×15	17%	
	6	6×15	100%	

Fig. 1. Parallel opposed tangential breast fields with a separate internal mammary field and a single small-boost cobalt-60 field to the area of the primary tumor bed. This effectively raises the dose in the primary tumor bed to 6000 rads (6100 maximum).

may be adequate, but the most successful series have included an additional 1500 rads or more by either external or interstitial means, raising the total tumor-bed dose to 6500–8000 rads. If axillary sampling is negative, and the patient had an outer-quadrant lesion, then the lymphatic irradiation could be excluded and only the breast need be treated.

The accompanying case and treatment plans demonstrate the modern dosimetry methodology and results.

Case Example: 47-year-old woman with 2-cm central breast mass. Excision was performed and the finding was infiltrating ductal carcinoma. No axillary dissection was performed. In this case, we wanted to treat the entire breast to 5000 rads uniformly and boost the dose to the excision site. The lymph nodes were also to be treated to 5000 rads. The procedure followed was as follows:

1. Reproduce the patient's anatomic cross section on paper through the use of ultrasound or solder-wire contour taking.

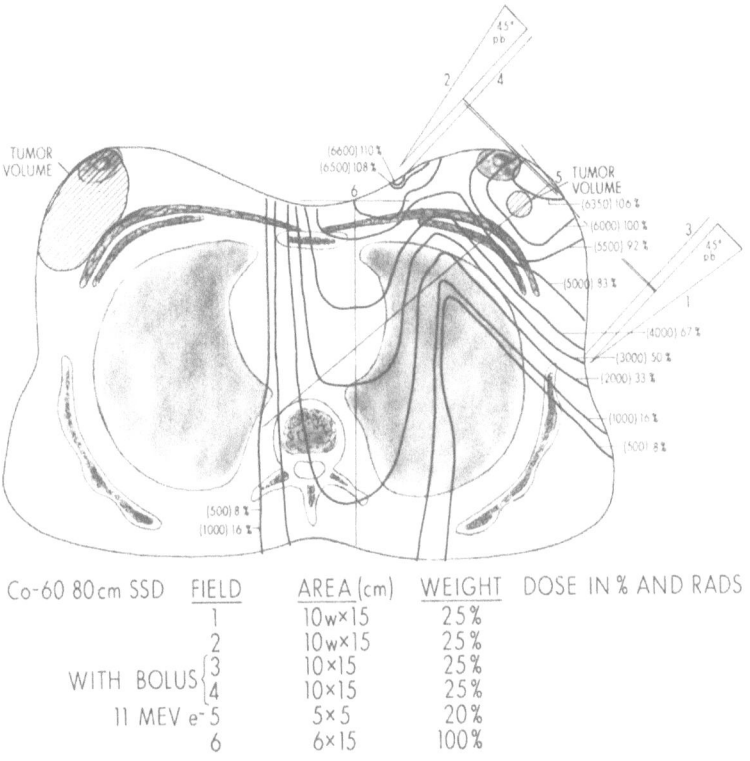

Co-60 80cm SSD	FIELD	AREA (cm)	WEIGHT	DOSE IN % AND RADS
	1	10w×15	25%	
	2	10w×15	25%	
WITH BOLUS	{3	10×15	25%	
	4	10×15	25%	
11 MEV e⁻	5	5×5	20%	
	6	6×15	100%	

Fig. 2. The same basic treatment scheme as in Fig. 1 is shown here. However, here the boost dose to the primary tumor bed is given with 11-MeV electrons. Again, 6000 rads is achieved in the tumor bed (6350 maximum). Because of the limited penetrance of the electron beam, a lower total lung dose is given in this case compared to Fig. 1.

2. Transpose the tumor volume and/or areas at risk for recurrence onto the cross-sectional contour.

3. Supply the treatment-planning team (medical physicist, dosimetrist, and technologist) with a prescription indicating what doses and dose variations are desired and acceptable. This must include any normal tissues with potentially dose-limiting radiation tolerance levels, and how much is acceptable there. (Example: Lung to receive not more than 2000 rads to 50% of lung.) The location of these structures should be indicated on the contours.

4. The treatment-planning team will then devise one or more plans from which the therapist can pick the best (Figs. 1–3).

The cosmetic result obtained in this patient one year after excisional biopsy is shown in Fig. 4.

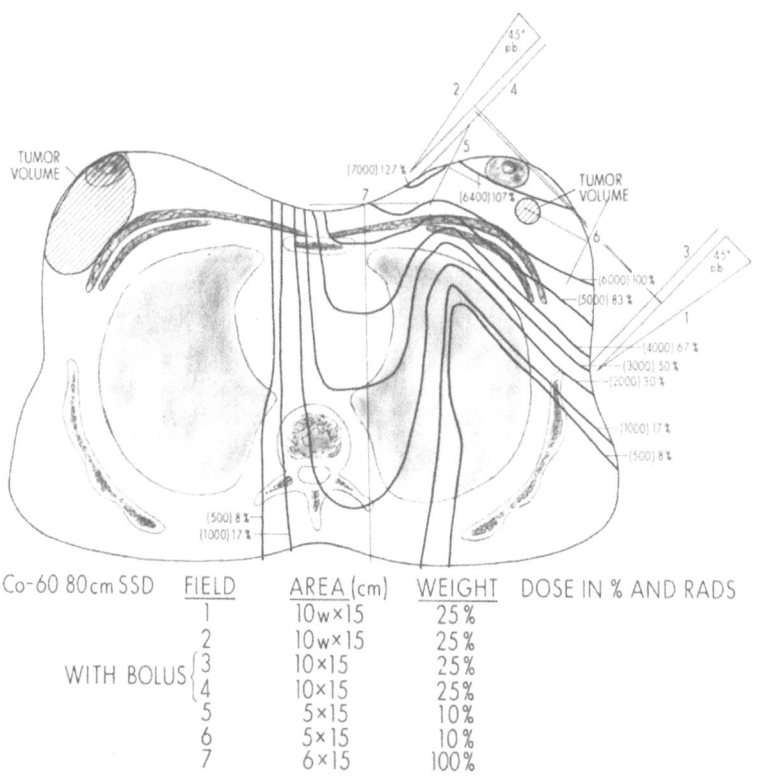

Co-60 80cmSSD	FIELD	AREA (cm)	WEIGHT	DOSE IN % AND RADS
	1	10w×15	25%	
	2	10w×15	25%	
WITH BOLUS {	3	10×15	25%	
	4	10×15	25%	
	5	5×15	10%	
	6	5×15	10%	
	7	6×15	100%	

Fig. 3. The use of small parallel opposed tangential fields to boost the primary-tumor-bed dose is shown. The boost fields do not contribute any additional pulmonary dose, and adequately raise the tumor-bed dose to 6000 rads (6400 maximum).

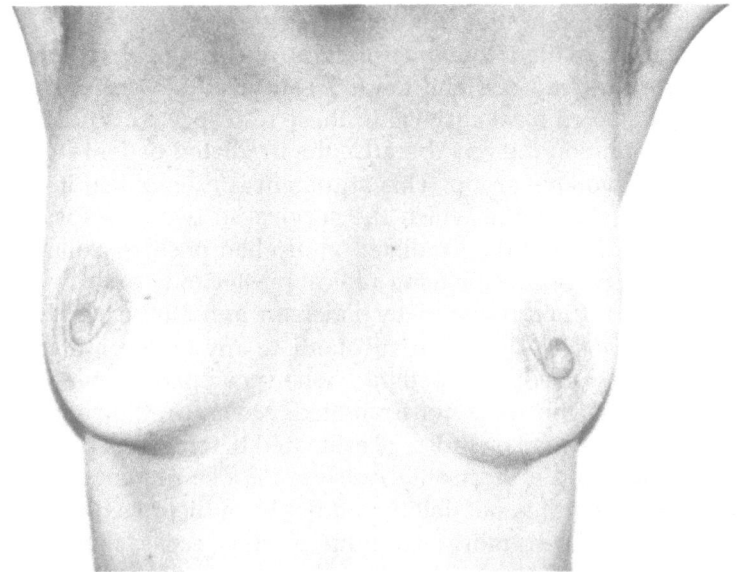

Fig. 4. This patient is shown one year after excisional biopsy of a 2-cm infiltrating ductal carcinoma from the mid-outer-right breast. Axillary staging was negative. The breast was treated as shown in Fig. 1. Physical examination and mammography are unremarkable.

3. Stage II

3.1. The Controversy

Statement of Controversy: Is there a role for postoperative radiation therapy in Stage II breast cancer in view of the advance in adjuvant chemotherapy? Does radiation therapy reduce rather than increase survival? Is radiation therapy of the chest wall and surrounding nodes systemically immunosuppressive? How is lymphopenia related to host resistance?

In the management of any malignancy, the first goal is to improve survival. The absence of appropriate randomized trials to specifically evaluate the influence of postoperative irradiation on survival led to the use of nonrandom retrospective data. Several such studies appeared to show a survival advantage of approximately 10% for those patients given postoperative irradiation,[16–18] as compared to those who were not treated. In fact, it was reasonable to expect that some patients would have occult residual local or regional disease without distant metastases, and this group would benefit from postoperative irradiation. Data from

Chu et al.[19] support this concept. They report that of 215 patients treated with radiation therapy for local and regional recurrence, 44 (20%) survived five years and ten (5%) survived ten years. It was also assumed that even *equal* survival in these retrospective studies favored the use of radiation therapy, because the irradiated patients were likely to be a less favorable group. This argument is exemplified in Table III, from Fletcher et al.,[20] in which the survival in two series is the same (62–63%), but 29% of the irradiated group had positive axillary nodes, compared to 9% of those having radical mastectomy only.

Controlled trials reported by Paterson and Russell,[21] Easson,[22] and Fisher et al.[23] all failed to substantiate any survival advantage in postoperatively irradiated patients when compared to comparably staged patients who were not irradiated. Raventos,[24] using statistical inference as suggested by Bross,[25] estimated that regional postoperative radiotherapy could at best only cause a 5% rise in "cure rates," and further stated that this possibility had not been disproved in any of the trials to date. Even more damning is the recent suggestion that radiotherapy decreases survival because of immunosuppression. This proposition by Stjernsward,[26] based on weak and contradictory evidence, will be dismantled later.

It seems reasonable to conclude that there is only a small proportion of patients with breast cancer whose survival can be improved by postoperative radiotherapy; that is, those patients with residual regional disease after surgery who do not have distant metastases. The survival argument may well not justify the routine use of postoperative irradiation in Stage II breast cancer.

Table III
Ten-Year Survival in Two Radical Mastectomy Series
at M. D. Anderson Hospital (January, 1955–December, 1967)[a,b]

Treatment	No. of patients	Percent of axillary nodes histologically positive	Percent survival
Radical mastectomy only[c]	246	9	63
Irradiation (peripheral lymphatics and breast) + radical mastectomy	419	29	62

[a]From Fletcher et al.[20]
[b]Age-adjusted survival rate: Berkson–Gage.
[c]These patients had primary lesions located in the outer half of the breast with histologically negative axilla. The 9% who had positive axillary lymph nodes should have had postoperative irradiation, but, for a variety of reasons, did not.

To analyze the effectiveness of surgery or irradiation, survival alone is not adequate; it reflects the natural history of the disease more than the effect of the treatment. Perhaps one can make judgments about the appropriateness of local forms of treatment based on survival, but, again, to judge effectiveness the local–regional control of disease in the treated volume should be studied. It is also logical to control the disease in the primary tumor (T) and the regional node (N) compartments as a prerequisite to the introduction of systemic agents to control the occult disease in the metastatic (M) compartment.

While many authors reported in retrospective studies that local and regional recurrences were lessened after postoperative irradiation, it was not until the "Manchester trial" that accurate data were available.[21] In this important study, patients with "operable" breast cancer were randomly assigned to have radical mastectomy alone, or followed by postoperative irradiation, as their initial treatment. Within the study, there were two separate series (1949–1952 and 1952–1954) in which the postoperative radiation was different. The patients who were randomly assigned to be watched were treated with irradiation when they developed recurrence. A total of 1461 cases were entered in the study.

The findings challenged the wisdom of routine postoperative irradiation. First, as mentioned earlier, there was no significant difference in survival, indicating that those patients who were to die of metastases already had occult hematogenous dissemination at the time of the original treatment. Second, the irradiated patients, regardless of which technique was used, had notably lower rates of recurrence in the flap, axilla, and supraclavicular areas. Table IV gives the actual data. The "quadrate" technique delivered adequate doses to the chest wall and axilla, and did not effectively treat the supraclavicular region. The recurrence rates reflect the dosimetric inadequacies of each technique.

The third question to which the protocol addressed itself was how effectively these recurrences could be treated once they occurred. From examination of their data, it is evident that about one-half of the recurrences in the "watched" patients were successfully managed once they occurred. There were fewer patients in the "treated" groups who died with recurrent disease present, but this difference is less striking than the initial recurrence rates.

This study has led to two opposing conclusions: first, that routine postoperative irradiation is not needed because the recurrences can be effectively managed when they appear, and, alternatively, that postoperative irradiation can effectively prevent recurrences and could do so to a greater extent with a better technique combining the strong points of both the "quadrate" and "peripheral" techniques.

Table IV
Local and Regional Recurrences in Breast Cancer Patients—
Results of the "Manchester Trial"[a]

	Quadrate		Peripheral	
Recurrence site	Treated	Watched	Treated	Watched
Percent recurrence:				
Operation flap	11.0	19.9	16.2	19.9
Axilla	3.1	10.9	5.7	7.3
Supraclavicular	15.0	17.1	6.3	17.3
Percent with recurrence at death:				
Operation flap	9.8	11.7	9.8	12.2
Axilla	1.8	4.8	3.6	3.0
Supraclavicular	8.0	9.7	4.3	7.4

[a]From Paterson and Russell.[21]

In the initial design of the "quadrate" technique, very little attention was paid to the internal mammary nodes. In fact, Handley and Thackray[27] were the first to clearly identify the internal mammary lymph node areas as a common site of metastatic spread from carcinoma of the breast. It became apparent in radical mastectomy series that there was a significant incidence of involved internal mammary nodes, which was as high as 48% of all cases with positive axillary nodes.[28] Haagensen *et al.*[29] reported an overall incidence of 32.5% internal mammary node metastases for 1007 patients treated by radical mastectomy: 19.6% for those with negative axillary nodes, 33.5% for those with axillary disease of less than 2.5 cm in diameter, and 50.2% for those with axillary disease larger than 2.5 cm in diameter. These represent selected biopsies in those patients in whom they felt there was a higher than average risk of internal mammary involvement and therefore the percentages are inflated. However, Handley and Thackray,[30] have reported that the incidence of internal mammary node metastases also varied considerably with the location of the tumor in the breast. Outer-quadrant lesions with axillary metastases had a 23% incidence, central lesions a 49% incidence, and medial-quadrant lesions a 54% incidence of internal mammary lymph node metastatic disease by biopsy. The importance of these findings is that except for the relatively few advocates of supraradical mastectomy with internal mammary lymph node dissection or chestwall resection, these lymph nodes, proven to be tumor-bearing in a relatively high percentage, go untreated when only radical mastectomy is employed. This information was a major stimulus for the use of routine postoperative radiation therapy in patients with positive axillary lymph nodes or with medial and central lesions in the breast. While the incidence of internal mammary lymph node metastases on biopsy is high, the incidence of parasternal or clinical internal mammary lymph node recurrence is relatively low. Haagensen *et al.*[31] reported only 24 parasternal recurrences in patients followed for ten years, out of a total series of 626 patients (less than 3%). This incidence of recurrence rose to as high as 10% in those patients with central or inner-quadrant lesions, as reported by Urban.[32] Perhaps this is due to a deep spread of internal mammary lymph nodes into the mediastinal nodes and dissemination from this focus, rather than superficial appearance as parasternal nodules.

In this country, the National Surgical Adjuvant Breast Project (NSABP) clinical trial addressed the question of the role of postoperative irradiation.[23] However, there are some major objections to the study,[33] such as a very high exclusion of patients receiving radiotherapy; i.e., 48.6% of the patients assigned to receive postoperative irradiation were excluded for various reasons. The data, however, tend to support the Manchester conclusions. There was no apparent survival advantage, but local and regional recurrences were reduced (Table V). This study has been redone and data should become available to either substantiate this issue or disprove it.

Two other series are worth including here. First, Chu, Lucas, Farrow, and Nickson[34] analyzed 790 patients in terms of patterns of failure after surgery alone and surgery plus postoperative irradiation. As in the previous studies, this was orthovoltage radiation to lower doses than are currently used. When comparing patients with similar stages of disease, they found no significant difference in survival or in local recurrence rates, with the exception of marked reduction in supraclavicular recurrences in irradiated patients with positive axillary dissections (10% versus 23% for the unirradiated group).

Perhaps the best demonstration of the effectiveness of modern megavoltage radiotherapy given in adequate doses to prevent local and regional recurrences is from M.D. Anderson Hospital as presented by Nelson and Montague.[35] Their figures show that supraclavicular and parasternal recurrences can be eliminated altogether by postoperative irradiation. Elective treatment of the chest wall in high-risk patients is also shown to be effective in reducing the recurrence rate from the 25–45% reported by others[34,36,37] to 10% or less. Table V summarizes data from a number of reports on recurrence and survival rates in breast cancer patients.

All of the data presented thus far have compared radical mastectomy to radical mastectomy plus radiation therapy. McWhirter[17] demonstrated that simple mastectomy plus postoperative radiotherapy was at least as effective as radical mastectomy. This led to the adoption of

Table V
Influence of Postoperative Irradiation on Recurrence and Survival in Patients with Axillary Metastases

Author, year	No. of patients		Chest-wall recurrence (%)		Regional recurrence (%)		Recurrence-free survival (%)		Dose (rads)
	XRT	No XRT	XRT	No XRT	XRT	No XRT	XRT	No XRT	
Robbins et al., 1966[38]	224	200			13[a]	26[a]	29	38	3500
Jackson, 1966[39]	709	752			11[a]	20[a]			3500
Host and Bernhovd, 1975[40]	109	92	8	15	2.8	14.1	53	50	2500–3500
Chu et al., 1967[34]	170	219	24	23	10	23	44[b]	47[b]	3500
Paterson and Russell, 1959[21]									
Quadrate	327	393	11	20	15	17	55	56.5	
Peripheral	382	359	16	20	6	17	57.1	61	
Fisher et al., 1970[23]	124	139	7	25	1	3	38	32	5000
Archambault et al., 1964[41]	168	—	4	—	2	—	54	—	4500–6000
Fletcher, 1972[6]	273	—	—	—	1.3	—	—	—	5000–5500

[a] Supraclavicular recurrences only.
[b] Absolute survival (not recurrence-free).

less radical operations by many surgeons, combined with the use of postoperative irradiation. It seems reasonable to expect that modified radical mastectomy, total mastectomy, or simple mastectomy would have increased local and regional recurrence rates without adjuvant radiotherapy.

This consideration becomes germane now that the trend is away from elective irradiation and toward adjuvant chemotherapy. This is the last portion of the postoperative irradiation controversy. It remains to be seen how effective these systemic agents are in preventing regional recurrences.

The preliminary and highly publicized data pertaining to results from the use of adjuvant systemic chemotherapy in advanced Stage II (four or more positive nodes) carcinoma of the breast raise further doubts as to what the role of postoperative radiation therapy is or should be in these patients. There have been few recurrences reported in a recent paper by Bonadonna et al.,[42] but follow-up is very short and more than half the patients were still being treated with multiple drugs at the time of the report. In the NSABP report, using Melphalan, there does not appear to be an excessive number of local recurrences in the premenopausal group, although there were indeed some patients who manifested local recurrence as the first sign of failure in the postmenopausal group.[43] Should the frequency of local recurrence remain low, a strong argument could be made for eliminating postoperative irradiation. Time, rather than verbal debate, is required to solidify computerized, projected survival curves years beyond the median follow-up time of the study.

Relatively few clinical trials under way will help clarify the role of radiation therapy in Stage II carcinomas of the breast; however, the recurrence rates from the various adjuvant chemotherapy protocols may clarify the situation.

Perhaps the most damaging type of criticism against the use of postoperative radiation therapy is the depression of local and systemic immunity, allowing the cancer to spread and reduce survival. The major current protagonist for this viewpoint has been Stjernsward.[26] Simplistically, he has theorized, based on anecdotal case observations, that the lymphopenia following irradiation is related to the host resistance to contain the cancer. Based on one case analysis, the major lymphocyte depression is that of the T-cell lymphocytes, again implying that these cells are responsible for immunologic defense in breast cancer patients. His further effort to establish this link was made utilizing the Mantel–Haenzel statistical procedure in examining data from the clinical trials concluding that an increased mortality occurred in irradiated patients. Refutation of this hypothesis by recently accumulated data follows.

Numerous investigations have shown that lymphopenia follows locoregional-field radiation therapy. Lundell demonstrated that patients receiving pre- or postoperative radiation therapy have a reduction in peripheral lymphocytes.[44] There is evidence that both T- and B-cell lymphocytes are affected, as measured by use of the transformation response. A prospective study done by a group of investigators at the Radiumhemmet* in a controlled clinical trial studying the value of preoperative radiation versus postoperative radiation versus mastectomy alone has correlated lymphocyte counts, transformation tests, metastasis formation, and survival. Local radiotherapy, given pre- or postoperatively, reduces peripheral lymphocytes to 50%.[41] Unlike Stjernsward's[26] observation, Blomgren et al.[45] have shown that mainly B-cell lymphocytes were affected, while T cells were increased. The relative responsiveness of lymphocytes to purified protein derivative of tubercle bacillus (PPD) in vitro was significantly reduced, but to the nonspecific mitogen phytohemaglutinin (PHA) or pokeweed mitogen (PWM) remained unchanged. The capacity of patients to maintain their natural serum antibody level to the common viruses as herpes simplex, cytomegalic virus, or morbilli, was unaffected.

More recent studies by Baral et al. have shown a more rapid repopulation of B-cell than T-cell lymphocytes in irradiated early breast cancer patients. This correlated with similar studies in seminoma patients.[46] Although there is a long-lasting peripheral lymphopenia, with recovery not fully achieved at two years, the PPD reactivity has reached original levels at five months postirradiation. The important observation is that metastases occurred equally in this aforementioned controlled trial in arms of the study at 18 to 36 months follow-up interval. Furthermore, the incidence of lymphopenia was significantly lower in patients with the discovery of metastases than in those patients without metastases. This suggests that the metastases are due to a loss of host resistance which in turn reflects, rather than causes, the loss of immunity.

The argument by Papatestas and Kark[47] suggests that there is a relationship between survival and the pretreatment lymphocyte count. In a study of 305 patients, they found that patients in all stages who remained free of metastases during the first five postmastectomy years had significantly higher pretreatment counts than those who did develop metastases or second primaries. Interestingly, while mean peripheral lymphocyte counts did not vary significantly among Stages I, II, III, and IV, and pretreatment, the separation of patients into disease-free recurrence groups during the first five years effectively separated two populations of patients on the basis of pretreatment lymphocyte

*The institution at which Stjernsward wrote his original paper.

counts. Again, there was little difference among the various stages in terms of lymphocyte count within those two groups. While Stjernsward and others have interpreted such data as an effect of treatment, it is the conclusion of Papatestas and Kark that the difference in lymphocyte counts in patients with breast cancer may be completely independent of treatment and could rather be attributed to the true stage of disease.

Other studies, more sophisticated in the extent to which they study immune reactivity, have found that, in fact, lymphocyte function as tested by the PHA test is intact. Roberts and Jones-Williams[48] postulate that "blocking factors in the serum interfere with the expression of lymphocyte sensitivity." In contradistinction are the papers by Gross et al.,[49] in which assessment of delayed hypersensitivity by dinitrochlorobenzine (DNCB) was not impaired in the majority of patients after radiation therapy, and by McCredie et al.,[50] in which PHA responsiveness of lymphocytes did not change or was increased in patients for the period of 11 months after treatment with radiation therapy.

The crux of the issue appears to be that there are a variety of measurable changes that occur in blood lymphocyte levels and in functional assays of systemic immune response. Whether or not any of these have any clinical significance when altered by a specific mode of therapy is unresolved at the present time. Nonetheless, there is concern among responsible radiation therapists that such influences on immunity may be detrimental to patients and further study is definitely warranted in this regard.

The mere argument that patients who present with depressed immunity have a poor prognosis does not imply that therapeutically altering some aspects of the immune response necessarily changes the prognosis. The immune response can improve if the cancer is controlled by irradiation. This is noted in two papers from the Albert Einstein College of Medicine[51,52] in which a delayed hypersensitivity reaction in patients treated with radical radiation therapy was evaluated relative to their ultimate response. The general result was that those who were able to mount a strong pretreatment hypersensitivity response to DNCB or croton oil proved to be better responders to radiation therapy and had longer survival. This corroborates other data suggesting that those patients who inherently have a stronger or more complete immune reactivity are able to handle their malignancy better and are more favorable responders to therapy, regardless of its direct effect on immune response.

A summary of the whole argument regarding potential negative effects of radiation therapy or immune suppression is presented in a brief paper by Stjernsward.[26] In this paper, a series of studies from Manchester, Copenhagen, Edinburgh, and the NSABP, one of which demonstrated significant differences in survival between those patients having surgery alone and those having surgery plus postoperative radiation therapy, are added together in such a way that the combined data suggest a negative effect of radiation on survival. There is serious question as to the validity of the simple addition of patients from a variety of different studies in which the stage and treatment techniques were vastly different and for which only one end point is being compared. Even if one were to accept the statistical result suggesting increased mortality among the patients given postoperative radiation therapy, the offered explanation that this survival difference is secondary to negative effects on the host immune response is without direct evidence.

3.2. Indications for Radiation Therapy

The indications for the selective use of postoperative irradiation should not be changed in light of currently available information. Such treatment, in skilled hands, using modern equipment, is effective in reducing local and regional recurrences, is well tolerated by the patients, and is without significant adverse side effects.

The situations in which the risk of chest-wall and surrounding lymph node recurrence are high enough to warrant this treatment are:

1. Simple or total mastectomy in patients with axillary node metastases.
2. Radical mastectomy with four or more positive axillary nodes.
3. Central or medial lesions with any axillary disease.

There are two other situations when the nodal status is uncertain in which postoperative node irradiation is indicated:

1. Central and medial lesions without axillary disease. (Treat the internal mammary and supraclavicular nodes.)
2. Simple mastectomy in patients without axillary dissection. (Here, again, the surrounding lymphatics should be irradiated.)

In time, the use of systemic adjuvant chemotherapy in controlled trials may demonstrate that local and regional recurrences can be effectively prevented. It is too early in the use of these programs to make such a judgment now.

3.3. Techniques of Treatment

The process of arriving at a treatment technique decision is basically the same here as for Stage I. The radiation oncologist must determine what volumes of tissue are at sufficient risk of recurrence to warrant treatment. This information must then be translated into a three-dimensional representation of the patient's anatomy so that individualized treatment planning can be done.

As indicated in Section 3.2, there are two distinct situations in which treatment is given. In one, apical axillary, supraclavicular, and internal mammary lymph node areas are to be treated. This is usually accomplished by cobalt-60 or similar-energy machinery with a straight anterior field shaped like an "inverted L." The second treatment situation is that in which there is a higher risk of chest-wall recurrence, and the decision is made to treat the operative site and the surgical scar, as well as surrounding lymphatics. This can be accomplished in two basically different ways. One is a modification of the "McWhirter technique" using tangential or glancing fields to treat the chest wall, while sparing the underlying lung. This may be combined with the inverted-L-shaped field discussed above. The second technique makes use of the limited range in tissue of high-energy electrons.[53] There are several advantages to this technique:

1. The thickness of the chest-wall tissues can be accurately determined by the use of diagnostic ultrasound (Fig. 5).

2. Electron-producing linear accelerators can produce a variety of electron energies, each with its own effective range in tissue. The energy which produces the optimal dose distribution can then be selected.

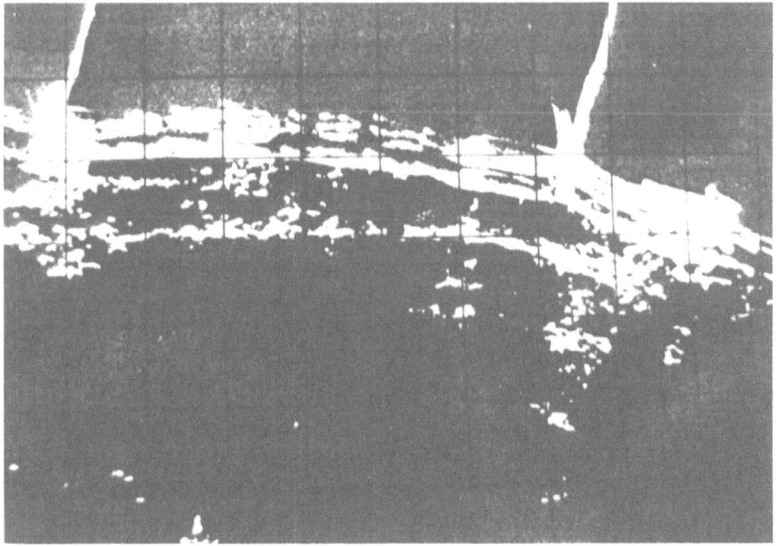

Fig. 5. There are many uses for diagnostic ultrasound in radiation therapy treatment planning. Here, the thickness of the chest wall is demonstrated, allowing accurate planning for chest-wall irradiation.

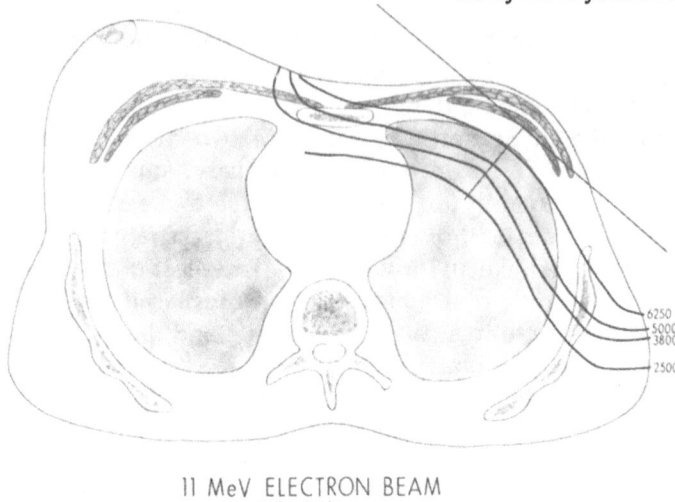

11 MeV ELECTRON BEAM
(20×25) cm

Fig. 6. A single, angled 11-MeV electron beam is used here to treat the chest wall and internal mammary lymph nodes. Note the rapid dose falloff with depth in tissue.

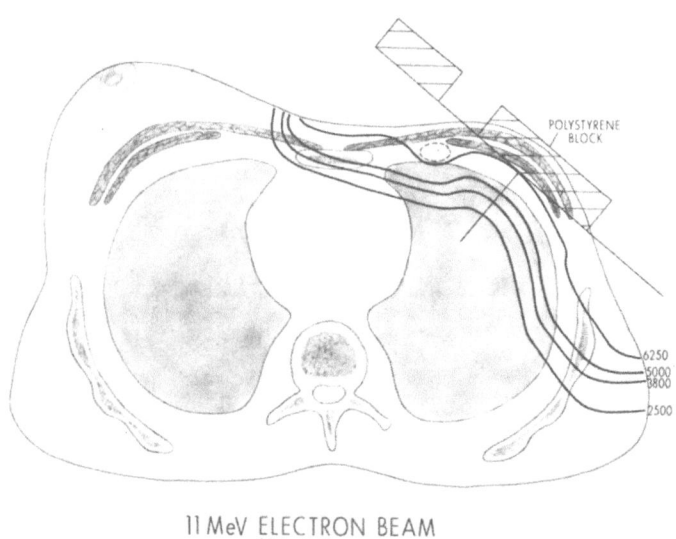

11 MeV ELECTRON BEAM
(20×25) cm

Fig. 7. The same electron beam as in Fig. 6 is shown here. Polystyrene blocks are used to modify the depth of penetration to more accurately conform to the chest-wall thickness, but still allow adequate treatment of internal mammary nodes.

3. Electron fields can be relatively easily shaped to conform to the areas at risk. Furthermore, by the use of tissue-equivalent absorbent materials, the depth at which effective radiation is delivered can be modified as clinically indicated.

4. The ability to treat the chest wall and relatively superficial lymph nodes without treating mediastinal structures allows us to avoid the radiation-induced lymphopenia discussed in Section 3.1. This should permit the simultaneous or sequential use of radiation and chemotherapy without competitive and additive leukopenia.

Examples of the way in which electron-beam therapy can be tailored to deliver the desired dose distribution are shown in Figs. 6 and 7.

4. Stage III

4.1. The Controversy

Statement of Controversy: Can radiation therapy alone really control huge advanced breast cancers when its ability to control occult disease is questioned? Can surgery be utilized after full-dose irradiation? Has preoperative irradiation ever proven itself, and what is meant by irradiation surgery? Inflammatory carcinoma is a contraindication to surgery, but has radiation therapy ever successfully ablated this type of breast cancer? What role, if any, does chemotherapy play with irradiation?

There are considerable data related to control of advanced breast cancer. The studies actually claiming success focused upon survival following successful irradiation. However, more so than in early breast cancer, survival rates are misleading, since locoregional control is the most accurate measure of effective irradiation. The evidence lies in two types of experience: the incidence of sterilization of breast cancer converted to operability after a good response to radiation treatment, and the observation of locoregional control after high-dose, often combined external and interstitial treatment. The gradual demonstration that aggressive local treatment can be successful requires further modification with the advent of effective chemotherapy regimens such as "CMF." The impact of chemotherapy in augmenting local control, as well as its ability to reduce the incidence of metastases, are the essential new approaches in protocols.

In 1952, Smithers[54] published the results of treating a series of 1467 breast cancer patients, 281 of whom were Stage III. These patients were treated primarily with radiation therapy, with the addition of limited surgery in some cases, and achieved an absolute five-year survival rate of 10% with a 15% recurrence-free rate. This is contrasted to other earlier reports in the literature by Cade[55] and by Haagensen and Stout[56] on management of Stage III carcinoma of the breast by surgery alone. In their series, the survivals were 9% and 4%, respectively, at five years; Haagensen and Stout reported no five-year patients without recurrence, along with a 40% local recurrence rate.

Many series, however, including those by Baclesse[57] and Bouchard,[58] contained mixtures of advanced patients and early patients in whom the unifying factor is treatment by radiation therapy alone. The Bouchard series had 109 patients treated primarily with radiation, 87% of whom had advanced and late-stage disease. The results are further complicated by the fact that 23% of these patients had eventual mastectomy. In fact, only 60 of these patients were Stage III and only 38 of the 60 had histologic proof, either by biopsy (23), mastectomy (12), or autopsy (3). An additional 17 patients did have clinical evidence of recurrent, progressive, or late metastatic disease to indicate that they had malignant disease. Eighteen of the Stage III patients had postirradiation mastectomies on the basis that they had complete resolution of apparent tumor and were clinically operable at that time. Six of these contained no residual tumor. Twenty-four of the 60 Stage III patients survived five years (40%) and 17 were free of disease (28%). The survival rate and disease-free survival rate were higher in those patients subjected to postirradiation mastectomy, indicating the degree of selection upon which that procedure was based. Removing those cases in which there was only presumptive clinical evidence of carcinoma without biopsy or eventual progression (5) does not significantly alter the results obtained.

The point in presenting the data from this paper in such detail is first, to demonstrate the proven efficacy of radiation therapy with or without subsequent mastectomy in controlling Stage III carcinomas of the breast locally, and, secondly, to indicate the complexity of such analyses caused by inclusion of patients in many stages, degrees of histologic clarification, etc. This is further compounded in many series by a variety of treatment techniques, variations in dose by as much as 200%, etc.

Some of these difficulties beset the paper by Hochman and Robinson,[59] in which a series of 82 patients treated with radiation therapy alone is reported. Thirty-five of these patients were Stage III, 60.1% of whom were alive at three years (21 patients), 20.1% alive at five years (7 patients), and only two patients (5.7%) alive at eight years; all patients were dead by ten years. Of the entire 82 patients, biopsy was evident in only 28 cases, with an additional 48 cases being confirmed as malignancy on the basis of metastases. The remaining six patients were lost to follow-up immediately after treatment, and were counted as dead. Although the authors comment on the late radiation effects on the breast, they do not provide data on the degree of tumor control obtained within the total area.

An interesting series of patients is reported by Ruth Guttmann.[16] This series of 174 patients was composed of those found to be inoperable by lymph node biopsy as performed by Haagensen. There were 62 patients with involvement of the internal mammary lymph nodes and apical axillary lymph nodes, 63 patients with involvement of the internal mammary lymph nodes alone, and 49 patients with involvement of the apical axillary lymph nodes alone. She obtained a 60% five-year survival in the 148 patients who had been followed as long as five years. This gradually fell to a 30% ten-year survival, although six patients did die during that interval of other causes. It is interesting to compare these survival figures with the positive-node patients in other studies such as the National Surgical Adjuvant Breast Project[43] and the Milan studies by Bonadonna et al.[42] In those studies, patients with high axillary lymph node involvement had a 25% disease-free survival at anywhere from two to five years. Of course, disease-free survival is not directly comparable to absolute survival, although the correlation is very strong. Guttman also compares her figures favorably to those published by Urban and Martani,[60] who performed extended radical mastectomy. While comprehensive local control data are not included, autopsy could demonstrate no tumor in the breast area in 20 patients, 17 of whom were cancer-free systemically.

Many authors consider the use of radiation therapy alone to be the standard treatment for locally advanced carcinoma of the breast, because many of these patients are not suitable for any operative intervention. An early paper by Baclesse[57] reported a series of patients treated at the Curie Foundation from 1936 to 1945. Fifty-eight patients were treated with radiation plus radical surgery and achieved an 88% local control rate. These represented Stage II and Stage III patients, with the distinction between the two stages being that Stage II represents tumor up to 6 cm in diameter but without deep fixation, ulceration, or extensive scirrhous carcinoma. Skin involvement is included in Stage II, but edema, *peau d'orange*, or skin nodules would place the patient into Stage III. Considerable information is presented summarizing the result of treatment of 130 patients from 1936 to 1945 who had Stage II, III, or IV (Stage IV being those with distant metastases or inflammatory carcinoma) carcinoma of the breast. Treatment was given with extended fractionation over anywhere from four weeks to more than 14 weeks, with the best results being reported in patients receiving orthovoltage treatment extended beyond 10 weeks in a fractionated fashion. The data are not presented in a way which makes comparison with previously mentioned studies for local control possible; however, overall, 79 patients obtained complete regression of tumor. This certainly indicated a potential for treating extensive local disease with radiation therapy only, and many subsequent studies reaffirmed this. Fletcher and Montague[61] report a 72% local control rate using the prolonged fractionation technique of Baclesse in 273 patients, and, in the same publication, reported 167 patients treated by radical radiation preceded by simple mastectomy with an identical 72% local control rate.

Our own experience has convinced us that these locally advanced tumors can be effectively treated by radiation alone in many cases. We have treated 50 such patients using primarily radiation. At the time of treatment, some patients had metastases and some did not. The survival curves for Stages III and IV are identical. Some patients' survival was too short to allow evaluation of local treatment effectiveness. However, there is a clear distinction between two groups of patients. Those treated to conventional doses (4000–6000 rads) had a poor local control rate, whereas the 22 patients treated to more than 7000 rads experienced an 82% rate of local and regional control[62] (see Section 4.4). Table VI summarizes much of this data.

A number of authors have advocated planned preoperative irradiation and surgery for these patients.[65,66,69,70] The rationale and benefits of preoperative irradiation in this group of patients have been emphasized by the Toronto and M.D. Anderson groups. Preoperative irradiation has been advocated in head and neck cancers and colorectal cancers as well. The arguments for its use are basically the same in all areas. These are:

1. Radiation can kill individual cancer cells.
2. Even those cells not killed may lose their reproductive capacity and, hence, be unable to act as sources of local–regional or distant recurrence.
3. Intraoperative dissemination of cancer cells may be prevented by reactionary fibrosis and contracture around lymphatics, etc.
4. A relatively greater effect can be obtained from radiation to undisturbed tumor because of better oxygenation secondary to intact blood supply.
5. Tumor regression after preoperative irradiation may transform an inoperable tumor into one where surgery is possible without cutting through tumor.
6. The delay in surgery offers the tumor a chance to declare its biologic activity; that is, cancers already metastatic may become manifest and alter the overall aim of treatment.

While preoperative irradiation has had its advocates, it has never proven itself to be superior to other approaches. An early paper by

Table VI

Results of Radiotherapeutic Management of Locally Advanced Stage III Breast Cancer

Author, year	No. of patients	Local control (%)	Survival (%)	Treatment technique	Dose range/time
Atkins and Horrigan, 1961 [63]	39	13	31.7 (3 yr)	Mainly orthovoltage	4000–5000 rads/3–4 weeks
Griscom and Wang, 1962 [64]	50	35	19.5 (5 yr)	Orthovoltage	4000–6000 rads/5–6 weeks
Bouchard, 1963 [58]	60	43	40 (5 yr)	Orthovoltage	6000+ rads/75–100 days
Delarue et al., 1965 [65]	266	—	28.5 (5 yr)	Preoperative irradiation and surgery	4500 rads/4 weeks
Guttmann, 1967 [16]	174	High	60 (5 yr)	Conventional irradiation	4000–7000 rads/5–7 weeks
Fletcher et al., 1970 [66]	273	72	27.1 (5 yr)	Protracted fractionation	6000–8000 rads/>12 weeks
	167	72	39.8 (5 yr)	Simple mastectomy and postoperative irradiation	5000–7000 rads/5–7 weeks
Stoker and Ellis, 1972 [67]	24	87	—	Preoperative irradiation and surgery	5000 rads + boost/5–6 weeks
Brown et al., 1974 [68]	189	88	45.5 (5 yr)	Surgery + postoperative irradiation	5000 rads + boost/5–6 weeks
Keys and Rubin, 1976 [62]	22	82	13 (5 yr)	External + interstitial	>7000 rads/8 weeks

Frank Adair[71] (originally presented in 1935) reported considerable experience with the use of preoperative irradiation in primary, operable cancer of the breast. The definition of "operable" at that time included many locally advanced patients with lymph node metastases. His series consisted of 117 patients treated preoperatively with low-energy orthovoltage radiation or external radium-pack treatment (neither of which would be considered adequate in the modern era by any stretch of the imagination). Of interest, however, was the fact that the primary tumors were seen to be either reduced in size or completely eliminated clinically in all of the patients, and 60% or more of the enlarged lymph nodes were seen to regress partially or completely. As the patients were subsequently operated on, histologic confirmation of the effectiveness of even this relatively low-dose irradiation was obtained, and in 25% of the tumors, the most careful histopathologic examination was unable to demonstrate residual tumor. Overall, 51% of the patients had gross axillary involvement clinically, and, disappointingly, only 8% of these had microscopic elimination of tumor. The latter effect is clearly related to inadequate dose recognized even at the time of publication.

While the theoretical groundwork had not been laid at that time to understand the potential value of preoperative treatment, the results there certainly indicated some promise. However, it was many years later before careful evaluation of the role of preoperative treatment, especially in more advanced local tumors, was undertaken. Lumb[72] found similar reduction in clinical tumor size but did not report prevention of local recurrence. Windeyer[73] recommended preoperative irradiation for Stage II carcinoma of the breast and postulated that its greater effectiveness would be secondary to the improved blood supply present in the region of the tumor prior to mastectomy.

In 1962, White et al., from M.D. Anderson Hospital, reported experience with preoperative irradiation for a group of patients with surgically disturbed and/or borderline operable carcinomas of the breast.[70] This was a total of 193 patients, 23 of whom had borderline or debatable operable lesions. Thirty-one additional patients had biopsy prior to referral to M.D. Anderson Hospital, but because of small, clean, and dry biopsy wounds, did not receive preoperative treatment. Slightly less than half the patients had clinically positive lymph nodes. While the local recurrence rates are encouragingly low for the preoperative irradiation group, their staging is not entirely clear.

Papers reporting on the use of preoperative irradiation followed by mastectomy for strictly locally advanced series of patients include those of Woods[74] and Stoker and Ellis.[67] Both series reported local control rates of approximately 87% of 110 and 24 patients, respectively. With

relatively short follow-up periods, neither study claimed to have significantly affected long-term survival.

Delarue *et al.*, in a paper tabulating clinical and histopathologic
clues to predict biologic activity of carcinoma of the breast, noted that
their patients with locally advanced carcinoma had surprisingly good
five- to ten-year survival.[65] Using a biological classification of their own,
the survival rates are 71% for Stage III-A and 33% for III-B. The distinction between Stage III-A and III-B is the presence of movable or fixed
supraclavicular lymph nodes in Stage III-B, whereas III-A is a tumor of
greater than 5-cm size with or without axillary nodes.

In a number of series where patients were treated with radiation
therapy for locally advanced tumors, those that became clearly resectable after a good response to radiation were then operated on. While these
were not planned preoperative treatment in the sense of the previous
reports, radiation therapy followed by postirradiation surgery is advocated by Vaeth *et al.* when possible.[75] They reported on 27 patients,
with the earliest staged patient being T_2, N_2, and the majority of patients
being T_3 or T_4, with or without lymph node involvement. Eleven of these
were inflammatory carcinomas and will be mentioned subsequently. In
16 of the 27 patients, there was sufficient response to make surgery possible (11 radical mastectomies and 5 simple mastectomies without axillary dissection). Ten of these 16 patients were treated to intermediate
doses ranging from 4500 to 5200 rads, which correspond to the preoperative doses recommended in other studies. Local control was achieved
in 14 of the 16 patients receiving radiation plus surgery and in 8 of the 11
patients treated by radiation alone. It should be noted that this is a selective series in which the better responders were subjected to the combined procedure, making the control rate by radiation only quite re-
spectable. The patients treated by radiation only (11) generally received
higher doses ranging from 5100 rads to more than 6500 rads. Control of
positive regional nodes was also good in both groups: 13 to 16 patients
whose axillary treatment was radiation only and 10 of 11 who were
treated in combined fashion. The doses employed here were generally
lower than for the primary tumor. One interesting finding in this study
was that of those patients subjected to surgery after radiation, there was
no correlation with microscopic clearance of tumor and dose. This reflects the fact that the series is rather small in terms of the number of
cases and that patients were selected for surgery on the basis of response, suggesting that the total dose of those good responders who
received lower irradiation doses and then surgery was lower than that of
the poorer responders who were continued on radiation to higher levels.
It would be expected that a large series treated without selection to a

variety of doses would demonstrate a rather noticeable dose–response curve, with higher doses showing greater sterilization rates.

An alternative to preoperative radiation is the use of preradical-radiation surgery (similar to surgery and postoperative irradiation). This is advocated by Montague for patients with large masses and pendulous breasts where a simple mastectomy prior to radiation "seems a logical solution to the problem."[76] She reports on 196 patients treated in this fashion who were not candidates for primary surgery alone because of signs of local advancement, involvement of skin, ulceration, or inflammatory tumors. The overall local control rate was 78%, which is similar to the results of preoperative series previously mentioned. Treatment was locally about as effective as other forms of management for these advanced tumors, with the exception that 13 of the 33 ulcerative tumors recurred locally either in the chest wall, axilla, or both. This is a poorer overall control rate than would have been anticipated, and the author also reports local failure in 16 of 55 ulcerative tumors treated with a protracted radiation-therapy-only technique. This suggests that surgery should not be performed first for extensively ulcerated tumors, and a similar finding is noted in patients with inflammatory tumors. However, in this particular series, the inflammatory carcinomas were locally con-

Table VII
Local Control[a] of Late Stage II UICC Breast Carcinoma
(Unlimited Follow-Up)
(January, 1955–December, 1969)
Analysis: January, 1972[b,c]

Site of recurrences	Free of disease after simple mastectomy and irradiation (lesion technically suitable for radical mastectomy)	
	January, 1955–December, 1963 (103 patients)	January, 1964–December, 1969 (86 patients)
Chest wall	88% (91/103)	95% (82/86)
Axilla	88% (91/103)	99% (85/86)
Supraclavicular	93% (96/103)	99% (85/86)
Parasternal	99% (102/103)	100% (86/86)

[a]A patient may have a recurrence in more than one location.
[b]From Brown et al.[68]
[c]Survival rates (modified life-table method): 5 yr—45.5%; 10 yr—21.5%.

trolled after mastectomy and postmastectomy irradiation in 10 of 13 patients.

A later analysis (January, 1972) by Brown *et al.* of some of the same patient material from M.D. Anderson Hospital is of interest, although not entirely comparable to those patients mentioned previously.[68] In this study, patients with locally advanced tumors which were technically suitable for radical mastectomy were treated with simple mastectomy and radiation therapy. The local control figures for two different time intervals in this study are presented in Table VII and demonstrate from 88 to 99% local control in the early group and 95 to 100% in the more recent group of 86 patients. One difference in procedure in the more recent period has been the resection of low axillary lymph nodes along with the breast as part of the simple mastectomy. This may be partly responsible for the considerable increase in the axillary control rate. A higher dose was used in the supraclavicular regions (minimum 5000 rads and as high as 7000, depending on the size of the involved lymph nodes), and may be reflected in a higher control rate in that region as well.

4.2. Inflammatory Carcinoma

There are several reasons to consider "inflammatory" carcinomas separately. First, primary surgical attack is widely held to be contraindicated.[77,78] Second, survival is dismally poor; five-year survivors are rare, regardless of the type of primary management employed. However, the high local failure rate and poor survival are found in all breast cancers with extensive skin involvement, regardless of whether they show the clinical picture of inflammation or the microscopic picture of dermal lymphatic tumor plugging.[79,80]

Approximately one-third of these patients present with distant metastases,[81,82] and, in some series, nearly all had clinical evidence of axillary disease.[83,84] The type of local treatment cannot be expected to significantly alter survival where 80 to 100% of patients are dead within two years.[81-85] Several series reflect the inadequacy of surgery alone to control these tumors locally.[77,85] Early orthovoltage-treated series were only partially successful in local control, with 25% freedom from local recurrence.[81] While some combined radiation-surgery series are equally ineffectual,[85] Vaeth *et al.* (in a small group of 11 patients) reported 4 out of 6 local controls with radiation therapy followed by surgery, but only 2 out of 5 local successes with irradiation only.[75]

Wang and Griscom, however, reported 50% local control with radiation (supervoltage) only.[81] Barker *et al.*, in a recent series from M.D. Anderson Hospital, found overall 38% local failure in the breast treated by irradiation only, but 53% with combined surgery and radiation. Axillary recurrences increased these figures to 46% and 65%, respectively.[82]

Our own experience is that inflammatory cancers can be controlled most of the time with adequate doses of irradiation. While we have no recurrence-free survivors, seven of nine patients treated to high doses remained locally and regionally controlled, two for over five years.[62]

There is uncertainty about the role of systemic chemotherapy in this stage of disease, and this discussion is most relevant to inflammatory cancers. Should chemotherapy await the appearance of distant metastases, or should its use be begun primarily for its effect on the local disease and as an adjuvant form of treatment, and what combination of systemic treatment and local treatment is likely to be most effective in this disease? Here, there are little data. The effectiveness of single- and multiagent chemotherapy as an adjuvant to earlier-staged disease has been discussed elsewhere in this book. The fact that a relatively ineffective drug such as Melphalan can have as dramatic effect as is suggested in the NSABP study[43] is an interesting and important discovery. Multiple-agent chemotherapy such as CMF (Cytoxan, methotrexate, and fluorouracil) has been shown to produce complete and partial remissions in about 50% of patients who had not previously been treated with chemotherapy. However, this is in all types of metastatic disease, and combines complete and partial effects.[86] It is reasonable to assume that a combination such as CMF which is reasonably effective against metastatic disease would also have beneficial effects on local tumors as well. However, as has been pointed out, local control, while a challenge, is achieved in a sizable majority of patients by currently available means, and the more important need is for adjuvant therapy to improve the poor survival seen in this group of patients. Little data exist on the elective use of combination chemotherapy on locally advanced tumors, although institutional and cooperative group protocols are being designed and piloted along this line at the present time. If the early gains reported by Bonadonna et al.[42] for Stage II carcinoma of the breast can be translated into similar advances in Stage III, a major advance in the care of breast cancer patients will have occurred.

In summary, for inflammatory carcinomas:

1. Survival is poor and local therapy cannot alter it.
2. Surgery with or without radiation does not improve local results for most patients.
3. Biopsy followed by radical radiation therapy is indicated for most patients.
4. Adjuvant chemotherapy may improve survival.

4.3. Indications for Treatment

Optimal local management for Stage III carcinoma of the breast requires the use of radiation therapy for essentially all patients. The local recurrence rate, the extensiveness of the local recurrences, and the unfortunate sequelae of such consequences after surgical management alone make this form of therapy considerably less desirable. Under certain circumstances, such as in patients with large masses in pendulous breasts, technically difficult to treat by radiation therapy alone, preradiation mastectomy may offer a technical advantage. Also, as mentioned in previous sections, some patients with large masses may show enough response to preoperative doses of radiation therapy for the masses to become technically resectable, and for that select group of patients, the local control rate may be best with the combined form of treatment. However, for the remaining Stage III patients, the use of radiation

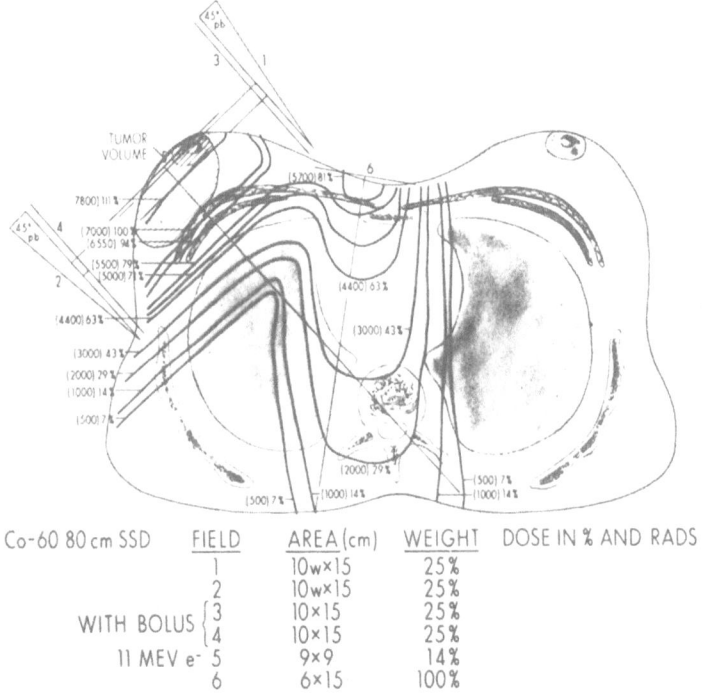

Co-60 80 cm SSD	FIELD	AREA (cm)	WEIGHT	DOSE IN % AND RADS
	1	10w×15	25%	
	2	10w×15	25%	
WITH BOLUS	3	10×15	25%	
	4	10×15	25%	
11 MEV e⁻	5	9×9	14%	
	6	6×15	100%	

Fig. 8. Treatment planning for Stage III breast cancer. Parallel opposed tangential breast fields equally weighted between wedges and bolus are supplemented here with a direct electron-boost field to raise the entire tumor-bearing area to a dose of 7000 rads. Field no. 6 is a separate internal mammary field.

therapy alone appears to offer excellent local control rates and not adversely affect survival.

4.4. Radiation Therapy Techniques, Doses, and Treatment Plans

Radiation therapy is given very similarly to patients with locally advanced disease as was described for the Stage I and II patients previously. The major difference is, first, that the tumor dose must be higher if the tumor is going to be controlled with radiation therapy alone, simply because it is a larger tumor. Second, the area over which the higher dose is applied must be greater because of the presence of involved lymph nodes being treated primarily with radiation. Several alternatives are available for raising the tumor dose to the required levels, including the use of smaller external-beam boosting fields, interstitial implantation of radioactive sources, or higher-energy electron-boosting fields.

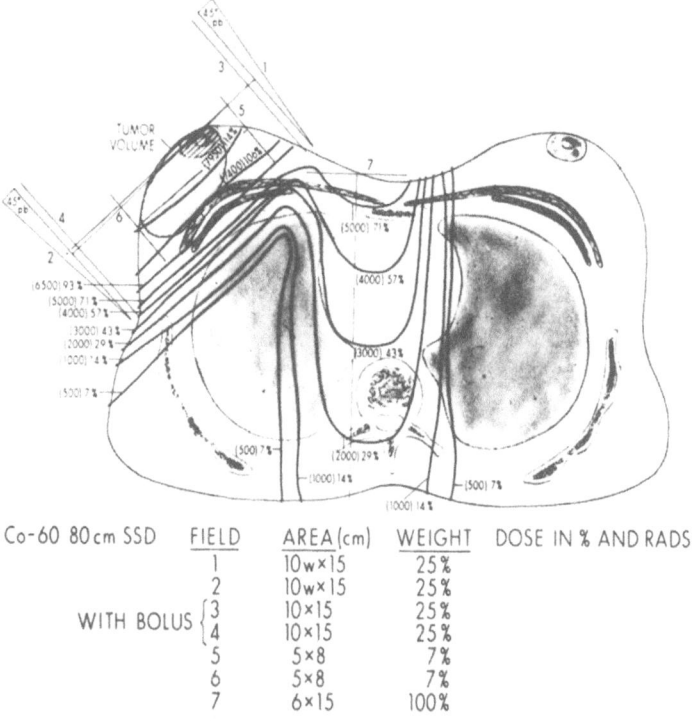

Co-60 80 cm SSD	FIELD	AREA (cm)	WEIGHT	DOSE IN % AND RADS
	1	10w×15	25%	
	2	10w×15	25%	
WITH BOLUS {3	3	10×15	25%	
WITH BOLUS {4	4	10×15	25%	
	5	5×8	7%	
	6	5×8	7%	
	7	6×15	100%	

Fig. 9. Treatment planning for Stage III breast cancer. Here, the basic treatment shown in Fig. 8 is supplemented by smaller parallel opposed boost fields to raise the dose to the primary tumor to above 7000 rads.

4.4.1. Advantages of Interstitial Techniques

There are several advantages in using interstitial techniques for raising the dose to residual masses of tumor. First, the low-dose rate of continuous irradiation provided by such methods may be biologically more effective than conventional external irradiation. Perhaps more important is the physical advantage of being able to concentrate rather high doses in the immediate area of concern with relative sparing of other tissues. With modern interstitial sources such as iridium-192 seeds or wire, afterloading methods can be used which allow greater control and flexibility in dose distribution and less radiation exposure to personnel. This approach can be used to implant a small residual area of induration, or as much as the entire breast and axillary nodes.

A variety of dosimetry plans are presented in Figs. 8–12. The desired dose to gross areas of tumor is 7000–8000 rads, with areas at risk for subclinical disease receiving 5000 rads. Because of skin infiltration, it is

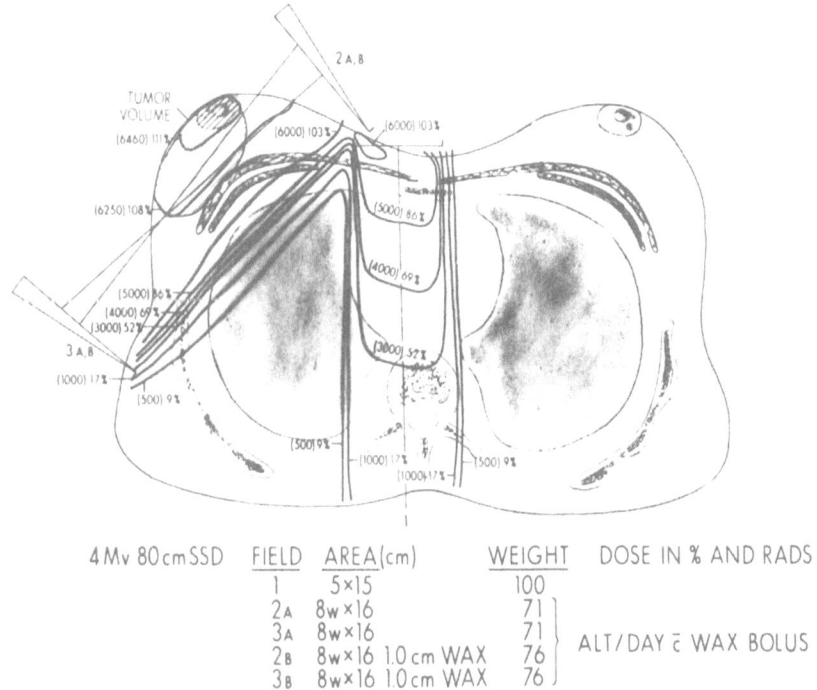

4 Mv 80 cm SSD	FIELD	AREA (cm)	WEIGHT	DOSE IN % AND RADS
	1	5×15	100	
	2ᴀ	8w ×16	71	
	3ᴀ	8w ×16	71	ALT/DAY c̄ WAX BOLUS
	2ʙ	8w×16 1.0 cm WAX	76	
	3ʙ	8w×16 1.0 cm WAX	76	

Fig. 10. Treatment planning for Stage III breast cancer. Here 4-MV X rays are used in an array of four oblique wedged fields biased slightly toward bolus (76 versus 71 weighting). This basic treatment would be supplemented as in Figs. 8 and 9. Figs. 11 and 12 show other alternatives.

often necessary to reduce the skin-sparing characteristic of high-energy treatment beams and give the same high dose to the skin of the breast as to the underlying tumor mass. This will frequently produce a moist skin reaction and late skin changes (see Fig. 16). The examples presented in Figs. 13–16 illustrate the combined use of external and interstitial irradiation.

4.5. Studies Under Way and Future Protocols Needed

The major area which requires investigation in Stage III carcinoma of the breast is the use of adjuvant chemotherapy along with primary management as outlined above. Local control is the appropriate index of success of local therapy, but in these patients, the life-limiting disease is the frequency of metastatic dissemination, and extrapolating the apparent effectiveness of adjuvant chemotherapy in Stage II carcinomas to Stage III suggests that some gain in survival should be seen with the routine use of adjuvant therapy there. Studies are under way to determine what is the best combination of local and systemic therapy, and to what extent each form of therapy should modify the other. One example of such a study is the use of systemic chemotherapy prior to radiation therapy in inflammatory carcinoma of the breast at M.D. Anderson Hospital. This form of induction chemotherapy shows some

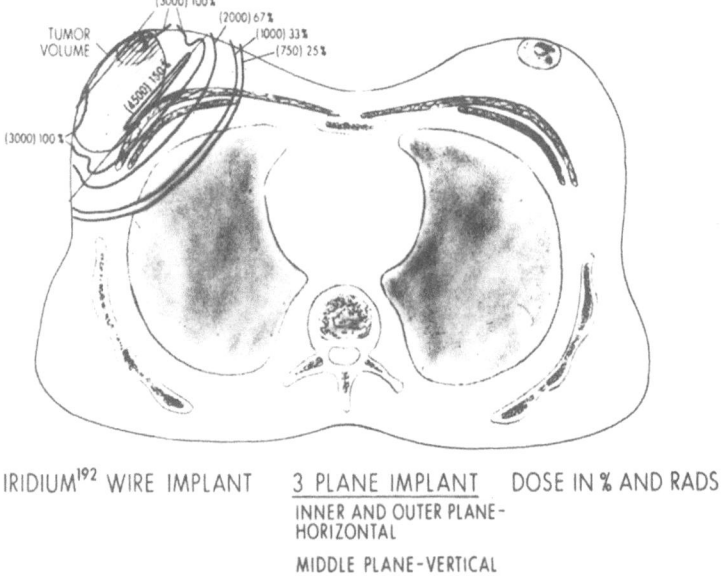

IRIDIUM¹⁹² WIRE IMPLANT   3 PLANE IMPLANT   DOSE IN % AND RADS
                            INNER AND OUTER PLANE-
                            HORIZONTAL
                            MIDDLE PLANE-VERTICAL

Fig. 11. Treatment planning for Stage III breast cancer. An interstitial implant can be useful to boost the dose through primary tumor areas (see text). Here, a three-plane iridium-192 wire implant is shown giving 4500 rads to the tumor mass.

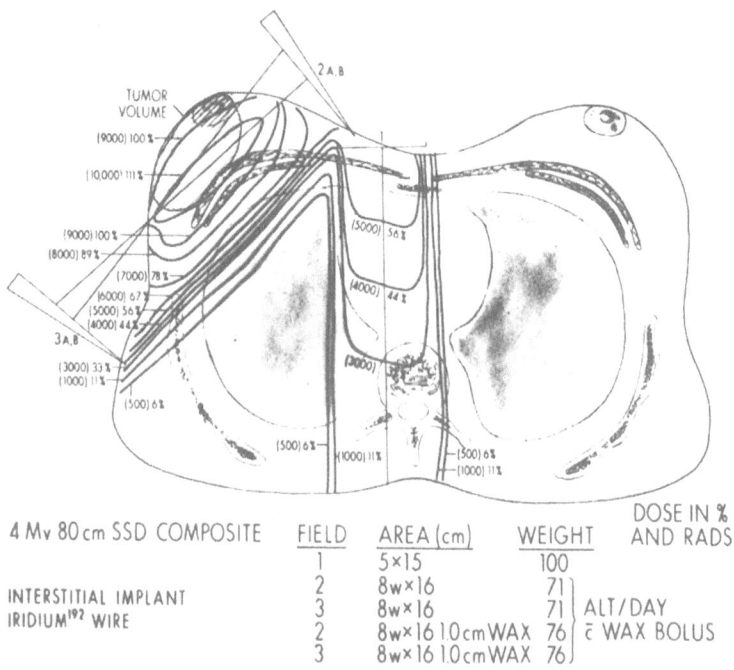

4 Mv 80 cm SSD COMPOSITE	FIELD	AREA (cm)	WEIGHT	DOSE IN % AND RADS
	1	5×15	100	
INTERSTITIAL IMPLANT IRIDIUM¹⁹² WIRE	2	8w×16	71	ALT/DAY
	3	8w×16	71	
	2	8w×16 1.0cmWAX	76	c̄ WAX BOLUS
	3	8w×16 1.0cmWAX	76	

Fig. 12. Treatment planning for Stage III breast cancer. This is the composite total dose distribution that would occur if the external treatment from Fig. 10 and the interstitial implant shown in Fig. 11 were both used. The entire tumor volume would receive more than 9000 rads.

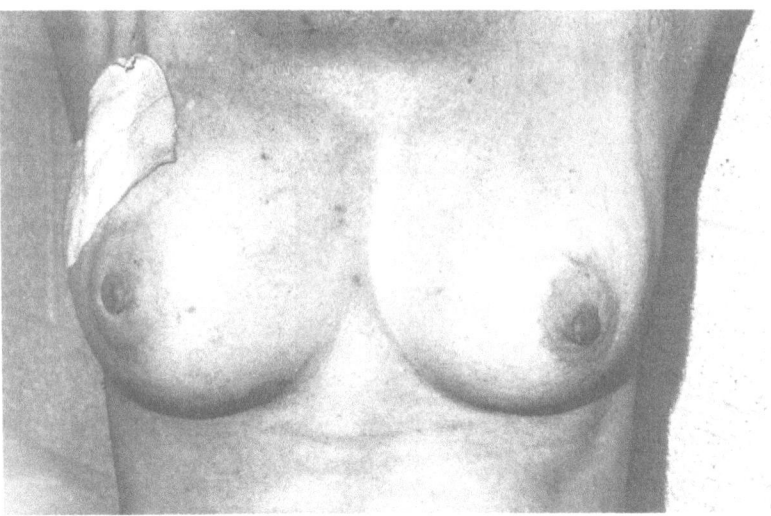

Fig. 13. This 42-year-old woman presented with inflammatory carcinoma of the breast with small palpable axillary nodes. The patch covers breast and skin biopsy site. Treatment was begun with external-beam radiation similar to the basic plan shown in Figs. 8 and 9 (without the boost field).

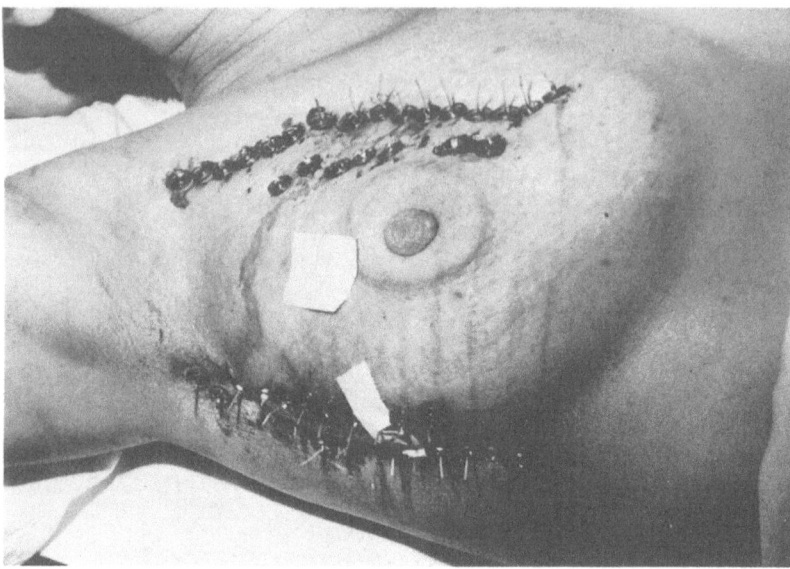

Fig. 14. The same patient shown in Fig. 13 is seen here after completing 5000 rads external treatment. An iridium interstitial implant was performed, with two planes through the breast and the deeper plane extending through the lower axilla.

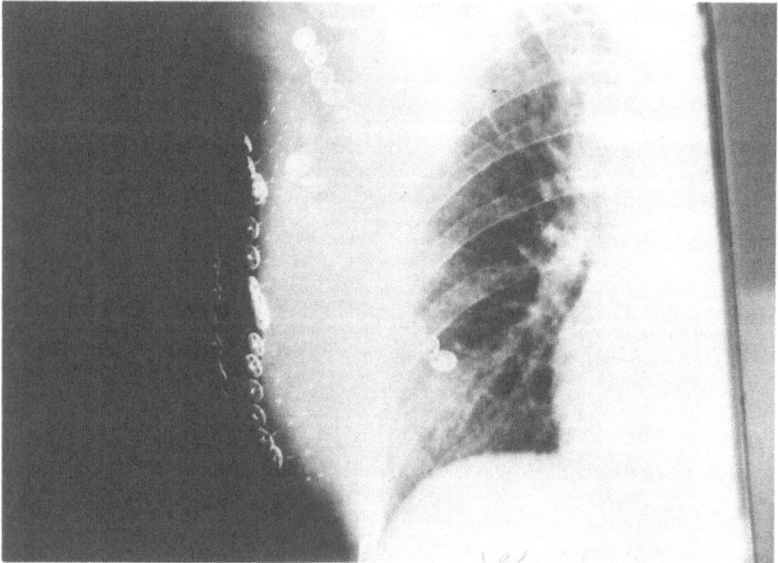

Fig. 15. This is one of the X rays taken for dose calculation of the iridium implant shown in Fig. 14. Identification of each short wire segment is necessary for accurate dosimetry. Note the uniform distribution of sources.

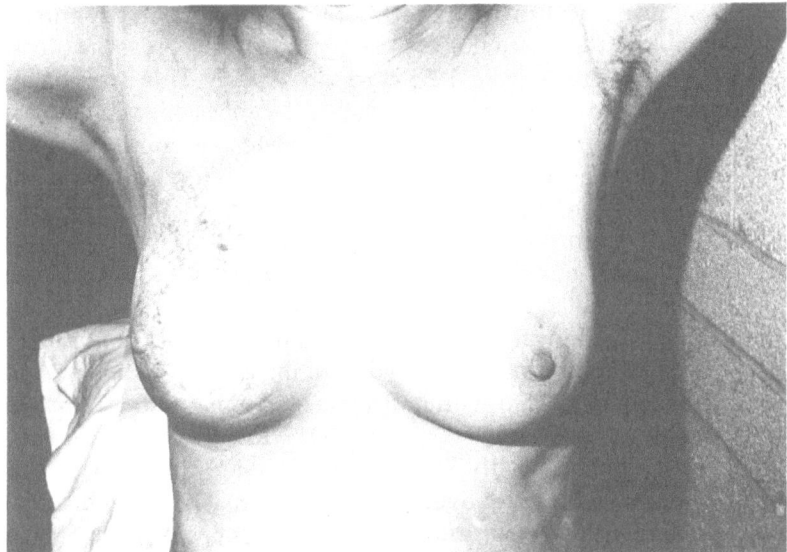

Fig. 16. The same patient shown in Figs. 13–15 is seen here two years after treatment. Examination reveals increased firmness generalized throughout the breast with some subcutaneous thickening. Mammography demonstrates those changes described in Table II. The patient died of disseminated metastatic disease at three years without local or regional recurrence.

promise in its effect on the local tumor as well as in its hope for success in preventing clinical appearance of distant metastases. Other questions to be answered in this stage of disease include: To what extent can chemotherapy replace radiation therapy because of the smaller number of cells to be killed? Can neutron-irradiation of bulky breast carcinomas and bulky involved lymph nodes improve the local control rate when compared with conventional gamma- or X-irradiation? And, finally, if systemic chemotherapy is effective in prolonging survival, will local recurrences of patients treated with radiation therapy for the primary lymph node disease become more common as the patients live longer?

5. Stage IV

5.1. The Controversy

Statement of Controversy: Does radiation therapy produce rather than prevent chest-wall and pulmonary metastases (Dao hypothesis)? What is the new role of radiation therapy in metastatic cancer in view of advances in chemotherapy?

In 1962, Dao and Kovaric reported on a series of 354 patients who were evaluable after treatment for carcinoma of the breast at Roswell Park Memorial Institute from 1954 through 1958. [87] This was a strictly retrospective study of patients treated in different fashions, comparing the results of radical mastectomy, radical mastectomy and irradiation, simple mastectomy, and, finally, simple mastectomy and irradiation. There is no indication in this study as to the basis for selection of specific treatment aside from the fact that patients having simple mastectomy tended to be a more elderly group. This study reported to show that the incidence of skin metastases in the irradiated field and lung metastases on the ipsilateral side was increased in patients who received radiation as compared to the incidence observed in nonirradiated patients. A total of 213 patients were treated with radical mastectomy, with a 17.5% incidence of pulmonary metastases and an 11% incidence of skin metastases. This is compared with 30 patients receiving radical mastectomy followed by irradiation, with a striking increase to 53% incidence of ipsilateral pulmonary metastases and 47% incidence of ipsilateral skin metastases. Figures for simple mastectomy are 38 patients with 13% pulmonary and 8% skin metastases; 73 patients received simple mastectomy and irradiation, with a doubling to 27% pulmonary and 16% skin metastases (Table VIII).

There is an obvious bias in this comparison, as the frequency of nodal metastases is grossly dissimilar in the various groups: 90% of the patients irradiated after radical and 63% irradiated after simple mastectomy; the figures for the unirradiated patients were 45% after radical mastectomy and 50% after simple mastectomy. Clearly, patients with more advanced disease will have a higher incidence of recurrence and metastases.

An attempt is made to select similar groups on clinical and pathologic grounds so that valid comparisons of recurrence rates can be made. Patients with axillary metastases were matched using all of the node-positive patients except for the radical mastectomy group. In that group, only 35% of 96 patients with positive axillary nodes were included in their comparison (Table IX). The authors then tabulated ipsilateral skin and lung metastases, concluding that the radiation increased the number of skin recurrences in the field and pulmonary metastases on the side where some lung tissue was exposed to irradiation. However, when ipsilateral *and* contralateral skin and pulmonary metastases are analyzed, the conclusions are different. Their data are presented in this way in Table IX. In patients whom the authors feel are comparable, radical mastectomy alone has the highest incidence of pulmonary metastases, the two irradiated groups slightly better, and simple mastectomy alone, the best overall result. Skin recurrences were

Table VIII

Pulmonary and Skin Metastases in Women with Breast Cancer in the Entire Series[a]

Type of treatment	No. of patients	Percent lung metastases	Percent skin metastases	Percent negative axillary nodes
Radical mastectomy	213	17.5 (37/213)	11 (24/213)	55
Radical mastectomy and radiation therapy	30	53 (16/30)	47 (14/30)	10
Simple mastectomy	38[b]	13 (5/38)	8 (3/38)	50
Simple mastectomy and radiation therapy	73[b]	27 (20/73)	16 (12/73)	37

[a]Data abstracted from Dao and Kovaric.[87]
[b]Axillary nodes biopsied at the time of mastectomy.

Table IX

Pulmonary and Skin Metastases in Women with Clinically and Pathologically Comparable Breast Cancers[a]

Type of treatment	No. of patients	Percent skin recurrence	Percent lung metastases	Percent total metastases
Radical mastectomy	35	34 (12/35)	45 (16/35)	57 (20/35)
Radical mastectomy and irradiation	27	52 (14/27)	44 (12/27)	56 (15/27)
Simple mastectomy	19	16 (3/19)	21 (4/19)	21 (4/19)
Simple mastectomy and irradiation	46	26 (12/46)	41 (19/46)	50 (23/46)

[a]Data abstracted from Dao and Kovaric.[87]

most common (52%) in radical mastectomy plus postoperative irradiation, with radical mastectomy alone, simple mastectomy plus irradiation, and simple mastectomy alone following in order of decreasing frequency. This incidence of local and regional recurrences with or without postoperative radiation therapy is much higher than in many series published (see Section 4). Whether the unexpectedly poor results presented by Dao and Kovaric reflect inadequate surgery and irradiation, or unusually advanced disease, is unclear. However, further analysis is illuminating.

Despite the fact that these patients are presented as being clinically and pathologically comparable, the survival in this more limited group suggests, in fact, that they are not. Looking at survival of three years or longer, 23% survived with radical mastectomy, versus only 7% survival for those with radical mastectomy and irradiation. Simple mastectomy had a 47% survival and when followed by irradiation, this dropped to 28%. As is usually the case in nonrandomized series of patients with malignancy where a portion received postoperative treatment, these survival figures and recurrence figures strongly suggest that the patients who received postoperative radiation therapy had more advanced disease.

Other studies have been published to test the hypothesis presented by Dao and Kovaric. Perhaps the most similarly analyzed series is that presented by Chu et al. from Memorial Hospital in New York.[34] They retrospectively analyzed patients treated during each of two two-year periods. These were time intervals during which policy dictated essentially that no patient receive prophylactic postoperative radiation therapy for carcinoma of the breast (1950–1951) and when nearly all patients were treated postoperatively (1953–1954). They wound up with a total of 790 patients, of whom 116 had to be excluded for a variety of reasons, 98 of them for a second malignancy previously, simultaneously, or subsequently. They very carefully analyzed patients on the basis of comparable staging. The result of survival analysis, as in the paper by Dao and Kovaric, showed no statistically significant differences between irradiated and unirradiated patients, with the exception that Chu et al. found that patients with the axillary apical lymph node involved had a 17% increase in survival when irradiated postoperatively (39% five-year survival versus 22% for the unirradiated group). This was significant at the 0.05 P-value level. Furthermore, the incidence of pulmonary metastases—ipsilateral, contralateral, bilateral, and undetermined—was identical in irradiated and unirradiated patients.

The incidence of local recurrence in the skin of the chest wall in patients with positive axillary nodes was 24% total for those who received postoperative radiation therapy and 23% total for those who received no postoperative radiation therapy. About two-thirds of the irradiated patients' skin recurrences were within previously irradiated fields and one-third outside. There were no chest-wall recurrences in patients with negative nodes who received postoperative radiation, and only three (1%) in patients without postoperative radiation therapy. The incidence of nodal metastases in dissected axillae and internal mammary regions was identical in irradiated and unirradiated groups, but there was a 2% incidence of supraclavicular metastases in the negative-axillae unirradiated group, as opposed to none in the irradiated group with negative axillae. Further, there was a 23% incidence of supraclavicular metastases (50 out of 219) in patients with mastectomy only and positive nodes, versus 10% (17 out of 170) in those who received postoperative radiation therapy. They concluded thus: "it can be stated conclusively that radiation therapy does not increase the possibility of lung, pleural, or skin metastases."

5.2. Indications for Irradiation

There are many situations in patients with metastatic breast cancer in which appropriate application of radiation therapy is beneficial. The challenge is to balance economy of the patient's time and treatment expense, minimization of treatment morbidity, competition for hematologic reserve with systemic chemotherapy and effective, lasting, palliation of the symptomatic situation.

The most common indication for irradiation is painful bone metastases. Most often involved and symptomatic are the proximal femurs, pelvic bones, and vertebral column. While a variety of treatment techniques and dose schedules can be employed, the results are encouraging. Approximately 90% of patients obtain significant relief of symptoms.[88]

Another common problem is the presence of symptomatic brain metastases. With or without the use of simultaneous steroid medication, there is unquestionable objective and subjective improvement in the majority of patients who complete their course of treatment.[89,90] Usually, the whole cranial contents are treated, and some authors recommend boosting the dose in the areas of unknown metastatic disease.[89] A randomized study performed by the Radiation Therapy Oncology Group (RTOG) suggests that a dose of 3000 rads in ten fractions over two weeks is as effective as higher doses and longer fractionation, and hence, may be preferable, as it is more efficient.[91]

Pulmonary metastases only rarely require irradiation. However, when bronchial obstruction is apparent or imminent, then local treatment may be beneficial. More commonly, mediastinal disease may produce compression of the esophagus, superior vena cava, etc., which can have devastating effects. Acute superior vena caval obstruction should be treated as a radiotherapeutic emergency. We advise using high-dose fractions at first (e.g., 300–400 rads daily for three days). This is followed by reduced fractional size (200 rads) up to a total dose of 4000–5000 rads.[92]

Hepatic metastases are very common in breast cancer patients and occasionally warrant palliative irradiation. When a painfully distended hepatic capsule is disabling, the entire liver may be treated. This is not uniformly successful, but may provide significant relief for some patients. Marked improvement of grossly abnormal liver function occasionally occurs. Two techniques have been tried: large single-dose treatment (600–1000 rads in one day) and fractionated treatment (200 rads daily up to 2000–2400 rads total). Platelet counts should be monitored carefully during and after such treatment.[93]

Another uncommon site of metastasis is the choroid of the eye. It is worth mentioning, however, because appropriate radiotherapeutic management can prevent loss of vision and often restore vision when retinal distortion has altered it. A single posteriorly-angled lateral field can be used to deliver 3000–4000 rads in two to three weeks. Alternatively, combinations of anterior and lateral fields are used when more uniform treatment of the entire eye or orbit is desired.

Nodal metastases (or recurrences) require high doses of irradiation to control. It is important to recognize that such tumor deposits often have considerable depth. This is especially true when dealing with internal mammary recurrences, which often present with parasternal skin involvement and may be mistaken for chest-wall disease. In fact, they have substantial retrosternal masses and a high likelihood of mediastinal nodal involvement.[94]

One other clinical situation occurs often enough to be worth mentioning: the development of epidural tumor causing spinal cord compression can present a neurological emergency. Radiation therapy can effectively control the tumor, but the rate of regression is slow. Therefore, if spinal cord function is to be preserved, prompt identification of the area of compression by myelogram, followed by surgical decompression, is a must. Furthermore, unless radiation therapy is added, there is a high risk of recurrent compression with transection of the cord function.

6. Conclusions

The radiation oncologist should be an integral part of the team involved in evaluating and managing breast cancer patients. If this team approach works properly, then many situations will be recognized in which judicious use of radiation therapy can improve the quality of the patient's life. Coordination of this treatment with the necessary systemic hormonal or chemical therapy requires close cooperation among the oncologic specialists involved. This can result in better patient care and progress toward more effective cancer therapy.

ACKNOWLEDGMENTS

The authors wish to thank Mr. Bowen Keller for his assistance with the treatment planning and dosimetry illustrations. We also thank Mrs. Roberta Carter for her dedication and help in preparing this chapter.

7. References

1. H. Atkins, J.L. Hayward, D.J. Klugman, and A.B. Wayte, Treatment of early breast cancers: A report after ten years of a clinical trial, Br. Med. J. **2,** 423–429 (1972).
2. J.H. Farrow, A.A. Fracchia, G.F. Robbins, and E.L. Castro, Simple excision or biopsy plus radiation therapy as the primary treatment for potentially curable cancer of the breast, Cancer **28,** 1195–1201 (1971).
3. P.M. Rissanen, A comparison of conservative and radical surgery combined with radiotherapy in the treatment of Stage I carcinoma of the breast, Br. J. Radiol. **42,** 423–426 (1969).
4. M.V. Peters, The role of local excision and radiation in early breast cancer, in: Breast Cancer: Early and Late (M.D. Anderson Hospital, ed.), pp. 171–189, Year Book Medical Publishers, Inc., Chicago (1970).
5. L.R. Prosnitz, R. Leonard, and I.S. Goldenberg, Radiation therapy as primary treatment for early stage carcinoma of the breast, Cancer **35,** 1587–1596 (1975).
6. G.H. Fletcher, Local results of irradiation in the primary management of breast cancer, Cancer **29,** 545–551 (1972).
7. S. Hellman, Personal communication (1976).
8. E. Weber and S. Hellman, Radiation as primary treatment for local control of breast cancer, J. Am. Med. Assoc. **234,** 608–611 (1975).
9. S. Mustakallio, Conservative treatment of breast carcinoma—Review of 25 years follow-up, Clin. Radiol. **23,** 110–116 (1972).
10. P.J. Fitzpatrick, The radiotherapy of early breast cancer, To be published in Radiology (Presented at RSNA Meeting, Chicago, 1975).
11. L. Wise, A.Y. Mason, and L.V. Ackerman, Local excision and irradiation: An alternative method for the treatment of early mammary cancer, Ann. Surg. **174,** 392–401 (1971).
12. G.H. Fletcher, Clinical dose–response curves of human malignant epithelial tumors, Br. J. Radiol. **46,** 1–12 (1973).
13. W.D. Bloomer, A.L. Berenberg, and B.N. Weissman, Mammography of the definitively irradiated breast, Radiology **118,** 425–428 (1976).
14. National Research Council, Advisory Committee on the Biological Effects of Ionizing

Radiations, The Effects on Populations of Exposure to Low Levels of Ionizing Radiation, BEIR Report, Washington, D.C., National Academy of Sciences—National Research Council (1972).

15. G.H. Seydel, The risk of tumor induction in man following medical irradiation for malignant neoplasm, Cancer 35, 1641–1645 (1975).
16. R. Guttmann, Radiotherapy in locally advanced cancer of the breast, Cancer 20, 1046–1050 (1967).
17. R. McWhirter, Simple mastectomy and radiotherapy in the treatment of breast cancer, Br. J. Radiol. 28, 128–139 (1955).
18. R. McWhirter, Cancer of the breast, Am. J. Roentgenol. 62, 335–340 (1949).
19. F.C. Chu, F.-J. Lin, J. Kim, S. Huh, and C.J. Garmatis, Locally recurrent carcinoma of the breast, Cancer 37, 2677–2681 (1976).
20. G.H. Fletcher, E. Montague, and A.J. Nelson III, Combination of conservative surgery and irradiation for cancer of the breast, Am. J. Roentgenol. 126, 216–222 (1976).
21. R. Paterson and M.H. Russell, Clinical trials in malignant disease, Part III, Breast cancer: Evaluation of post-operative radiotherapy, J. Fac. Radiol. 10, 175–180 (1959).
22. E.C. Easson, Post-operative radiotherapy in breast cancer, in: Prognostic Factors in Breast Cancer (A.P.M. Forrest and P.B. Kunkler, eds.), pp. 118–135, William and Wilkins Co., Baltimore (1968).
23. B. Fisher, N.H. Slack, P.J. Cavanaugh, B. Gardner, and R.G. Ravdin, Post-operative radiotherapy in the treatment of breast cancer: Results of the NSABP clinical trial, Ann. Surg. 172, 711–732 (1970).
24. A. Raventos, Post-operative radiation therapy, Cancer 28, 1651–1653 (1971).
25. I.D.J. Bross, Predictive statistical approaches in evaluating surgical procedures, Cancer 28, 1637–1646 (1971).
26. J. Stjernsward, Decreased survival related to irradiation post-operatively in early operable breast cancer, Lancet 2, 1285–1286 (1974).
27. R.S. Handley and A.C. Thackray, Invasion of the internal mammary lymph glands in carcinoma of the breast, Br. J. Cancer 1, 15–20 (1947).
28. R.S. Handley, Further observations on the internal mammary lymph chain in carcinoma of the breast, Proc. R. Soc. Med. 45, 565–566 (1952).
29. C.D. Haagensen, C.R. Feind, F.P. Herter, C.A. Slanety, and J.A. Weinberg, The Lymphatics in Cancer, pp. 381–382, W.B. Saunders Co., Philadelphia (1972).
30. R.S. Handley and A.C. Thackray, Invasion of the internal mammary lymph nodes in carcinoma of the breast, Br. Med. J. 1, 61–63 (1954).
31. C.D. Haagensen, C.R. Feind, F.P. Herter, C.A. Slanety, and J.A. Weinberg, The Lymphatics in Cancer, p. 357, W.B. Saunders Co., Philadelphia (1972).
32. J.A. Urban, Clinical experience and results of excision of the internal mammary lymph node chain in primary operable breast cancer, Cancer 12, 14–22 (1959).
33. J.A. del Regato, Radiotherapy as a post-operative surgical adjuvant in the management of cancer of the breast, Radiology 98, 695–698 (1971).
34. F.C. Chu, J.C. Lucas, Jr., J.H. Farrow, and J.J. Nickson, Does prophylactic radiation therapy given for cancer of the breast predispose to metastases? Am. J. Roentgenol. 99, 987–994 (1967).
35. A.J. Nelson and E.D. Montague, Resectable localized breast cancer—The rationale for combined surgery and irradiation, J. Am. Med. Assoc. 231, 189–191 (1975).
36. C.D. Haagensen and A.P. Stout, Carcinoma of the breast. II. Criteria of operability, Ann. Surg. 118, 859–870; 1032–1051 (1943).
37. J.S. Spratt, Locally recurrent cancer after radical mastectomy, Cancer 20, 1051–1053 (1967).

38. G.F. Robbins, J.C. Lucas, A.A. Fracchia, J.H. Farrow, and F.C.H. Chu, An evaluation of post-operative prophylactic radiation therapy in breast cancer, *Surg. Gynecol. Obstet.* **122**, 979–982 (1966).

39. S.M. Jackson, Carcinoma of the breast: The significance of supraclavicular lymph node metastasis, *Clin. Radiol.* **17**, 107–114 (1966).

40. H. Host and I. Bernhovd, Combined surgery and radiation therapy versus surgery alone in primary mammary carcinoma, *Acta Radiol. Ther. Phys. Biol.* **14**, 25–32 (1975).

41. M. Archambault, M.I. Griem, and D.J. Lochman, Results of ultrafractionation radiation therapy in breast carcinoma, *Am. J. Roentgenol.* **91**, 62–66 (1964).

42. G. Bonadonna, E. Brusamolino, P. Valagussa, A. Rossi, L. Brugnatelli, C. Brambilla, G. Tancini, E. Bajetta, R. Musumeci, and U. Veronesi, Combination chemotherapy as an adjuvant treatment in operable breast cancer, *N. Engl. J. Med.* **294**, 405–410 (1976).

43. B. Fisher, P. Carbone, and S.G. Economon, L-Phenylalanine mustard (L-PAM) in the management of primary breast cancer, *N. Engl. J. Med.* **292**, 117–122 (1975).

44. G. Lundell, Effects of radiation therapy on blood-borne leukocytes in patients with mammary carcinoma, *Acta Radiol. Ther. Phys. Biol.* **13**, 307–312 (1974).

45. H. Blomgren, R. Berg, J. Wasserman, and U. Glas, Effect of radiotherapy on blood lymphocyte population in mammary carcinoma, *Int. J. Rad. Oncol. Biol. Phys.* **1**, 177–188 (1976).

46. E. Baral, H. Blomgren, B. Petrini, and J. Wasserman, Blood lymphocytes in breast cancer patients following radiotherapy and surgery, *Int. J. Rad. Oncol. Biol. Phys.* **2** (1977), in press.

47. A.E. Papatestas and A.F. Kark, Peripheral lymphocyte counts in breast carcinoma, *Cancer* **34**, 2014–2017 (1974).

48. M.M. Roberts and W. Jones-Williams, The delayed hypersensitivity reaction in breast cancer, *Br. J. Surg.* **61**, 549–552 (1974).

49. L. Gross, O.L. Manfredi, and A.A. Protos, Effect of cobalt-60 irradiation upon cell-mediated immunity, *Radiology* **105**, 653–655 (1973).

50. J.A. McCredie, W.R. Inch, and R.M. Southerland, Effect of post-operative radiotherapy on peripheral blood lymphocytes in patients with carcinoma of the breast, *Cancer* **29**, 249–256 (1972).

51. J.L. Bosworth, N.A. Ghossein, and T.L. Brooks, Delayed hypersensitivity in patients treated by curative radiotherapy, *Cancer* **36**, 353–358 (1975).

52. N.A. Ghossein, J.L. Bosworth, and R.E. Bases, The effect of radical radiotherapy on delayed hypersensitivity and the inflammatory response, *Cancer* **35**, 1616–1620 (1975).

53. F.C.H. Chu, L. Nisce, A.S. Baker, A. Sattar, and J.S. Laughlin, Electron-beam therapy of cancer of the breast, *Radiology* **89**, 216–223 (1967).

54. D.W. Smithers, P. Rigby-Jones, D.A.G. Galton, and P.M. Payne, Cancer of the breast, *Br. J. Radiol. Suppl. 4*, 1–90 (1952).

55. S. Cade, Treatment and results in carcinoma of the breast, *Am. J. Roentgenol.* **62**, 326–327 (1949).

56. C.D. Haagensen and A.P. Stout, Carcinoma of the breast: Results of treatment, 1935–1942, *Ann. Surg.* **134**, 151–172 (1951).

57. F. Baclesse, Roentgen therapy as the sole method of treatment of cancer of the breast, *Am. J. Roentgenol.* **62**, 311–319 (1949).

58. J. Bouchard, Advanced cancer of the breast treated primarily with irradiation, *Radiology* **84**, 823–841 (1963).

59. A. Hochman and E. Robinson, Eighty-two cases of mammary cancer treated exclusively with Roentgen therapy, *Cancer* **13**, 670–673 (1960).

60. J.A. Urban and M.A. Martani, Significance of internal mammary lymph node metastases in breast cancer, *Am. J. Roentgenol.* **111**, 130–136 (1971).

61. G. Fletcher and E. Montague, Radical irradiation of advanced breast cancer, *Am. J. Roentgenol.* **93**, 573–583 (1965).
62. H.M. Keys and P. Rubin, Unpublished data presented at the Annual Meeting of the American Society of Therapeutic Radiologists, Atlanta, Georgia (October 13–16, 1976).
63. H. Atkins and W.D. Horrigan, Treatment of locally advanced carcinoma of the breast with Roentgen therapy and simple mastectomy, *Am. J. Roentgenol.* **85**, 860–864 (1961).
64. N.T. Griscom and C.C. Wang, Radiation therapy of inoperable breast carcinoma, *Radiology* **79**, 18–23 (1962).
65. N.C. Delarue, C.L. Ash, V. Peters, and R. Fielden, Preoperative irradiation of locally advanced breast cancer, *Arch. Surg.* **91**, 136–153 (1965).
66. G. Fletcher, E.D. Montague, and E.C. White, Role of radiation therapy in the primary management of breast cancer, *Prog. Clin. Cancer* **4**, 242–256 (1970).
67. T.A.M. Stoker and H. Ellis, Post-irradiation toilet mastectomy in the management of locally advanced carcinoma of the breast, *Br. J. Radiol.* **45**, 851–854 (1972).
68. G.R. Brown, J. Horiot, G.H. Fletcher, E.C. White, and D.W. Ange, Simple mastectomy and radiation therapy for locally advanced breast cancers technically suitable for radical mastectomy, *Am. J. Roentgenol.* **120**, 67–73 (1974).
69. W.C. Powers, Breast cancer—pre-operative and post-operative radiation therapy, *Cancer* **24**, 1301–1306 (1969).
70. E.C. White, G.H. Fletcher, and R.L. Clark, Surgical experience with pre-operative irradiation for carcinoma of the breast, *Ann. Surg.* **155**, 948–953 (1962).
71. F.E. Adair, The effect of pre-operative irradiation in primary operable cancer of the breast, *Am. J. Roentgenol.* **35**, 359–370 (1936).
72. G. Lumb, Changes in carcinoma of the breast following irradiation, *Br. J. Surg.* **38**, 82–93 (1950).
73. B.W. Windeyer, Clinical aspects of radio-resistance, *Acta Radiol. Suppl. 116*, 108–119 (1954).
74. W. Woods, Locally advanced breast cancer and pre-operative radiotherapy, *Med. J. Aust.* **1**, 561–567 (1972).
75. J.M. Vaeth, J.C. CLark, J.P. Green, A.F. Schroeder, and R.O. Lowy, Radiotherapeutic management of locally advanced carcinoma of the breast, *Cancer* **30**, 107–112 (1972).
76. E.D. Montague, Physical and clinical parameters in the management of advanced breast cancer with radiation therapy alone, *Am. J. Roentgenol.* **99**, 995–1001 (1967).
77. G.F. Robbins, J. Shah, P. Rosen, F. Chu, and J. Taylor, Inflammatory carcinoma of the breast, *Surg. Clin. North Am.* **54**, 801–810 (1974).
78. N. Treves, The inoperability of inflammatory carcinoma of the breast, *Surg. Gynecol. Obstet.* **109**, 240–242 (1959).
79. S.L. Saltzstein, Clinically occult inflammatory carcinoma of the breast, *Cancer* **34**, 382–388 (1974).
80. D.L. Ellis and S.L. Teitelbaum, Inflammatory carcinoma of the breast—A pathological definition, *Cancer* **33**, 1045–1047 (1974).
81. C.C. Wang and N.T. Griscom, Inflammatory carcinoma of the breast, *Clin. Radiol.* **15**, 168–174 (1964).
82. J.L. Barker, A.J. Nelson, and E.D. Montague, Inflammatory carcinoma of the breast, *Radiology* **121**, 173–176 (1976). (Presented in part at the RSNA Meeting, Chicago, 1975.)
83. K.W. Barber, M.B. Dockerty, and O.T. Clagett, Inflammatory carcinoma of the breast, *Surg. Gynecol. Obstet.* **112**, 406–410 (1961).
84. B.F. Byrd and S.E. Stephenson, Jr., Management of inflammatory breast cancer, *South. Med. J.* **53**, 945–947 (1960).
85. T.L. Dao and J.D. McCarthy, Treatment of inflammatory carcinoma of the breast, *Surg. Gynecol. Obstet.* **105**, 289–294 (1957).

86. M. De Lena, C. Brambilla, and A. Marabito, Adriamycin plus vincristine compared to and combined with cyclophosphamide, methotrexate, and 5-fluorouracil for advanced breast cancer, *Cancer* **35**, 1108–1115 (1975).

87. T.L. Dao and J. Kovaric, Incidence of pulmonary and skin metastases in women with breast cancer who received post-operative irradiation, *Surgery* **52**, 203–212 (1962).

88. F.R. Hendrickson, W.H. Shehata, and A.B. Kirchner, Radiation therapy for osseous metastases, *Int. J. Rad. Oncol. Biol. Phys.* **1**, 275–281 (1976).

89. M. Deutsch, J.A. Parsons, and R. Mercado, Jr., Radiotherapy for intracranial metastases, *Cancer* **34**, 1607–1611 (1974).

90. S.E. Order, S. Hellman, C.F. Von Essen, and M.M. Kligerman, Improvement in quality of survival following whole brain irradiation for brain metastases, *Radiology* **91**, 149–153 (1968).

91. Radiation Therapy Oncology Group (RTOG), Unpublished data (in preparation for publication).

92. P. Rubin, J. Green, and G. Holzwasser, Superior vena caval syndrome, *Radiology* **81**, 385–387 (1963).

93. H.P. Schultz, E. Glatstein, and H. Kaplan, Management of presumptive or proven Hodgkin's disease of the liver: A new radiotherapy technique, *Int. J. Rad. Oncol. Biol. Phys.* **1**, 1–8 (1975).

94. P. Rubin, S. Bunyagidj, and C. Poulter, Internal mammary lymph node metastases in breast cancer: Detection and management, *Am. J. Roentgenol.* **111**, 588–597 (1971).

Immunology and Immunotherapy of Human Breast Cancer

RECENT DEVELOPMENTS AND PROSPECTS FOR THE FUTURE

JORDAN U. GUTTERMAN, GIORA M. MAVLIGIT,
EVAN M. HERSH, GABRIEL HORTOBAGYI, AND
GEORGE BLUMENSCHEIN

1. Introduction

The discovery of tumor-specific antigens and tumor-specific immune responses in both animals and humans with malignant disease has increased understanding of the host defense mechanisms in the etiology and pathogenesis of cancer. However, before these tumor-specific immunological phenomena were clearly documented in man, it was strongly suspected that host defense mechanisms or their failure played a role in the etiology and pathogenesis of tumors. As these tumor-specific immune mechanisms were discovered in man, the concept of immunological surveillance was developed. [1]

Several well-known clinical phenomena have suggested the exis-

JORDAN U. GUTTERMAN, GIORA M. MAVLIGIT, EVAN M. HERSH, GABRIEL
HORTOBAGYI, AND GEORGE BLUMENSCHEIN · Departments of Developmental
Therapeutics (J. U. G., G. M. M., and E. M. H.) and Medicine (G. H. and G. B.), The
University of Texas System Cancer Center, M. D. Anderson Hospital and Tumor Institute,
Houston, Texas. This work was supported by Contract NO1-CB-33888 from the National
Institutes of Health, Bethesda, Maryland; a grant from Burroughs Wellcome Co., Research
Triangle Park, North Carolina; and a grant from the Cancer Research Institute, New York,
New York. Drs. Gutterman and Mavligit are the recipients of Career Development Awards
(CA 71007-03 and CA 00130-02, respectively) from the National Institutes of Health,
Bethesda, Maryland.

tence of this relationship. Spontaneous regressions of cancer have been observed both in patients with solid tumors and in patients with acute leukemia. [2] These have sometimes been associated with infectious complications, suggesting an immunological mechanism. Pathologic observations made almost 50 years ago revealed that some solid tumors were associated with lymphocytic infiltration; the presence of lymphocytic infiltration in a primary tumor was recognized as a good prognostic indicator. [3] Although there are many exceptions, the age relationships of cancer have also been used as evidence for host defense and immunological surveillance. [4] An important clinicopathologic observation is the very high incidence of *in situ* cancers and the low incidence of related invasive cancers. Two sets of observations made recently indirectly support the concept that immunological deficiencies are involved in the etiology and pathogenesis of cancer. First, there is an increased incidence of malignancy associated with immunological deficiency disease. [4] The second observation is the recent finding that there is an increased incidence of malignant disease in patients undergoing chronic immunosuppressive therapy for the maintenance of organ allografts. [4] It is conceivable that the genetic basis for immunological deficiency is also the basis for an increased susceptibility to malignancy and that the reduced host defense mechanisms have nothing to do with the pathogenesis. In spite of these reservations, the concept of immunological surveillance was developed during the last several years. This concept was first given expression by Thomas in a discussion on the general aspects of delayed hypersensitivity. [5] Burnet has greatly expanded this concept in a series of lectures and papers. [6] Direct evidence to support this surveillance hypothesis has come from a variety of animal experiments. Of prime importance are the studies of the immunological consequences of chemical or viral carcinogenesis in mice. [4] Susceptible mice subjected to either chemical or viral carcinogens undergo moderate to profound immunological suppression during the latent period before the development of identifiable tumors. This immunological incompetence involves both cell-associated and humoral immunity, and tends to recover as the primary tumors first appear. There is a general and not a tumor-specific immune defect. Specific types of immunosuppressive treatment also influence the incidence and rate of development of tumors. These include neonatal thymectomy and treatment with antilymphocyte serum or immunosuppressive drugs. These treatments also accelerate the rates of local growth and metastases of already established tumors.

Recently, there has been a body of evidence tending to negate the concept of immunological surveillance. [4,7] These arguments have been presented elsewhere and will not be reviewed here. (A discussion on the evidence for stimulation of tumor growth by the immune system will be developed later in this review.) Suffice it to say that the original concept of immunological surveillance probably needs a redefinition in the light of recent experiments. However, it has been extremely useful to begin to understand the host–tumor relationship. The precise role of the immune system in the prevention (and perhaps stimulation) of tumor growth will hopefully be more accurately defined over the coming years.

Immunological deficiency is involved not only with the etiology but also with the pathogenesis and entire natural history of the malignant process. Now that we are in the era of systemic treatment, recent studies indicate that the immunological mechanisms are involved in the response to conventional nonimmunological treatment. This will be expanded in the sections below. The immunological deficiency associated with cancer is of two types. First, there is a nonspecific immunological deficiency which becomes severe as the disease disseminates. Second, there is a tumor-specific immunological deficiency related to the release of tumor antigens which operates to suppress local host defenses. This may be one of a number of reasons why primary cancers disseminate even when the host is immunocompetent. Immunological deficiency associated with cancer was first observed in patients with lymphoid malignancies[8] and more recently in patients with solid tumors. Levin and co-workers demonstrated that patients with metastatic solid tumors had impaired development of new delayed hypersensitivity and impaired local inflammatory responses.[9] This immunological deficiency was apparently caused by the tumor, in that it was not found in patients free of disease after surgery. Although Levin and co-workers did not identify a defect in the antibody response to viral antigens, several investigators have found that patients with solid tumors had an impaired primary antibody response to a variety of antigens.[10] In addition, patients with advanced solid tumors show impaired *in vitro* lymphocyte blastogenic responses to a variety of mitogens. This is due in part to a serum factor that can inhibit lymphocyte blastogenesis.

A second type of immunological deficiency, associated with metastatic tumors, which is tumor-specific, has been described in animal systems. The tumor mass inhibits the immune response to the tumor either locally or systemically, while other immune responses and overall immunocompetence in general are normal. Alexander and Hall noted that the lymphoblast response of a lymph node to an injection of tumor antigen is completely inhibited if an actively growing tumor of the same type is present in the lymphatic drainage of the stimulated lymph node.[11] Stjernsward reported that tumor-specific immune responses are suppressed in animals that have recently had a large tumor removed.[12] This immunosuppression is probably due to the release of relatively large amounts of tumor antigen which inactivate the immunological response.

This chapter will describe the immunology of patients with malignant breast cancer. We will review the evidence for nonspecific immune deficiency as well as the evidence for a tumor-associated immune response. The second part of the chapter will be devoted to a review of advances in immunotherapy of human cancer, including breast cancer, which have been made during the last few years.

As noted above, the overwhelming experimental evidence supports the notion that animal and human cancer cells express foreign antigens and that these antigens evoke an immune response by cancer patients. The science of tumor immunology is very young and methods to detect these tumor-associated antigens are, at best, inexact. We will review the evidence that a tumor-associated immune response(s) exists. Several techniques, including histopathologic analysis of biopsy and autopsy specimens, have been applied in the study of tumor immunology. General immunocompetence has been evaluated by a variety of techniques. In order to assess the humoral component of the immune response, serum immunoglobulin levels and antibody responses to new antigens are measured. *In vitro* techniques to assess the cell-associated immune response include lymphocyte stimulation by mitogens and antigens as well as mixed lymphocyte culture reactivity. *In vivo* tests of cellular immunity include delayed cutaneous hypersensitivity reactions to recall antigens or to primary antigens; measurement of peripheral-blood lymphocyte counts and lymphocyte subpopulations, including T and B cells; measurement of an inflammatory response; and measurement of the function of the reticuloendothelial system (RES).

2. Histologic Evidence for Host Immune Response

Although Chapter 2 is devoted to the histopathology of breast cancer, the host immune response as assessed by histology is important enough to warrant a short review here.

Infiltration by lymphoreticular cells is a common feature of many human malignant neoplasms. Such infiltrates are a prominent feature of some tumors, such as seminoma of the testis and medullary carcinoma of the breast. Virchow, as early as 1863, commented on the stromal response to tumors. [13] When spontaneous regressions of human tumors were recognized at the turn of the twentieth century, an intense interest developed in the host response to the tumors. For example, Handley, in 1907, suggested that "round cell infiltration" in melanoma indicated a "regression process." [14] Wade, in 1908, commented that tumors can be "borne away on a lymphocyte tide." [15]

The prognostic importance of the lymphocytes to human tumors was suggested by their positive association with good prognosis. In 1921 and 1922, MacCarty and co-workers commented on this association, particularly in breast cancer[16] Other workers in the early 1920s, such as Greenough in 1925, made this association. [17] Moore and Foote, in 1949, associated good prognosis in medullary carcinoma of the breast with lymphoid infiltration. [18]

The importance of structural characteristics of breast cancer and prognosis was further strengthened by important studies by Bloom in England in the 1950s[19] and by Black and co-workers beginning in the middle 1950s.[20] These studies suggested that the biologic behavior of breast cancer could be correlated with the differentiation of the primary tumor. Black and co-workers, in 1953, reported that the regional lymph nodes draining breast cancers demonstrated a variety of reactive and degenerative changes. They noted a specific lymph node pattern called "sinus histiocytosis" (SH) which indicated a favorable prognosis. Thus, the importance of the lymphoreticuloendothelial (LRE) system in the biologic behavior of breast cancer was clearly determined.

It is important to briefly summarize the classic studies of cell-mediated reaction to early *in situ* as well as advanced cancer. Intraepithelial lymphocyte accumulation in the region of *in situ* carcinoma is less prominent or absent as compared to accumulation in normal ducts. In contrast to a decrease in the number of intramucosal lymphoid cells in areas of *in situ* carcinoma, accumulation of lymphoid cells is seen in the stroma around the cancer-containing ducts. [21]

Invasive breast cancer, however, has been shown to be associated with reactive and degenerative changes in regional lymph nodes and the primary tumor. Such changes are qualitatively similar to those seen in response to *in situ* carcinoma. While the LRE responses to invasive cancer are similar, other reactions, including lymphoid cell infiltration and SH, are less frequent in response to invasive as compared to *in situ* carcinoma. [22] Less than 40% of patients with invasive carcinoma show evidence of significant lymphoid infiltration in their primary tumors or SH responses in their axillary lymph nodes. However, Black and co-workers have shown a strong correlation between the LRE response at the time of mastectomy and subsequent survival. [23] Thus, it appears that lymph node response reflects an immunological response to the tumor and probably is the *in vivo* or histologic correlate of cellular hyper-sensitivity.

Hamlin, in 1968, performed a detailed study of cellular infiltration in 272 tumors. [24] There was a strong correlation between the host resistance and prognosis and between cell reaction and tumor grade. In addition, Berg reported that a peripheral plasma cell infiltrate in poorly differentiated carcinomas was associated with an improved survival rate. [25] In contrast, Champion and associates found that this type of reaction was associated with a poor prognosis. [26] Other discerning notes were published by Scarff and Torlomi in 1968[27] and by Sommers, [28] who failed to find any difference between the cell reaction in intraductal carcinoma and the invasive type.

Although the findings of Black and co-workers demonstrating favorable survival with the SH response have been confirmed by some, but not all, investigators, Silverberg *et al.* demonstrated that only patients with moderately or poorly differentiated primary breast tumors and patients with at least one, but not greater than eight, tumor-involved axillary lymph nodes showed a correlation between SH response and good prognosis. [29] Hamlin reported on an extensive index of host defense reactions which includes mononuclear cell infiltration in the primary as well as regional lymph nodes. [24] Zelen also reported on a multifactorial relationship, including histologic as well as immunologic factors which correlate with prognosis. [30]

Several workers, including DiRe and Kister and their associates, [31,32] have failed to support any correlation between SH and good prognosis. In his original publication in 1956, Berg [33] failed to find a relationship between SH and good prognosis. However, more recently, he has succeeded in demonstrating such a relationship. [34] Fisher and co-workers demonstrated that there was no prognostic significance for SH in patients with four or more positive nodes as well as in patients who relapsed within one year of surgery. [25,36] However, the presence of marked SH was associated with an absence of nodal metastases.

Applying our present-day understanding of the distribution of different lymphoid cells in lymph nodes, Tsakraklides and associates correlated the ten-year survival in a group of 227 women with breast cancer. They noted that the best prognosis was associated with what was characterized as a lymphocyte-predominant pattern in the regional lymph nodes. The worst prognosis was measured in those patients with lymphocyte-depleted regional lymph nodes. An intermediate prognosis was noted in patients with a germinal center or an unstimulated pattern. [37] Hunter and co-workers have recently published interesting results correlating regional lymph node histology with prognosis. [38] In a review of the histologic sections of lymph nodes removed during surgery, 16 of 17 patients in whom SH was the dominant lymphoid reaction were alive with no evidence of cancer five or more years after operation. Five of six patients in whom germinal center hyperplasia was the only significant reaction died of cancer in less than five years. Patients with both SH and germinal center hyperplasia had a survival that was intermediate, with 17 of 25 patients alive and free of cancer. These data would certainly suggest that a B-cell proliferation, as demonstrated by histologic classification, is not associated with as good a prognosis as the SH reaction, which may represent activated macrophages and/or a T-cell reaction.

Fisher and co-workers [35,36] failed to confirm the interesting findings of Tsakraklides and co-workers. In contrast, Fisher's results failed to reveal any relationship between a particular nodal pattern and short-term treatment failure. Longer follow-up may be needed to demonstrate such a relationship. As a matter of fact, a lymphocyte-predominant pattern in regional nodes was found by Fisher *et al.* to be associated with absent lymphoid cellular reaction within the tumor.

Thus, it is clear that a variety of immunological reactions, demonstrated by histologic features, can be shown both in the primary tumor as well as in the regional lymph nodes of breast cancer patients. However, the precise significance of these reactions remains to be determined and further work will need to be carried out. (For a detailed description of the histopathologic features of breast cancer, see Chapter 2.)

3. General Immune Competence

3.1. Delayed Cutaneous Hypersensitivity

Delayed-type hypersensitivity detected by skin testing with recall or primary antigens involves complex mechanisms. [39] When an antigen to which the individual is sensitive is injected, a proportion of the antigen remains in the localized area of the basal layers of the epidermis and the upper layers of the dermis. Sensitized lymphocytes with specific reactivity to the antigen arrive at the area and recognize the antigen. Recognition is mediated, presumably, through monocytes and macrophages. Thus, the first step may be the uptake of the antigen and its processing by fixed tissue macrophages, after which it is brought into contact with sensitized lymphocytes. These lymphocytes undergo blastogenic transformation and produce soluble factors including vasoactive substances, macrophage chemotactic factor, migration inhibiting factor, macrophage activating factor, and so forth. [40] The net result is the accumulation of lymphocytes, their associated blastogenic transformation, and an accumulation of monoocytes which transform at the local site to macrophages. These events produce the clinical features of delayed-type hypersensitivity, including erythema due to vasodilation and induration due to local edema and the perivascular accumulation in the dermis of large numbers of lymphocytes, lymphoblasts, monocytes, and macrophages. If the antigens are ingested and destroyed by the macrophages, the phenomenon is self-limiting, gradually disappearing within 48 to 96 hours. [41] Anergy or unresponsiveness to recall skin-test antigens has been demonstrated in a variety of infectious and autoimmune diseases as well as in cancer and immunodeficiency diseases.

Anergy can also develop with advancing age, which is associated with a decline in immunological reactivity.

3.1.1. Primary Antigens

It has been demonstrated that a substantial percentage of cancer patients have varying defects in the ability to mount a delayed hypersensitivity reaction to new or primary antigens such as DNCB and KLH. [42] In a study reported by Eilber and Morton, 90% of cancer patients who were DNCB-positive at the time of surgery were operable and remained free of disease at six months. In contrast, 90% of patients who were unable to respond to DNCB were found to be inoperable or recurred within six months of surgery. [43] In general, patients with adenocarcinomas (such as breast cancer) have a lesser deficiency of DNCB responsiveness as compared to patients with squamous cancer. [44] Actually, many studies carried out in breast cancer patients suggest that these patients have only minimal defects in the ability to express delayed hypersensitivity to nonspecific antigens until late in the disease. For example, Bolton and co-workers showed that among early breast cancer patients, there was a minimal decrease in DNCB responsiveness as compared to a control group. Greater impairment was seen in advanced cancer patients. [45] Pinsky and co-workers also demonstrated a decrease in DNCB responsiveness among breast cancer patients with advanced disease. [46] Wanebo *et al.* showed that only patients with nodal metastases demonstrated a slight, but statistically insignificant, impairment of DNCB responsiveness. [47] Surprisingly, patients with negative nodes or advanced disease showed no impairment in DNCB responsiveness. [47] Golub and associates detected a modest degree of DNCB impairment in advanced breast cancer patients. [48] Cunningham and co-workers correlated DNCB-induced delayed cutaneous hypersensitivity reactions with the course of disease in patients with recurrent breast cancer. [49] Patients with strong delayed cutaneous reactions to DNCB were characterized by a significantly higher probability of surviving and a longer median survival time as compared to those with weak or negative responses. Additionally, there was a greater probability of responding to therapy with strong, as compared to weak or negative, responses. It was also suggested that patients with Grade III tumors with a dense lymphocyte infiltrate had more frequent strong delayed reactions to DNCB than did patients with few lymphocytes. [49]

3.1.2. Recall or Established Antigens

The early breast cancer patient has few defects in responding to recall antigens. Only late in the disease do defects arise. Roberts and

Williams reported minimal depression of reactivity in early breast cancer patients but a significant decrease in the response to varidase among 99 patients with disseminated carcinoma of the breast. [50,51] Bolton and co-workers found no significant decrease in the *in vivo* response to recall antigens among early patients. However, there was a significant decrease in reactivity among disseminated breast cancer patients as compared to normal controls. [52] Of interest, Bolton and co-workers showed that skin-test reactions were diminished to a greater degree in patients with carcinoma of the colon and rectum and stomach cancer as compared to breast cancer patients. [45] They emphasized that response to the varidase skin test was particularly decreased in patients with advanced breast cancer, suggesting perhaps some specificity for this skin-test antigen among breast cancer patients. We have previously suggested that certain recall antigens may detect immunological defects in specific histologic types of cancer. For example, the dermatophytin skin test is a very sensitive indicator of immunological deficiency in patients with acute leukemia and malignant melanoma, [53] while the candida skin test is very sensitive in detecting immunological impairment among lung cancer patients. [54] Finally, Nemoto *et al.* found virtually no impairment of responsiveness to recall antigens in patients with localized breast cancer, but a great deal of deficiency in patients with advanced disease. [55]

3.2. Lymphocyte Counts in Breast Cancer

Recent reports suggest that the number of circulating peripheral lymphocytes may be useful as a prognostic index in patients with breast cancer. Krant and co-workers [56] and Riesco [57] reported a significant correlation between the number of peripheral lymphocytes and the cure rate among 589 cancer patients, including a large number with breast cancer. Others have also shown that lymphocyte counts are useful as a prognostic indicator. [58] Recently, Papatestas and co-workers reported that patients with early breast cancer had higher pretreatment lymphocyte counts than did patients with advanced tumors. The five-year survival among patients with pretreatment counts above 2000/mm³ was 87% in Stage I, 67% in Stage II, and 57% in Stage III. The comparable figures for patients with lower counts were 82%, 51%, and 29%, respectively. [59]

Enumeration of subpopulations of lymphocytes is now possible with the distinction of T and B lymphocytes. Various studies have demonstrated that the numbers of T cells and/or B cells may either be decreased or even increased in cancer patients. Wybran and Fundenberg demonstrated that the number of circulating T cells, as measured by the E-rosette assay, is frequently decreased in advanced breast cancer patients.[60] There is also evidence that B cells, as enumerated by complement receptors or surface immunoglobulin, are, respectively, decreased or increased in advanced breast cancer patients.[47] One must take into account the influence of chemotherapy and radiotherapy in these assays (see below).

It should be emphasized at this stage in the review that patients with myasthenia gravis who have low lymphocyte counts have an increased incidence of breast cancer. Since experimental thymectomy results in a decreased incidence and delayed appearance of breast cancer, and because the presence of the thymus is essential for the development of experimental breast cancer (see below), the role of the thymic lymphocytes and the thymus in breast cancer must be carefully evaluated.[61,62]

3.3. *In Vitro* Tests

The evaluation of *in vitro* lymphocyte reactivity to mitogens has yielded varying results in patients with breast cancer. For example, many studies have shown essentially no decrease in reactivity to mitogens such as phytohemagglutinin (PHA).[45,50,51,63] Other investigators, including Robinson,[64] Knight,[65] Miller,[66] Whittaker,[67] and their associates, observed a variable decrease in lymphocyte reactivity. Nemoto *et al.*[55] showed that reactivity to mitogens only decreased in the terminal stages of breast cancer.

Golub and co-workers studied the *in vitro* and *in vivo* immunocompetence of eight patients with metastatic breast cancer. These patients primarily exhibited defects in so-called recognition assays. The primary skin-test response to DNCB and the *in vitro* response in the mixed leukocyte culture were markedly reduced in most carcinoma patients.[48] In contrast, the proliferative capacity of these patients' lymphocytes—that is, the ability to respond to recall antigens and to mitogens such as PHA and concanavalin A—was less impaired as compared to lymphocytes of melanoma patients. These authors suggested that the lymphocytes of melanoma patients have a defect primarily in proliferation and that carcinoma patients, including those with breast cancer, exhibit defects in primary *in vitro* recognition. It was of interest that concanavalin A was more sensitive in detecting impaired immunity than was PHA. Thus, these findings may have relevance to some of the "normal" studies reported by other workers.

Wanebo *et al.*[47] demonstrated that lymphocyte responses to mitogens were generally normal for breast cancer patients. However, there was a significant depression of lymphocyte responses to *Candida albicans* and *Escherichia coli*. Certain responses actually produced a "V-shaped" pattern, demonstrating maximum depression in patients with Stage I cancer and then an increase in patients with Stage II and Stage III cancer. Wanebo speculated that the higher responsiveness to certain mitogens and antigens in patients with Stage II and Stage III disease may represent a stimulation of peripheral-blood lymphocytes in patients with nodal metastases and locally advanced breast cancer analogous to the stimulation of regional lymph node lymphocytes (see below). Similar results were reported by Whitehead and co-workers, who found a significant depression of T-cell levels in patients with Stage I and Stage II breast cancer; in Stage III patients, however, the values had returned to the normal range. [68]

Several workers have studied the capacity of regional lymph node lymphocytes to respond to mitogens *in vitro*. Fisher and co-workers[69,70] showed that cells of all regional lymph nodes from breast cancer patients respond to PHA stimulation. The response of stimulated and nonstimulated regional lymph node cells from patients with negative nodes was significantly greater than that of cells from women with positive nodes. When lymphocytes from peripheral blood and from regional lymph nodes of the same breast cancer patients were exposed to undiluted PHA, the response of the former was significantly greater than that of the latter. While both types of cells were less stimulated by diluted PHA, the response of regional lymph node cells was significantly greater than that of peripheral blood cells. The lymph node lymphocytes from patients with colon cancer responded similarly to those from breast cancer patients. All nodes responded to PHA stimulation, but the response was greater when the lymphocytes came from negative- rather than positive-node patients. The PHA responsiveness of these regional nodes was increased primarily in patients whose carcinomas were of low nuclear grade and contained only mild degrees of lymphoid infiltrate. There was no relationship between SH and lymphocyte transformation. Finally, the location of the nodes correlated with *in vitro* responsiveness, the low axillary nodes responding better *in vitro* than the high axillary nodes. These nodes thus behave similarly to the peripheral-blood lymphocytes.

Ambus and co-workers studied the regional and peripheral lymphocyte responsiveness to PHA and to allogeneic leukocytes in eleven breast cancer patients. [71] In this study, the response of peripheral blood cells to PHA tended to be greater than that of lymph node lymphocytes. In contrast, the lymph node lymphocytes tended to be more responsive to allogeneic leukocytes (MLC response) than were the peripheral blood lymphocytes. An inverse correlation was noted between the response of peripheral-blood and lymph node lymphocytes to tumor cells (to be described in later sections). It should be noted that Fisher *et al.* reported the identical finding that with undiluted PHA, the response of peripheral-blood lymphocytes was greater than that of lymph node lymphocytes. The finding that lymph node lymphocytes were more responsive to allogeneic leukocytes is of great interest. It may reflect their important role in the primary immune recognition of foreign tissue antigens. [71] Jubert and co-workers [72] have also demonstrated a trend for greater reactivity in the mixed leukocyte cultures of lymph node lymphocytes and appendix lymphocytes as compared to peripheral blood lymphocytes. The reactivity of regional cells in tumor-associated assays will be described and summarized below.

Although several workers have demonstrated that the serum or plasma from cancer patients depresses the response of normal lymphocytes to antigens and mitogens, others have failed to confirm these results. For example, Whittaker and co-workers found that lymphocytes from patients with disseminated breast cancer responded normally to PHA when cultured in the presence of normal serum. [67] However, serum taken from cancer patients decreased the *in vitro* response of normal lymphocytes to PHA. There have been several studies demonstrating a serum inhibitory effect in breast cancer patients. [67,68,73–75] Although most studies have demonstrated inhibitors in the serum of patients with advanced breast cancer, some have failed to find serum inhibitors. [76,77] These differences may be explained by the use of different PHA in different concentrations, different time course for culturing lymphocytes, etc.

Several substances have been implicated as the major source of inhibitor material. The α-2-globulin, which is a regulatory molecule, has been implicated. A low-molecular-weight peptide bound to several plasma proteins and present in smaller amounts bound to α-globulin has been partially characterized. [78] Substances including IgG, C-reactive protein, and prostaglandins and other materials have also been implicated. [79] Some workers, such as Blomgren and associates, [77] showed potentiation of response with the serum of breast cancer patients. Whitehead and co-workers [68] found that the number of E-rosette-forming T cells in breast cancer patients was reduced only because such cells were coated with serum materials. Other workers have shown a complete lack of correlation between the depression of lymphocyte function and the degree of lymphocyte serum inhibition.

4. Tumor-Associated Antigens

Tumor cells appear to have on their surfaces tumor-associated antigens which are capable of inducing rejection responses in their hosts.

Tumor-associated antigens have been demonstrated on most cells of induced and spontaneous tumors of animals. Tumor-associated antigens can be divided into those found on tumors induced by chemical or physical agents and on tumors induced by DNA and RNA viruses. Classically, chemically induced tumors appear to have distinct antigens with no cross-reactivity between them. In contrast, viral tumors possess antigens which appear to cross-react extensively within the group induced by the same virus (reviewed in reference 80). Murine mammary tumors in general, are induced by RNA viruses and resistance to these tumors can be transferred with lymph node or peritoneal cells. In addition to the common cross-reactive antigens of spontaneous mammary tumors in mice, another class of tumor-associated antigens exist which are unique to each tumor and are not associated with virus.

Tumor cells also demonstrate the expression of antigens normally present in embryonic tissues. These fetal antigens are usually expressed only during fetal life. During the neoplastic process, genes become reactivated and their products appear in the transformed cells.

Despite the evidence for the presence of tumor-associated antigens and immune surveillance, the precise nature of the immune response and its relationship to tumor growth is complicated.

Prehn[81,82] questioned the role of immune surveillance in the development of cancer. Although it is well accepted that a strong immune response can bring about the destruction of early tumor, a weak immune reaction may not be beneficial and may thereby stimulate tumor growth. The possible promoting effect of weak immunity on experimental mammary tumors is now rather firmly established in the literature. Prehn has formulated the concept of immunostimulation to account for the "sneaking through" whereby tumors can escape recognition and destruction and grow in immunocompetent hosts, particularly if the initial tumor inoculum is small. The concept of immunostimulation may explain some paradoxical findings in experimental breast carcinogenesis. For example, some experiments in which the immune reactivity of animals is reduced will yield a decrease in the incidence of breast tumors. Furthermore, neonatal thymectomy and other maneuvers decrease the incidence of spontaneous breast cancer.[83-88]

A similar host–tumor relationship exists in pregnancy. It appears that an immune reaction caused by a maternal–fetal histoincompatibility gene difference stimulates the growth of the placenta.

As mentioned in the introduction, the spontaneous regression of human tumors provides strong evidence for the involvement of some immune mechanisms in the destruction of tumor cells. In the original report by Everson in 1964,[2] five of the 130 patients with spontaneous tumor regression were patients with breast cancer. The common finding of *in situ* tumors at autopsy is frequently quoted as evidence of immune containment of tumor. Although this has not been documented in human breast cancer, Hutter and Kim[89] and other workers have documented the high incidence of bilaterality and multicentricity of *in situ* lobular breast carcinoma, which far exceeds the clinical incidence of this type of cancer.

In addition, as is well known, the natural history of breast cancer shows that a disease-free state can be maintained for many years in the presence of disseminated cancer. Patients have survived for years despite the presence of circulating cancer cells in their blood prior to therapy.[90] Circulating cancer cells have been identified in a majority of patients with tumors confined to the breast, and many of these patients are still cured.[91] Edwards and co-workers demonstrated in 1972 that palpable axillary lymph nodes in some breast cancer patients regressed spontaneously following simple mastectomy. Seventy-five percent of patients with Stage II disease showed regression of axillary lymph nodes following this surgical procedure. Many of these nodes must have contained tumor.[92] The evidence for tumor-associated immune reactivity by regional lymph nodes will be presented below.

The international differences in histology and survival in breast cancer support the importance of the host immune response. However, although survival rates for breast cancer patients in Japan are higher than in the United States, the relationships of histologic type and lymphoid infiltrate to survival could not be determined.

Finally, patients having a previous history of *in situ* cancer were found to have a more favorable stage and survival characteristics than those with breast cancer preceded by benign lesions and invasive cancers. These findings have suggested cross-reacting immunologic responses in patients with *in situ* breast cancer.

4.1. Skin-Test Assays to Detect Antigens in Breast Cancer

There are a variety of *in vitro* and *in vivo* techniques to clarify and identify tumor-associated immune reactivity in breast cancer patients. Skin tests with delayed hypersensitivity measurements have been used for studying the cell-mediated immune response of breast cancer patients to tumor-associated antigens. Hughes and Lytton performed studies with crude cytoplasmic fraction of tumors.[93] Five of 20 breast cancer patients reacted to autologous tumor extracts. Stewart reported that approximately 20% of patients with cancer of the breast reacted to crude autologous extracts.[94] Interestingly, there was an inverse correlation between positive skin tests and survival in that study. Alford and co-workers reported studies with crude membrane extracts and partially separated, soluble sonicated extracts of breast tissues.[95] Patients with breast cancer reacted not only to soluble fractions from autologous and allogeneic breast tumors, but also to comparable fractions from control breast tissues. Six of 13 patients had a delayed hypersensitivity reaction to breast cancer membrane extracts but not to normal breast membranes derived from either the same mastectomy specimen or from the breast tissue of patients with cystic disease. Patients with other types of cancer did not react to these preparations. Membrane preparations appeared to be tumor-specific but soluble membrane fractions gave less specificity. The breast cancer patients were as reactive to soluble breast fractions derived from normal tissue as to the breast cancer fractions. Thus, this reactivity appeared to be detecting organ-specific antigen in soluble fractions. Subsequent studies by Hollinshead and co-workers have further clarified this reactivity.[96] Soluble membrane antigen was separated by gradient polyacrylamide gel electrophoresis (PAGE) and the various gel regions were tested and separated. The crude unfractionated extracts did not evoke a positive reaction. However, after chromatography on Sephadex G-200, a skin-reactive antigen was found in fraction 2. The nonreactivity of the crude extracts appears to be due to inhibitory factors which Hollinshead and co-workers have described for other tumors. Fraction 2 was then further separated by PAGE and a tumor-associated antigen appeared in region 2B. In addition, there appeared to be other skin-reactive antigens in region 2A that were probably tissue-associated antigens, since they were found in breast tumors and also in benign breast tissue. Allogeneic as well as autologous fractions evoked positive reactions. This could be due to common antigens because of viral association with the tumor. However, other causes of common antigenicity would include fetal antigens and tissue-associated antigens. Other patients with early breast cancer reacted to tissue antigens, as evidenced by the reactions to Sephadex fraction 2 of benign breast tissues and by the reactions to PAGE region 2A antigens. There was also some reactivity to the more specific 2B antigens. In contrast, the Stage IV patients seemed to react only to associated antigens, giving negative reactions to control breast materials and to region 2A antigens. The reason that patients with localized disease reacted to breast tissue antigen, but patients with advanced disease did not, is not clear at this time.

4.2. Lymphocyte Stimulation by Breast Cancer Antigens

The *in vitro* lymphocyte blastogenic resonse to breast cancer cells or solubilized extracts has also revealed the reactivity of patients' lymphocytes. Several workers have observed the capacity of patients' lymphocytes to respond *in vitro* to these materials from patients with various solid tumors. [97–99] We have shown that solubilized antigen can stimulate autologous lymphocytes from breast cancer patients. [97] In addition to the reactivity of peripheral-blood lymphocytes, there is evidence that regional lymph node lymphocytes can also respond to breast cancer antigens. Ambus *et al.* reported on the *in vitro* blastogenic response of peripheral-blood leukocytes and lymph node leukocytes of cancer patients which were examined simultaneously in paired studies. [71] The lymph nodes were obtained at the time of surgical tumor extirpation from the area draining or adjacent to the tumor. There was an inverse relationship between the responses of peripheral-blood lymphocytes and lymph node lymphocytes to tumor cells. In those subject whose peripheral-blood lymphocytes responded to tumor cells, the response of lymph node lymphocytes was usually negative and/or significantly lower. In contrast, in those subjects whose lymph node lymphocyte response to tumor cells was positive, the peripheral-blood responses were usually negative and/or significantly lower. A positive response by lymph node lymphocytes to tumor cells *in vitro* correlated with a significantly higher mixed leukocyte culture response among lymph node lymphocytes as compared to peripheral blood lymphocytes. The response of lymph node lymphocytes to autologous tumor cells was much greater than that of the respective peripheral-blood lymphocytes. This goes along with previous reports by some, but not all, investigators showing the immunocompetence of regional lymph nodes in breast cancer.

A direct technique suggesting interaction of lymphocytes and tumor cells has been described. Richters and Sherwin described the coexistence of lymphoid cells and tumor cells in fresh surgical specimens. [100] There is increasing evidence along this line that the nature and degree of mononuclear cell infiltration of human primary metastatic tumors is complex. We recently studied the mononuclear content of human solid tumors. Both primary and metastatic solid tumors, including lymph node metastases, were studied from 45 patients. Six patients had breast adenocarcinoma. Primary tumors tended to contain a greater number of lymphocytes than did metastatic tumors. Interestingly, however, the lymphocyte responses to mitogens and antigens tended to be greater among metastatic tumors than primary tumors, suggesting that the lymphocytes were already precommitted to tumor antigens in the primary tumors.

Deodhar and co-workers described the interaction between tumor cells and lymphocytes in a tissue culture system. [101] Ten patients who had no nodal or other metastatic involvement showed a significant tumor cell–lymphocyte interaction. Four patients with extensive involvement of the axillary lymph nodes showed no interaction. In six patients with no nodal involvement, both the nodal lymphocytes and the peripheral lymphocytes were available for study. In all instances, the nodal lymphocytes showed a greater degree of reactivity than the peripheral lymphocytes.

4.3. Cytotoxicity

Perhaps the most frequently applied and complicated technique is the cytotoxicity assay. This test detects the capacity of peripheral-blood lymphocytes to kill target cells. Its initial application was in counting or visual observation of target cells. Sensitized lymphocytes killed target cells or inhibited the outgrowth of target cells into colonies. Because the colony-inhibition test is complicated and the measurements are difficult, it is rarely used, and most laboratories now apply a microcytotoxicity assay. Most tests use isotopic labels to count the target cell survival. The target cells are prelabeled with an isotope. The effector cells are added, and, after appropriate incubation, the isotope remaining in the target cells is counted as a function of the number of surviving cells. There have been many reviews of this technique and it will not be the purpose of this chapter to review the pros and cons of the various aspects of these tests.

The Hellstroms and their associates first noted that lymphocytes from cancer patients killed target cells of the same histologic type as the patients' disease.[102] In contrast, the lymphocytes from normal donors or from cancer patients with different cancers could not kill these specific tumor types. Fossati and co-workers also demonstrated specific cytotoxicity against breast cells.[103] Recent evidence, however, does not entirely support this specific cytotoxicity reactivity. It is quite clear today that lymphocytes from normal individuals or from cancer patients with different histologic types *can* kill the "inappropriate" tumor cell. Takasugi *et al.* demonstrated that normal donor lymphocytes can kill tumor target cells as effectively as lymphocytes from patients with specific tumor types.[104] Other workers have also demonstrated that peripheral lymphocytes from normal donors are effective in killing breast cancer target cells.[105, 106]

In addition to the problem with the effector cells, the choice of target cells is crucial for the tests. Target cells vary tremendously in antigenicity. There has been such a tremendous amount of controversy regarding these tests that it is difficult to know exactly what these tests are measuring. There seems to be no doubt that lymphocytes from cancer patients can kill tumor cells, including breast tumor cells. However, lymphoid cells from normal donors can also kill. This may not be a nonspecific finding and may represent sensitized lymphocytes due to tumor immunity or cross-reactive antigens [104-106] (see below).

4.3.1. The Role of Serum Factors

The Hellstroms [107] initially discovered that the sera of patients with growing or progressive tumors contained blocking factors that abrogated cell-mediated immunity as detected by the cytotoxicity assay. The blocking activity was removed by absorption with tumor cells. This activity appeared to reside in the immunoglobulin fraction of serum. Thus, they interpreted this as a blocking antibody. Later results by Sjogren and co-workers suggested, more appropriately, that the blocking was probably due to antigen–antibody complexes. [108]. In addition to these blocking materials, inhibition of lymphocyte function, due to circulating tumor antigen probably shed from the tumor cell membrane, prevented lymphocyte cytotoxicity. [109]

In addition to factors that block tumor cell killing, there are serum effects that may be able to potentiate the cytotoxic capacity of effector cells. Hellstrom and co-workers demonstrated that sera from patients who were free of disease, if mixed with blocking sera from patients with progressive disease, abrogated blocking of lymphocyte cytotoxicity. [110] They termed this "unblocking." The nature of these unblocking factors is unclear. Serum-potentiating cytotoxicity has also been termed antibody-dependent cellular cytotoxicity or lymphocyte-dependent antibody and K-cell cytotoxicity. There is a population of effector cells that can mediate a cytotoxic event once armed by a specific antibody againat target cells. Sera can promote or "arm" cytotoxicity of noncytotoxic normal lymphocytes. Breast cancer patients have been demonstrated to possess such serum promoting factors. [111] There has been no correlation between these antibodies and the clinical course of events, however. Many workers, including Levy, Avis, Heppner, and others have published extensively on cytotoxicity reactions. [112-114] However, not all reports have been able to confirm these results showing a positive correlation between the presence of blocking factors and *in vivo* tumor progression. The many problems involved with cytotoxicity assays have been reviewed recently. [115]

Lymphocyte-mediated tumor reactivity against breast carcinoma has also been used to identify reactivity among normal populations. In a recent paper by Byers *et al.*, normal patients and household contacts of disease-free carcinoma patients showed similar cytotoxicity values. [116] Similarly, Yonemoto and co-workers reported that specific cellular immunity among sisters and daughters of breast carcinoma patients could be shown in a significant percentage of cases.[117]

Microcytotoxicity tests have been applied to demonstrate antigenic cross-reactivity between cancer of the breast and fibrocystic disease. Avis and co-workers have demonstrated in a series of studies[113,118] that peripheral lymphocytes obtained from 12 of 13 patients with fibrocystic disease of the breast were specifically cytotoxic to breast cancer cells as measured *in vitro*. Sera from six women with active fibrocystic disease or metastatic breast cancer could specifically block the cytotoxicity of lymphocytes from either population of patients against cancer cells. This implied extensive antigenic cross-reactivity between benign and malignant hyperplastic disease of the breast. Sera from four individuals clinically free of fibrocystic disease or fibroadenoma neutralized the blocking activity of the sera of patients with metastatic breast cancer. A similar implied cross-reactivity was reported with peripheral lymphocytes from men with benign prostatic hyperplasia which were capable of destroying prostatic cancer cells. Since individuals with a history of fibrocystic disease of the breast have two to three times the chance of developing breast cancer over the normal female population, there appears to be some biologic characteristic of fibrocystic disease that predisposes the patient to future breast malignancy.

4.4. Measurement of Lymphokines

A number of soluble materials are released by immune lymphocytes with recognition of antigen. These materials have been classified as lymphokines. The lymphokine that has been most extensively investigated by *in vitro* assays is migration inhibitory factor (MIF), which inhibits the migration of macrophages. The inhibition of macrophage migration has been correlated with the *in vivo* cutaneous hypersensitivity reaction. The initial efforts apply an indirect MIF test; little has been published on the detection of breast cancer antigens by this assay. However, the so-called direct assay, in which leukocytes from cancer patients are tested for migration with and without tumor cells or tumor extracts, has been extensively applied in breast cancer. One of the first applications of this test in breast cancer was the inhibition of migration reported by Anderson and co-workers.[119] Eight of 22 patients with breast cancer exhibited inhibition of autologous leukocyte migration in the presence of breast cancer extracts. Nine patients with benign mammary lesions did not exhibit migration inhibition in the presence of autologous tissue. Segall and co-workers demonstrated similar findings in 8 of 13 patients with breast cancer.[120] A number of reports have confirmed these findings during the last several years. McCoy and co-workers showed that migration of leukocytes from 20 of 26 breast carcinoma patients was significantly inhibited by KCL extracts of breast carcinoma, [121] but not by KCL extracts of normal or benign breast tissue. Leukocytes that were obtained from patients with carcinoma other than that of the breast were rarely inhibited by soluble KCL extracts of breast cancer. However, allogeneic breast cancer tissue did induce inhibition of migration, suggesting that breast cancers share common tumor antigens. Thus, several tests, including the cytotoxicity assay as well as the leukocyte migration inhibition test, suggest a common antigen or antigens in breast cancer, implying a viral etiology as documented in the murine mammary tumor system by Blair and co-workers in 1968 (see below and reference 86). Cochran and co-workers, using the leukocyte-migration technique, examined the leukocytes of 138 breast cancer patients and 157 controls. [122] Fifty-four percent of breast cancer patients showed sensitization to tumor extracts, as compared to only 15% of control donors; both autologous as well as allogeneic combinations showed reactivity, and rarely were extracts of noncarcinoma material able to evoke a positive reaction. Patients with localized disease exhibited inhibition more frequently than did those with advanced disease. Reactions were as frequent in patients with no obvious nodal involvement as in those with axillary lymph node involvement.

Variability detected in sequential testing with leukocyte migration has been recently emphasized. It appears that most cancer patients will react 50% of the time, but of great interest is the fact that almost normal female controls have positive reactions approximately one of every four times. Although there is a greater reactivity among breast cancer patients as compared to normal women, the reactivity among normal women could be related to sensitization to tumor antigens.

Black has reported a similar technique to test the response of peripheral leukocytes to cryostat sections of autologous and homologous breast tissue. [123] Migration inhibition of leukocytes occurred infrequently when cancer or control patients were tested against normal mammary tissues. Similar findings were reported when the leukocytes from control women were tested against breast cancer tissues. In contrast, migration inhibition was found in all eight patients with *in situ* breast cancer tested against autologous *in situ* breast cancer. Four patients with both *in situ* and invasive breast cancer were also tested against sections of their *in situ* breast cancer. Two of these patients reacted positively. Thus, 10 of 12 patients tested against autologous *in situ* breast cancer tissue demonstrated positive reactivity. Tests performed against autologous invasive breast cancer tissue revealed that 45 of 114 tests (39%) had positive inhibition. In this group, patients with Stage I disease had 46% positive reactivity; patients with Stage II with less than six positive nodes, 40%; and patients with Stage II with six or more positive nodes, 24%. Thus, the data showed a decline in positive reactivity from *in situ* to invasive breast cancer. When leukocytes from breast cancer patients were tested against autologous *in situ* and invasive breast cancer removed from the same patient, migration inhibition was more consistently produced by the *in situ* lesions as compared to the invasive cancer (50% for the former and 18% for the latter). In addition, when leukocytes with a positive response to at least one homologous *in situ* cancer target were tested against autologous and homologous invasive cancer, less than one-third the number of positive responses were recorded, suggesting strongly that *in situ* breast cancer is associated with a greater antigenicity than invasive breast cancer.[123] Thus, in addition to supporting the concept that breast cancer tissues share common antigens, Black's studies have demonstrated a correlation of *in vitro* responsiveness with the clinicopathological characteristics of the tissues and the responsive leukocytes. Breast cancer patients' leukocytes were clearly more regularly cross-reactive to *in situ* as compared to invasive homologous breast cancer tissues. Leukocytes that were responsive to LRE-positive autologous breast cancer tissues were more regularly responsive to LRE-positive, as compared to negative, homologous breast cancer tissue. These findings indicate that LRE-positive breast cancer tissues in general, and *in situ* breast cancer tissues in particular, possess common antigenic characteristics.

Finally, the leukocyte-migration assay has been very important in understanding the responsiveness of regional lymph nodes as reported above with the blastogenic assay. Ellis and co-workers[124] reported on the immunologic competence of regional nodes among 24 patients undergoing radical mastectomy. The degree of sensitization to breast cancer extracts was compared using lymphocytes obtained from regional lymph nodes and circulating lymphocytes. Among the breast cancer patients, migration inhibition detected immunity much more significantly in the regional lymph node lymphocytes as compared to peripheral-blood lymphocytes. In the noncancer control group, there was no significant difference in the immunologic response to breast cancer antigen between regional lymph node lymphocytes and peripheral-blood lymphocytes. A significant *in vitro* response was found in 17 of 24 regional lymph nodes of the radical mastectomy group, as compared to 7 of 24 of the peripheral-blood samples tested in the same group. These data are very similar to those reported above by Ambus and co-workers using the lymphocyte blastogenic response to autologous tumor cells. [71] Thus, two laboratories have strongly suggested that lymph node lymphocytes draining the breast cancer tissue are more responsive to tumor extracts than are peripheral-blood lymphocytes.

Recently, a new assay called the leukocyte adherence inhibiton (LAI) test has been used for measuring immunity from sensitized lymphocytes. Halliday and associates[125] developed a rapid assay which was based on the finding that nonsensitized leukocytes from both cancer patients and control subjects adhere to glass. Leukocytes from cancer patients, but not from control subjects, when mixed *in vitro* with antigen extracts of tumors of the same histologic type, undergo a decrease in their normal adherence to glass surfaces. The authors suggested that the LAI assay may have an immunologic basis similar to that of the migration test and the lymphocyte cytotoxicity assay. Grosser and Thomson[126] reported on results with a modified LAI procedure first used by Holan and co-workers. [127] Peripheral-blood leukocytes from 40 of 47 patients with breast cancer responded to an antigen extract of breast cancer with significant leukocyte adherence inhibition. In contrast, only 2 of 32 controls showed a similar response. Seven patients with benign breast disease did not react to the breast adenocarcinoma extract, indicating that primarily breast cancer patients contain leukocytes sensitized to the breast cancer antigen by this assay. The cell-associated antitumor response of the breast cancer patients appeared to be dependent upon the stage of disease.

4.5. Human Tumor Serology

Many techniques have been used to detect antibodies to tumor antigens. These include complement fixation, complement-dependent cytotoxicity, direct and indirect immunofluorescence, and immunoprecipitation. More recently, radioimmunoassays have been applied. There are many problems associated with serological assays, particularly in regard to specificity. Since tissue culture cells are frequently used, the problem of expression of fetal antigens on cells grown in fetal calf serum as well as mycoplasma contamination must be kept in mind. Detection of HLA antigens and blood-group antigens must also be sorted out. Despite the demonstration that antibodies to fetal calf serum can detect the so-called heterologous membrane antigen, there seems to be little doubt that humoral antibodies reacting against tumor-associated antigens exist in the sera of breast cancer patients. Perhaps the most important question is the biologic role of these antibodies. First, it should be mentioned that reports of immunoglobulin levels in breast cancer patients are somewhat varied. For example, Rowinska-Zakrewska and co-workers suggested that IgA levels were elevated in a group of 29 breast cancer patients as compared to control patients with benign breast disease. [128] Hughes demonstrated, however, that IgA levels were normal in a large series of breast cancer patients. [129] Roberts and co-workers found that serum IgA was elevated and serum IgG reduced in all stages of breast cancer. [130] Other workers have even suggested that elevated IgA levels may predict a good prognosis.

The evidence for a tumor-specific humoral immune response to breast tumor antigens is herewith presented. Edynak *et al.* showed that 91% of 24 patients with localized breast cancer had sera which reacted by indirect immunofluorescence against cell lines of breast cancer. [131] Twenty percent of normal controls were positive as well.

Humphrey and co-workers reported on an antibody reaction to a breast cancer extract detected by immunodiffusion or complement fixation. [132] Antibody was found in 46% of sera from patients with breast cancer, 25% of sera from patients with fibroadenoma, and 34% of sera from patients with fibrocystic disease. The complement-fixation test proved to be more sensitive in detecting the antibody. Sera from 54 volunteers, which included 44 females without breast disease, were tested for antibody to the antigen by immunodiffusion; no positive reactions were demonstrated. It was of interest that 11 of 13 patients with positive axillary lymph nodes and negative antibody response developed recurrences within one year. In contrast, only 3 of 18 patients with positive axillary lymph nodes and positive antibody reaction had recurrences from one to two years postoperatively. Thus, serodiagnosis, as well as cell-associated immunity, appear to be associated in part with a good prognosis. The Kansas Breast Study Group has reported several studies correlating the presence of circulating antibody to breast cancer antigens with a good prognosis. [133] Histopathologic studies have demonstrated a positive correlation between the presence of a positive antibody and the degree of lymphoid infiltration in the tumor and SH in the regional lymph nodes. Since all these features have been associated with improved prognosis in patients with breast cancer, these studies support theories relating histologic features to host–tumor mechanisms.

Although breast cancer tissue culture lines have been difficult to establish, recent success in this endeavor has been useful as a source of material to detect antibodies. [134,135] Nordquist and co-workers have detected antitumor antibodies in most human breast cancer sera by a variety of techniques. The tests applied were important for specificity. A fixed cell immunofluorescence demonstrating intracellular antigens detected antibodies that appeared to be organ-specific, whereas the membrane fluorescence test detecting membrane antigens was more indicative of a tumor-associated immune response. [136]

Antibody responses have also been found in patients with benign breast disease. Patients with fibroadenoma or fibrocystic disease frequently have antibodies against breast-associated tumor antigens. Although the biologic role of these antibodies in these various studies is unclear, Baldwin and co-workers did report that 70% of breast cancer patients had complement-dependent cytotoxic antibodies in their sera which were directed against breast tumor cells grown in tissue cultures.[137] The tumor specificity of these antibodies needs to be further clarified and defined.

4.6. Other Evidence for Breast Cancer Antigens

Springer and co-workers have carried out a series of interesting and important studies on blood-group antigens in breast cancer.[138–140] Initially, they reported that active substances of blood groups A, B, and O occur in healthy and malignant human tissue. Two major antigens of the second human blood-group system—that is, the M and N antigens—occur in human mammary gland tissue in benign as well as in malignant lesions. However, a precursor T (Thomsen–Friedenreich) antigen, as determined with human sera, occurs regularly in cancerous breast tissue but not in benign breast tissue. The TN antigen, which is the precursor to the T antigen, was also found regularly with human antisera in cancerous breast tissue. Both antigens also occurred in *in situ* carcinoma. No trace of T antigen could be found in six benign mammary glands studied. The T antigen therefore appears to be a breast-cancer-associated antigen. Anti-T antibody, which is present in all human sera, was severely depressed in the large number of breast cancer patients as compared to controls. Among 98 patients with breast cancer, 40% had an extremely depressed anti-T titer as compared to controls. It is of interest that human anti-T interacts specifically with the spontaneous TA3 mouse mammary adenocarcinoma cells which possess a precursor antigen of the human blood-group MN system. It is also of interest that antibodies to the T antigen reappear in the majority of patients whose breast had been removed because of cancer. In addition, anti-T antibodies can increase after intradermal immunization with T antigens. Springer and co-workers have speculated that the anti-T antibody present in all humans beyond six months of age may result from continuous antigenic stimulation by an individual's own intestinal flora, much like the human anti-ABO blood antibodies. Springer has described that 18 of 34 gram-negative bacteria isolated from human stools carried the T active structures. Thus, immunization with various bacterial materials for immunotherapy may indeed increase anti-T antibodies.

Other antigenic structures have been described. For example, carcinoembryonic antigen (CEA) was elevated in most patients with cancer of the colon and was also elevated in a substantial percentage of patients with breast cancer. [141] In a study by Hansen and co-workers, 45% of patients with breast cancer had elevated CEA levels. [141] Schwarz reported that elevated plasma CEA was correlated with the extent of disease. [142] Elevated CEAs were measured in 16% of patients with no evidence of metastases. Thirty-six percent of patients with regional metastases and 68% of patients with distant metastases had elevated CEA levels. Patients with other breast pathology (16% of those with fibroadenoma and 17% of those with cystic mastopathy) also had elevated CEA levels. Similar results have been reported by other workers, including Chu. [143] Stewart and associates showed that there was a rapid fall in CEA levels in patients responding to various treatments. [144] They felt that serial assays may be useful to monitor patients.

In addition to CEA, ferritin has been described as a potential marker for breast cancer cells. Marcus and Zinberg reported on the presence of ferritin isolated from breast tumors. [145] Ferritin can also be detected in the serum. The concentration of circulating ferritin was measured in 250 normal adult women and 229 women with early breast cancer by Jacobs and co-workers from Wales. [146] Patients with breast cancer had higher levels than normal women. Those with an initial circulating ferritin concentration above 200 μg/liter had a higher tumor recurrence rate during the subsequent four years. Some investigators have demonstrated that ferritin may be an expression of fetal production by tumor cells. However, ferritin also reflects abnormalities in the RES system in patients with malignancy. Further studies need to be carried out.

Other evaluations of changes in the tumor cell surface come from the work of Gupta and Schuster, in which 85 specimens of breast tissue were investigated for the isoantigens A, B, and H by a mixed cell agglutination reaction. [147] Twenty-five benign lesions of the breast demonstrated these isoantigens. On the other hand, tissues from primary as well as metastatic breast cancers were invariably negative for these isoantigens. This tends to confirm previous studies by some, but not all, workers (see references 138–140) on the loss of antigens from cancerous tissue. [148]

The nature of the cell surface of tumor cells has been studied extensively. For example, Richman studied the immunofluorescence reactions of benign and malignant human mammary tissue. [149] In all tissues, immunohistologic localization of IgA and IgM was noted in patterns previously described for other secretory epithelial tissue. On the other hand, IgG was localized only on the tumor cell surface but was not associated with epithelial cells from normal breast tissue or benign breast lesions. All breast and benign lesions failed to react with anti-C3. The demonstration of IgG on the tumor cell is quite important. Irie and co-workers also detected the presence of antibody and complement on human tumor cells by using immune adherence and mixed hemadsorption tests.[150] Whether the IgG was bound by the Fab or Fc portion of the immunoglobulin molecule was open to question. However, Tonder and Thunold have strongly suggested that there are receptors for the Fc portion on human breast cancer cells.[151] The amount of the Fc receptor varies from tumor to tumor. Some show a strong reactivity while others show weak or little activity. Fc receptors could act as a site for attachment of macrophages to the cell surface.

Other work demonstrating immunoglobulin coating of human cancer cells comes from Witz's group.[152] There was a strong correlation between grading of the tumor cell and the presence of coating. Three of the four breast cancer specimens with high-grade malignancy showed coating, whereas only two of five with low grade showed coating. Thus, there appeared to be a positive correlation between the malignant potential of the tumor and the immunoglobulin coat. These workers suggest that the immunoglobulin coat may prevent killing of the tumor cells.

5. Immunological Evidence for Viral Antigens in Human Breast Cancer

It is not the purpose of this review to discuss the extensive literature on the viral association with breast cancer.[153-157] However, it is pertinent to discuss briefly the cellular as well as serological evidence that some of the reactivity demonstrated above may be directed against viral-associated antigens. Evidence for reactivity as well as tolerance to mouse tumor viruses has been extensively reviewed elsewhere. There is biochemical and immunological evidence for viral expression in human breast cancer that is closely related to the murine mammary tumor virus (MMTV). Whether this is involved in the etiology of breast cancer is not clear. In addition to biochemical and molecular-biologic evidence, there is strong evidence obtained by immunological techniques for the existence of a virus similar to the MMTV in human milk and breast tumors. Approximately 25% of all human sera tested showed a neutralizing effect on the MMTV, irrespective of whether the sera came from breast cancer patients or not.[153] Additional evidence that cross-reactive antigens exist in the two species is furnished by the work of Priori and co-workers, who found by immunofluorescence that 50% of the sera from breast cancer patients could react positively with mouse mammary tumor cells.[158,159] Muller and co-workers have confirmed these findings.[160] It is important to point out that many of these serological reactions could be due to heterophile antibodies in the sera. However, Bowen and associates have shown that a small number of sera contain antibodies apparently specifically directed toward the MMTV particles as determined by electron microscopy. [161] Other workers have suggested that all of the serological reactivity may be nonspecific. [162] Stutman and Herberman have recently discussed the evidence for and against this viral specificity. [163] Overall, the serological evidence does strongly suggest a serological reaction against MMTV by human breast cancer patients.

In addition to serological evidence, there is good evidence based on cellular assays that cross-reactions between breast tumor antigens and mammary tumor viruses (MTV) exist. The important work of Black *et al.* has revealed a high frequency of reactivity (by leukocyte migration inhibition assays) of breast cancer patients' lymphocytes to MMTV-containing materials. [164] This has been confirmed by the lymphocyte-stimulation assay. [165] In addition, Hollinshead and co-workers have found that partially purified skin-reactive antigens prepared from human breast cancer react with heterologous antisera against MMTV or against Mason–Pfizer virus. [166] Further important work is being done to clarify these points.

Before discussing immunological intervention and the potential for immunoprophylaxis of breast cancer, it is pertinent to summarize the previous discussion. There seems to be little doubt that by the currently used assays, few defects of general immunocompetence have been described for patients with early breast cancer. However, as the disease progresses, there is a gradual decline in the overall general immunocompetence. These tests have had prognostic significance, in that patients with intact immunity tend to live longer than those without intact immunity.

The evidence that the breast cancer patient mounts an immune response against the breast tumor cells is overwhelming. Certainly, histologic studies clearly demonstrate that a variety of immunological reactions occur both in the draining lymph nodes and in the primary tumor. The biologic significance of the various immunological reactions described by the numerous *in vitro* tests is not clear at this time. Many of the data are contradictory. Some correlate with prognosis while others do not. However, tumor immunology is a young science. Better tests are needed to clarify the host–tumor relationship. Whether T cells, B cells, K cells, macrophages, or combinations thereof are needed for effective cellular cytotoxicity is not clear. The role of antibodies in the host defense is also unclear, although antibodies certainly do play a role in preventing metastases and possibly in killing tumor cells. The significance of concomitant immunity in breast cancer needs to be clarified.

There are a variety of escape mechanisms which develop and prevent effective immunological control of tumor growth. Many of these are factors released into the serum and have been described above. The tumor cell also modulates itself and probably loses antigenicity as the tumor progresses. Many reviews have described the array of immunological and biological phenomena which occur. Certainly, before intelligent immunological intervention can take place, a better understanding of these complicated mechanisms must be reached. However, as will be described below, encouraging attempts at immunological intervention have already occurred and will certainly occur in the future before the complex host–tumor relationship in breast cancer is fully elucidated.

6. Effect of Hormones on Immunity

It has been known for years that estrogen compounds are potent stimulants of the reticuloendothelial system in animals.[167] These data are relevant to other experimental data showing a heightened resistance to tumors in female animals as compared to male animals.[168] Little knowledge concerning the mechanisms of action of estrogens on macrophages or RES activity is available. Magarey and Baum demonstrated that administration of stilbestrol can prevent the suppression of RES phagocytic activity following radiotherapy in breast cancer patients.[169] High doses of stilbestrol did not produce any effect and were less effective than smaller doses. Other estrogen compounds such as estriol and ethinylestradiol showed no ability to stimulate RES phagocytic activity.

Pentycross and co-workers administered adjuvant stilbestrol to postmenopausal women and the androgen phenylpropionate to premenopausal women. It was clear that hormone therapy protected against the immunodepression following surgery as measured by the *in vitro* lymphocyte response to PHA. In addition, postmenopausal but not premenopausal patients appeared to have less immunosuppression to PHA following radiotherapy.[170]

It is well known that steroids have a variety of effects on the immune system.[171–173] Not only are steroids lympholytic, but they have been shown to inhibit the function of the RES. There is evidence in the literature that steroids may influence the site of metastatic disease in patients with breast cancer despite their known antitumor effect. Iversen showed that the incidence of splenic metastases was higher in patients receiving steroids as compared to those not receiving steroids.[174] Sherlock and Hartmann studied the patterns of metastases in breast cancer patients. Patients receiving steroids had a significant increase in metastases to the lungs, liver, heart, opposite breast, spleen, brain, and gastrointestinal tract when compared to patients with disseminated breast cancer who did not receive steroids.[175]

7. Influence of Radiotherapy on the Immune Response

A great deal of controversy has evolved during the last several years concerning the influence of radiation on the human immune response. It seems unequivocal that irradiation does have an effect on some aspects of the human immune response. Several investigators have shown that local radiotherapy induces lymphopenia in treated patients. [176,177] Total lymphocytes can remain depressed for up to ten years after irradiation. Stjernsward and co-workers suggested that radiotherapy-induced lymphopenia resulted from a loss of circulating T cells as estimated by the E-rosette assay. [178] However, other studies have shown that the defect is primarily one of a decrease in circulating B cells. Blomgren and co-workers[179] demonstrated that the frequency of lymphocytes having membrane-associated receptors for activated complement was significantly decreased after radiotherapy. In contrast, cells binding sheep erythrocytes to their cell membranes (or T cells) actually increased. The reasons for these paradoxical findings are not clear at this time. However, the decreased frequency of the EAC or complement receptor cell may not have been due only to a reduction of B cells, since other cells such as monocytes and perhaps null lymphocytes also express the complement receptor.

Various *in vitro* and *in vivo* tests have also been influenced by radiotherapy. McCredie *et al.* showed that the *in vitro* lymphocyte response to PHA was decreased for 12 months after radiotherapy. [176] Similarly, Cosimi and co-workers showed that the PHA response as well as delayed hypersensitivity recall skin tests decreased after irradiation. [177] Blomgren and co-workers showed that the *in vitro* response to purified protein derivative (PPD) decreased after irradiation, but there was no change in the lymphocyte response to PHA and pokeweed mitogen. [179] This has led Alexander to maintain that the immunological consequences of irradiation may have been overplayed. [180] There is little doubt that irradiation is immunosuppressive, but the specific defects need to be elucidated. What is important (as will be discussed below) is that certain forms of immunopotentiation such as *Corynebacterium parvum* may actually potentiate the efficacy of irradiation therapy and prevent its immunosuppressive properties.

8. Immunotherapy

Immunotherapy of human cancer is not a new discipline. For over two centuries, physicians have reported dramatic regressions of cancer following acute bacterial infections. One of the first investigators to apply immunotherapy in a large series of patients was William Coley. After observing a spontaneous regression of an inoperable recurrent sarcoma following a bout of erysipelas, Coley injected a recurrent metastatic sarcoma of the tonsil with a living streptococcal culture.[181] He succeeded in inducing a severe infection which led to a complete regression of the tumor. In 1892, Coley combined the streptococcal bacteria with the gram-negative endotoxin *Serratia marcescens*. Over the course of the next 30 years, he and other workers treated hundreds of patients with this and similar vaccines. Nauts has attempted to put together the long-term results of therapy with these various Coley's toxins.[182] Detailed histories of 920 microscopically proven cases treated by these various products indicated that when a potent, stable, unfiltered vaccine was used, many types of neoplasms regressed after inoculation by the intratumor or systemic route. Although sarcomas of soft tissues and histiocytic lymphomas were the most responsive tumors, there were numerous incidences of carcinoma of the breast responding to immunotherapy. Inconsistency in the results, as well as a failure to apply modern quantitative methodology for evaluating the clinical effects, led, in part, to a decline of this approach.

In the late 1950s and early 1960s, several groups demonstrated that BCG and other microorganisms were active antitumor agents in experimental models. In the early 1960s, Edmund Klein at Roswell Park Memorial Institute applied small organic chemicals in the pioneering treatment of skin cancer (see reference 183). Materials that induced contact delayed hypersensitivity reactions in the skin were effective in the treatment of some skin cancers. Klein observed that the concurrent administration of two or more sensitizing agents synergistically potentiated the antitumor activity of cell-mediated immune reactions. In addition, chemotherapy and immunotherapy were often synergistic locally. Subsequent studies indicated that the principles derived from the therapeutic approaches with epidermal neoplasms extended to a whole spectrum of malignant diseases in man, including breast cancer.

In the discussion of immunotherapy of human breast cancer, it is important to review briefly the general approaches to systemic immunotherapy and review what has been accomplished in major tumors other than breast cancer. The various concepts of immunodeficiency as well as interference with immune destruction must be kept in mind in understanding the developing field of immunotherapy. The improved prognosis for several human cancers which has been accomplished with immunotherapy has already established this modality as a major therapeutic approach in some cancer centers. The major approaches to immunological intervention include active nonspecific immunotherapy, active specific immunotherapy, adoptive immunotherapy, passive immunotherapy, and local immunotherapy.

Active nonspecific immunotherapy refers to the use of adjuvants, usually of microbial origin, which can heighten general immunocompetence, activate macrophages, and increase the activity of the RES.

Active specific immunotherapy refers to the administration of tumor cells or tumor antigens which are designed to increase specific antitumor immunity.

Adoptive immunotherapy refers to the transfer of lymphocytes or cell products of immune lymphocytes from one donor to another.

Passive immunotherapy is the use of antitumor antibodies from an immune donor.

Local immunotherapy refers to the inoculation of a variety of immunotherapeutic materials directly into the tumor.

8.1. Local Immunotherapy

Klein and Holtermann have reported that seven of fourteen patients with intradermal breast metastases responded to local immunotherapy with a variety of materials that induced a delayed hypersensitivity reaction.[183] Similarly, Stjernsward and Levin have reported that DNCB sensitization was effective against breast lesions.[184]

Smith and co-workers studied eight patients with breast cancer who were treated with local BCG.[185] All eight apparently had some degree of antitumor response. Lesions became necrotic and occasionally noninjected lesions also appeared to react after local administration of BCG. Recently, Partridge and co-workers reported on the intratumor injection of BCG.[186] Ten patients were treated for chest-wall recurrence with intratumor inoculations. Glaxo strain BCG was administered by direct injection every two weeks until a complete response was noted or until it was apparent that BCG was having no effect. Regression of chest-wall lesions occurred in six patients, and five of these had no recurrence of chest-wall lesion for nine to fourteen months after intratumor injection of BCG. Mastrangelo *et al.* have also reported efficacy of BCG.[187]

Dimitrov and associates reported on the intralesional injection of *C. parvum*. Nine patients with local recurrences were treated, all of whom had previously had irradiation or chemotherapy. The dose was 2.8–4.2 mg given weekly. Apparently, all patients responded and no local recurrences were recorded for any patient at the site of intralesional injection during the first year of follow-up. Serial biopsies revealed an accumulation of mononuclear cells around the tumor tissue with central necrosis. Giant cells with granuloma were also observed.[188]

Glucan has also been used in one study by Mansell and associates, who noted regression of a soft-tissue mass in one patient with breast cancer. [189]

8.2. Active Nonspecific Immunotherapy

Most of the data thus far involve active nonspecific immunotherapy, generally with microbial immunomodulators such as BCG, extracts of BCG, and C. *parvum,* and synthetic materials (levamisole).

8.2.1. Chemoimmunotherapy for Disseminated Malignancy

BCG was reported to be active in prolonging remission and survival in childhood and adult acute lymphoblastic leukemia by Mathe and co-workers in 1969. [190] Work with BCG was then extended by our group and others to patients with disseminated solid tumors. A study which has become important for the development of immunochemotherapy studies in breast cancer was reported for patients with advanced malignant meloanoma. [191] When BCG was interspersed with intermittent chemotherapy for disseminated malignant melanoma, the following activity was observed: (a) although there was no overall increase in remission rates when BCG was added to chemotherapy, remissions were significantly increased for chemoimmunotherapy patients in whom the tumor was confined to regional lymph node areas; thus, we speculated that if the immunotherapeutic agent were administered into the vicinity of the tumor, potentiation of chemotherapy might occur; (b) the durations of remissions were significantly prolonged with BCG plus chemotherapy as compared to chemotherapy alone; (c) the survival of responding patients was significantly prolonged with immunochemotherapy as compared to chemotherapy; and (d) the overall survival of all patients entered in the study was significantly prolonged with immunochemotherapy as compared to chemotherapy alone.

BCG immunotherapy has similarly prolonged chemotherapy-induced remission durations and/or survival in other studies for patients with acute myeloblastic leukemia, [192-194] Hodgkin's disease, and non-Hodgkin's lymphoma. [195]

Another bacterial immunopotentiator, C. *parvum,* when given subcutaneously on a weekly basis interspersed with chemotherapy, produced similar results: prolongation of remission and survival for patients with a variety of solid tumors including breast cancer (Israel[196]). When BCG or C. *parvum* is given by the peripheral route of immunization on a weekly schedule, interspersed with single-agent or combination chemotherapy, remissions and survival of patients with disseminated cancer are significantly prolonged.

Based on this work with microbial immunoadjuvants, particularly BCG and C. *parvum*, preliminary work on chemoimmunotherapy has now been reported for patients with metastatic breast cancer. A regimen employing 5-fluorouracil, adriamycin, and Cytoxan (FAC) was combined with lyophilized Tice or Connaught strain BCG by scarification and given on a weekly basis interspersed between chemotherapy. The results of the FAC chemotherapy regimens have been reported previously by our group.[197] There was no overall increase in the remission rate with FAC plus BCG as compared to FAC alone. This is not surprising, considering that the patients with soft-tissue metastases have such a high remission rate with chemotherapy alone. Based on the principles developed in malignant melanoma, we would not have anticipated that BCG would be capable of increasing visceral remission rates when given by the intradermal or scarification route. However, the duration of remission for patients treated with FAC–BCG has been almost double that of FAC alone[198-200]: the median duration was 9 months for FAC alone and 14 months for FAC–BCG ($P = 0.008$). Most notable has been the prolongation of survival with chemoimmunotherapy: only 27 of 78 responders treated with FAC–BCG have died, with a median survival estimated between 22 and 24 months, whereas 21 of 32 responders treated with chemotherapy alone have died, with a median survival of 15 months ($P = 0.004$). The overall survival for all treated patients has also been significantly prolonged with chemoimmunotherapy: 45 of 105 patients on FAC–BCG have died, with a median survival of 22 months, and 31 of 44 patients on FAC alone have died, with a median survival of 15 months ($P = 0.017$). Israel[196] and, more recently, Pinsky and coworkers[201] have reported similar prolongation of survival with weekly subcutaneous C. *parvum* and combination chemotherapy.

8.2.2. Adjuvant Immunotherapy or Chemoimmunotherapy for Micrometastatic Disease

A second major approach of immunotherapy is in the micrometastatic situation, that is, in patients with minimal residual disease following cytoreduction with chemotherapy or surgery. The postoperative use of sufficient numbers of viable BCG organisms can prolong the postoperative disease-free interval and survival among patients with recurrent malignant melanoma of the trunk.[202-206]

Several principles have been developed from these studies. First, delivery of BCG into the regional lymphatics of the tumor-bearing area is important. Second, a sufficient number of viable organisms is required to achieve a therapeutic effect. Failure to apply these principles may explain some of the negative results reported in other trials. Similar results with immunotherapy or chemoimmunotherapy in prolongation of the postoperative disease-free interval and survival for patients with minimal residual disease have been reported for carcinoma of the colon,[207] lung cancer,[208] and malignant lymphoma.[209]

The application of chemotherapy in the adjuvant postoperative setting for patients with micrometastatic disease has been covered in Chapter 3.

Today, it would not be clinically indicated to attempt an adjuvant trial in breast cancer without chemotherapy. However, the rationale for chemoimmunotherapy trials seems very solidly based on the beneficial results already achieved for patients with disseminated disease. In 1974, we initiated an adjuvant chemoimmunotherapy study for patients with positive lymph nodes removed at the time of surgery. We selected for our regimen the FAC–BCG program because this was the best regimen for patients with advanced disease. To date, 130 patients with one or more positive nodes—75 of whom had four or more positive nodes— have been treated with FAC–BCG.[210] After adriamycin is given to a total dose of 320 mg/M^2, it is discontinued and the patients are maintained on Cytoxan, methotrexate, and 5-FU plus BCG for a total of 24 months of treatment. There have been only five recurrences in the treated group, with a median follow-up time of >13.5 months. Remarkably, only one of the 130 patients has died. These results have been compared to our past experience from 1971 to 1974 with surgery and radiotherapy alone. The results demonstrate a highly significant prolongation of the disease-free interval, particularly for patients with four or more positive lymph nodes, as compared to the surgical control series. Similarly, the survival has been significantly prolonged for the adjuvant-treated group. Both pre- and postmenopausal patients have benefited from this intensive adjuvant therapy. It will be important over the coming years to document the role of immunotherapy in the adjuvant breast cancer setting. It would seem almost certain that immunotherapy will play a major therapeutic role. In addition, many of the complications of long-term chemotherapy, including immunosuppression, possible second malignancies, etc., may be prevented or at least reduced in incidence by the concomitant administration of immunotherapy.

8.2.3. Purified Microbial Materials

Because BCG and C. *parvum* are complex heterogeneous materials containing multiple antigenic components, it is perhaps fortunate that therapeutic benefits have already been achieved. Several groups, including Ribi and co-workers,[211] Lederer and co-workers,[212] and Yamamura and co-workers,[213] have contributed greatly to the chemical and biological understanding of mycobacteria and other microorganisms. These investigators are now achieving a far better defined separation of biologically active components of these organisms. Hopefully, the use of these subcomponents of microorganisms will increase therapeutic activity in humans as it has in certain animal models. The most extensively studied of the nonviable fractions of BCG is the methanol-extracted residue of BCG (MER) pioneered by Weiss and associates. [214] This material, which is active as an immunoprophylactic and immunotherapeutic material in mouse mammary tumors, is now being applied clinically. Positive results in terms of prolongation of remission and survival have already been reported for patients with acute myeloblastic leukemia. [215,216] Perloff and co-workers have reported suggestive data that the prognosis of breast cancer patients was improved by the addition of MER to multidrug chemotherapy. [217] We have carried out comparative sequential studies of MER with BCG in combination with a chemotherapy regimen called VAC–FUM. [218] Results thus far indicate that MER given subcutaneously produces a prolongation of remission and survival equivalent to that achieved with the same chemotherapy combined with BCG. Due to the rather excessive toxicity associated with the subcutaneous route of MER, we are now evaluating the intradermal route, which has been utilized clinically and is probably a more optimal way to immunize patients. It appears that a nonviable partially purified extract of BCG can certainly simulate the activity of BCG. This allows for far greater flexibility in immunotherapy, since the route of administration can be varied.

It was stressed in the earlier part of this discussion that immunotherapy has rarely increased remission rates. Three years ago we began to evaluate C. parvum administered by the intravenous route. Milas and co-workers, working with C. parvum, [219] and Baldwin and associates, working with BCG, [220] have clearly shown that in murine models the intravenous route achieves a far greater therapeutic activity for pulmonary metastases as compared to subcutaneous administration. We have carried out a phase 1 study of intravenous C. parvum and have found that this material can be given safely in doses from 1 to 5 mg/M² weekly or daily. [221] The objective was to begin to administer immunostimulants by the intravenous route in order to affect visceral disease. Simultaneously, Israel et al. also began to evaluate intravenous C. parvum. They recently reported that C. parvum given intravenously in a dose of 4 mg/day could achieve an antitumor response in approximately 40% of patients with advanced solid tumors, including a patient with breast cancer. [222] Band and co-workers in Canada have also reported that intravenous C. parvum can achieve an antitumor response in patients with breast cancer. [223]

Thus, we have designed a study utilizing intensive intravenous C. parvum in patients with advanced breast cancer. The model for this study was based on results in patients with advanced malignant melanoma, which has been a useful predictor for the efficacy of immunotherapy in breast cancer. In an ongoing study, we demonstrated that the intravenous administration of *C. parvum* on a daily basis for two weeks prior to chemotherapy could potentiate remission rates with imidazole carboxamide (DTIC)–actinomycin D in patients with advanced melanoma. [224] In addition, intensive intravenous *C. parvum* in combination with chemotherapy has been associated with a significant prolongation of remission and survival as compared to chemotherapy alone and, particularly, as compared to chemotherapy plus BCG by scarification. Most important has been the demonstration that intravenous *C. parvum* is associated with a significant increase in remissions in the lung and liver, confirming the principles first established in animal models.

Therefore, we have begun to pretreat patients with advanced breast cancer with intravenous *C. parvum* prior to FAC chemotherapy. These results are too preliminary for further comment at this time. However, we have already observed two patients who achieved a partial remission of their disease prior to chemotherapy with the administration of intravenous *C. parvum* alone.

A variety of other bacterial products in addition to BCG and *C. parvum* have great potential for immunotherapy. Such bacteria as *Brucella abortus, Bordetella pertussis,* and a streptococcal preparation, OK432, [225] have antitumor activity. The bacterial endotoxins have great potential, as indicated above in the discussion on the work of Coley. In particular, the recent work of Ribi *et al.* using mutant endotoxins combined with components of mycobacteria further emphasizes the potential of these materials. [226] Perhaps most important in this regard is the recent work of Carswell and co-workers showing that the hemorrhagic necrosis induced by endotoxins is probably due, at least in part, to a circulating substance known as tumor necrosis factor. Animals presensitized with BCG or *C. parvum* or with other materials that activate macrophages, which are then challenged with very small doses of endotoxin, secrete a factor in their serum which causes tumor regression and rapid tumor necrosis. Tumor necrosis factor is a glycoprotein which is probably released by activated macrophages. [227]

In addition to bacteria, viruses have also been used in immunotherapy. Regressions of cutaneous lesions including breast cancer have been reported following intralesional injection of metastatic nodules. [228] A most important area for the future is the area of viral oncolysis, in which active tumor immunity may be increased by the combination of viruses with tumor antigens. [229]

Fungal extracts may also play a very important role in active immunotherapy. Zymosan has been used by a number of workers, including Martin *et al.,* in experimental chemoimmunotherapy of breast cancer. [230] Most recently, Glucan administered by the intralesional route has been shown to be active in human tumors. Patients with breast cancer have responded to intralesional injection of this high-molecular-weight polysaccharide extract of a fungus.

8.2.4. Synthetic Adjuvants

Another major agent which is being applied in breast cancer is a synthetic immunoadjuvant, levamisole. This imidazole compound is a prototype of immunorestorative agents. It has numerous actions on the immune system and seems to augment suppressed immune responses. It has been used for a long time as an antihelminthic agent. It increases tuberculin and DNCB reactivity among immunodeficient individuals, including cancer patients. Levamisole increases the lymphocyte blastogenic response to antigens and mitogens. The first clinical trial with levamisole reported by Amery showed that the postoperative disease-free interval among patients with lung cancer could be prolonged. [231] Rojas and co-workers from Argentina documented the therapeutic activity of levamisole for patients with Stage III breast cancer. [232] Patients with inoperable Stage III breast carcinoma were given 150 mg of levamisole by mouth for 3 days every 14 days, after being rendered clinically free of disease by radiotherapy. Twenty-three patients were in the control group and 20 patients were in the Levamisole group. There was a significant prolongation of the disease-free interval from 9 to 25 months with levamisole. Among the controls, 35% were alive at 30 months as compared to 90% of the levamisole-treated patients. In both of these studies, delayed hypersensitivity tests revealed boosting in the patients receiving levamisole.

We recently initiated a study of the addition of levamisole to our FAC chemotherapy regimen. This compound did not increase the remission rate achieved with FAC alone. However, there has already been a significant prolongation of remission as well as survival among responding patients as compared to our previous results with FAC alone. The results thus far appear identical to those achieved with BCG or C. parvum. [233]

The use of materials which induce interferon or interferon itself also has great potential for the treatment of breast cancer, particularly considering the probable association of viruses in the pathogenesis of breast cancer. The interferon system is a complex mechanism of cellular defense in immunity which involves the release of substances from cells infected with virus. [234] It is not the purpose of this review to summarize the interferon field. However, it should be noted that interferon and interferon inducers have a variety of immunological effects. Interferon itself augments cell-mediated cytotoxicity to target cells. In addition, the *in vivo* administration of interferon in mice can suppress the immunity in some systems. Interferon inducers have been noted to be potent adjuvants and stimulators of the immune response. Some clinical work has been done with these materials. For example, one of the interferon inducers, Tilorone, has been evaluated by Regelson. [235] Some antitumor effect has been reported with this material in metastatic breast cancer. Interferon itself has been studied in osteogenic sarcoma, where an antitumor effect may have been observed. [236] Habis has done a small amount of work with interferon in breast cancer, demonstrating some antitumor effect. [237]

8.3. Active Specific Immunotherapy

Active specific immunotherapy is defined as the administration of tumor cells, modified tumor cells, or tumor cell surface antigen preparations in order to boost various components of specific tumor immunity.

Methods for tumor cell modification to increase immunogenicity include a variety of procedures which have been reviewed elsewhere. [238] These include the infection of tumor cells with viruses, or so-called viral oncolysis, to increase immunogenicity. The use of modified or unmodified tumor cells has proven to be therapeutically beneficial in malignant melanoma, [239] acute myeloblastic leukemia, [240,241] and soft-tissue sarcoma, [242] and clearly these approaches can boost immunity in a variety of solid tumors and acute leukemia. [243-245] More recently, purified antigens described by Hollinshead have been used to increase immunity in acute leukemia and seem to provide therapeutic effects in early lung cancer. [246]

Several groups have used immunotherapy coupled with tumor cells. Czajkowski and co-workers coupled protein with autologous tumor cells by the BDB (bisdiazobenzidine) method. [247] Two of 14 patients with advanced metastatic disease apparently entered remission. The technique was applied by Cunningham and associates to a group of patients with advanced solid tumors including breast cancer. However, only one patient responded. [248]

Anderson reported on 16 women injected with irradiated cancer cell autografts after simple mastectomy and irradiation. Twelve patients had Stage II carcinoma and four patients had Stage III disease. The data showed a significant prolongation of survival in the immunotherapy-treated group at seven years (61%), as compared to a group of 90 non-immunotherapy-treated Stage II patients treated with surgery and irradiation, in which there was a 30% survival at seven years. [249] Humphrey *et al.* reported on a small pilot study with various vaccines with or without plasma exchange. Two patients of six appeared to show objective regression of established disease with this approach. [250]

Clearly, more work is required with tumor vaccines in breast cancer.

8.4. Adoptive Immunotherapy

Adoptive immunotherapy is defined as the transfer from an immune or immunocompetent subject to a nonimmune or immunodeficient subject of lymphoid cells or other host defense cells or their products which can prevent the growth of tumor. The fundamental basis for the concept of adoptive immunotherapy of cancer is the well-defined ability to transfer specific immunity from immune to nonimmune syngeneic animals with lymphoid cells. Adoptive immunotherapy has been studied extensively in animals.

Although some benefit has been reported for patients with malignant melanoma, little has been done for patients with breast cancer using this approach.

The subcellular fraction that has received a great deal of attention is the so-called immune RNA. Work with this material was initiated in 1967 by Alexander and co-workers. [251] Pilch and associates have studied it extensively in animal models and more recently have begun clinical studies. [252] The use of immune RNA alone may induce tumor regression in a variety of solid tumors, but this work has not yet been applied to breast cancer.

However, the use of transfer factor has shown promise in patients with breast cancer. Sherwood Lawrence discovered the ability of lysates of peripheral-blood leukocytes to tranafer cell-mediated immunity. [253] Reviews on transfer factor have been published extensively elsewhere. Patients with breast cancer could be the source of transfer factor. However, recent evidence clearly suggests that non-cancer-bearing patients may also be immune to breast cancer antigens. It has been shown that relatives of patients with neuroblastoma and sarcoma as well as melanoma can have varying degrees of sensitization to tumor antigens. Yonemoto and co-workers reported that breast-carcinoma-specific cellular immunity existed among sisters and daughters of breast cancer patients. [117] In addition, patients with benign breast disease can have varying degrees of sensitization to breast tumor antigens, as described above. Recently, Byers *et al.* reported on cell-mediated immunity that was specifically directed against breast carcinoma, but not against osteogenic sarcoma or other carcinomas. [116] Such immunity was found to occur in the household contacts of patients with active breast carcinoma, but not in the normal population nor in household contacts of patients with osteogenic sarcoma. It was also not found in household contacts of breast carcinoma patients who had been disease-free for two or more years. There have been varying reports, however. For example, Brandes and Goldenberg,[254] Avis and co-workers,[113] and Yonemoto and associates[117] have all reported that tumor-specific cellular immunity exists in breast carcinoma patients who are cured or who are in remission. At any rate, there appears to be a population of people, whether they be household contacts, relatives, or cured breast cancer patients, who could be sources of transfer factor for immunotherapy. Oettgen and co-workers used pooled transfer factor from normal women and showed clear-cut antitumor activity in at least one patient with breast cancer.[255] Smith and co-workers have also published suggestive evidence for an antitumor effect with transfer factor in melanoma.[185]

8.5. Immunotherapy with Lymphokines

Many mediators, or lymphokines, released by lymphocytes and macrophages have been described in the literature. These include macrophage-activating factor, lymphotoxins, blastogenic factor, chemotactic factors, and so forth. Experience with induced delayed-type hypersensitivity challenge reactions at tumor sites suggested that some common component of the reactions was primarily responsible for the antitumor effects. Thus, the use of noncellular mediators of the delayed hypersensitivity reaction—or so-called lymphokines—represents perhaps a final path for the reaction. Work in guinea pigs suggests that these materials may have significant antitumor effects. The work of Papermaster, Holterman, Klein, and others clearly shows that crude lymphokines have significant antitumor effects when injected with the tumor.[256] Significant antitumor effects have been reported for patients with soft-tissue breast cancer. The reader is referred to their publications for specific histologic studies of this interesting phenomenon. Over the coming years, research on the purification of specific lymphokines and the systemic use of these materials by the intravenous and other routes will be carried out.

8.6. Thymic Hormones in Immunotherapy

A number of laboratories have identified factors extractable from the thymus or present in the serum which have activity identified as associated with normal thymic function. One of these materials, thymosin, has been demonstrated to be active *in vitro* and *in vivo* in increasing some components of the cell-associated immune compartment.[257] What role these materials will play in terms of clinical immunotherapy of cancer is unclear. Although many cancer patients have deficiencies in circulating T cells, these materials can increase suppressor T-cell activity. They may not be indicated for cancer patients with solid tumors. In addition, it should be stressed that thymectomy may have a beneficial effect in the host–tumor relationship against breast cancer, so that thymic products must be used with caution in this disease.

8.7. Passive Immunotherapy

Passive immunotherapy refers to the administration of serologic components that have direct or indirect antitumor activity. Specific antibodies have been used in some cancer patients, coupled in part with various chemotherapeutic agents. Antitumor effects, particularly in melanoma, have been reported. This is an important area, particularly in regard to the removal of unwanted circulating materials such as antigen or antigen–antibody complexes, and needs further exploration in man. Occasional reports of partial responses have been made using repeated plasmapheresis.[258]

Thus, there are several exciting approaches to the immunotherapy of breast cancer which need to be investigated in clinical trials in man. As of 1976, BCG, C. parvum, MER, and levamisole all seem to have prolonged survival for patients with breast cancer. As we begin to dissect out the deficiencies of the host immune response in breast cancer, immunological intervention should become much more intelligent and the therapeutic results should improve. Let us give some examples. If selective deficiencies of the T-cell compartment of the immune system were to develop, for example, after radiotherapy or chemotherapy, could these be reversed by a thymic hormone such as thymosin? As indicated above, thymosin does have a capacity both in vitro as well as in vivo to restore circulating T cells as measured by the E-rosette assay. One must, however, remember the possible beneficial effects of thymectomy in breast cancer. Tolerance to breast cancer antigens and putative mammary tumor viruses could theoretically be broken or reversed by several approaches, including transfer factor, interferon, endotoxins, or other immunopotentiators. As mentioned above, interferon has already been suggestively beneficial in patients with osteogenic sarcoma and has been able to achieve therapeutic benefit in a limited number of breast cancer patients. Whether viruses are directly or indirectly involved with the pathogenesis and etiology of breast cancer is unknown. Clearly, interferon has exciting possibilities in the management of human breast cancer. The results with tumor vaccines have been scanty. The vaccines applied have been very crude. The work on the separation and characterization of purified subcomponents of the crude tumor antigen material as well as microbial materials should yield products with greater therapeutic activity and more specificity. The intensive use of systemic intravenous immunoadjuvants to reach visceral metastatic deposits extends the concepts of local immunotherapy to the point where intimate contact between tumor cell and immunostimulant achieves the greatest effect.

Finally, the removal of unwanted circulating factors by plasmapheresis, and perhaps the suppression of selected components of the immune system by chemotherapeutic modalities, must also be further explored.

8.8. Interactions of Chemotherapy and Immunotherapy

A great deal more work needs to be done in the study of the interactions of various chemotherapeutic agents with immunotherapy. Each class of chemotherapeutic agents has a variety of effects on the immunologic precursor cells, including effects on stem cells, the cortical dendritic macrophage, and the uptake of antigen. [259] In addition, drugs affect lymphocyte proliferation, lymphocyte blastogenic release, antibody formation, and circulating antibody levels.

The effect of various chemotherapeutic agents on the immune response depends on the timing of administration with the antigen. For example, most drugs do not affect the processing of antigens if administered prior to the antigen.

Although various drugs have differing effects on the immune response, it must be taken into account that not all chemotherapeutic drugs are immunosuppressive in man. For example, Bruckner and coworkers have demonstrated that imidazole carboxamide (DTIC) is minimally immunosuppressive in man. [260] DTIC did not interfere with induction of delayed hypersensitivity to DNCB, did not suppress the primary humoral response to VI antigen, and did not interfere with the secondary response to tetanus toxoid.

Selective inhibition of the immune response may have potential applicability in the therapy of human cancer. This is based on the possibility that some of the blocking factors described in patients with solid tumors may be related to antibody or antigen–antibody complexes. Studies reported by DiLorenzo and associates on the selective alterations of immunocompetence with drugs such as methotrexate, 5-FU, and Ara-C need to be extended to man. [261] Another example of a drug with selective effects on the immune response is the alkylating agent cyclophosphamide, which appears to have greater immunosuppressive effects on antibody-producing cells (thymic-independent cells) as compared to cell-mediated immunity (thymic-dependent cells). [262]

Interesting studies on the use of chemotherapy to augment cell-mediated immunity in mice were recently reported by Mackaness *et al.* [263] Delayed-type hypersensitivity of mice to sheep red blood cells was evaluated. As the antibody response to the sheep red blood cells increased, the delayed hypersensitivity to the sheep red blood cells decreased. Treatment with cyclophosphamide was shown to "release" T cells from the inhibitory influence of the humoral response and to cause enhancement of delayed-type hypersensitivity. The magnitude of this enhancing effect was dependent upon the timing of the treatment relative to the time of immunization. The authors suggest that cyclophosphamide given before antigenic stimulation has a long-lasting effect on antibody formation but no apparent detrimental effect on the precursors of activated T cells. After antigenic stimulation, T cells can also become susceptible to cyclophosphamide action. Mackaness and associates showed that the inhibition of activated T cells by products of the humoral immune response was almost abolished by systemic infection with BCG. Mice infected with BCG developed a high degree of delayed hypersensitivity to the sheep red blood cells. Comprehension of the interaction between chemotherapy and immunotherapy is greatly assisted by the demonstration that the antibody levels increased with BCG treatment, suggesting that the augmentation of delayed hypersensitivity with BCG was due to the clearance of antigen–antibody complexes. Cyclophosphamide given with BCG produced a synergistic effect on delayed hypersensitivity. Studies such as these on the interaction of chemotherapeutic drugs, adjuvants, and antigens (such as tumor antigens) will have enormous potential for the future design of immunochemotherapy trials in man.

A basic concept that must be considered in the design of rational immunochemotherapy protocols is the rebound phenomenon following immunosuppressive chemotherapy. [264] Today, most chemotherapeutic regimens are intermittent in order to allow for a recovery of the immune response. An overshoot of this rebound is associated with a good prognosis. It should be emphasized that prolonged intermittent chemotherapy may also be associated with a progressive decline in immunocompetence. This may be related, in part, to a return of disease, but it may also be related to the prolonged chemotherapy. Recently, Borella and Webster [265] demonstrated that following three years of chemotherapeutic maintenance of acute leukemia patients, there was a prompt recovery of antibody synthesis and the blastogenic response in antigen-sensitive peripheral-blood lymphocytes, as well as an increase in T and B cells. There was no significant change in the magnitude of response to PHA following cessation of long-term chemotherapy. Differences in the response of bone-marrow and peripheral-blood lymphocytes were observed.

The pharmacology and pharmokinetics of drugs may be markedly affected by immune modulators. We and others have shown, for example, that BCG or C. *parvum* can inhibit drug-metabolizing enzyme activity in the liver.[266,267] The metabolism of drugs such as DTIC and cyclophosphamide, which depend on liver microsome activation, can be modified by immunotherapy. Little or no knowledge on the interaction of immune stimulants and DNA is apparent. It is well known, however, that drugs such as bleomycin, adriamycin,[268] and actinomycin may be more active in the presence of heat. What is the effect of chronic immune stimulation and fever on cell membranes and tumor uptake of these drugs? Fisher and co-workers have demonstrated experimentally that C. *parvum* may have more activity when used with aklylating agents than with antimetabolites.[269] Thus, careful attention needs to be directed toward interactions between various classes of chemotherapeutic compounds and immunomodulators.

The various effects of chemotherapy on the immune response are recognized. Some drugs are more immunosuppressive than others. Some drugs may actually increase immunogenicity of tumor cells by affecting the tumor cell membranes. Eventually, chemotherapeutic drugs may be able to selectively suppress unwanted activities of the immune response such as suppressor T-cell activity. The effects of immune modulators on cell kinetics, stem-cell activity, and host immune defenses all need to be woven into the strategy of cancer treatment (reviewed in reference 270). Immunotherapy cannot be merely "tagged" onto chemotherapy protocols without careful consideration of these biologic variables. The interspersion of immunotherapy with chemotherapy has to be thought out carefully. For example, some experimental work has demonstrated that immunotherapy prior to chemotherapy may result in enhancement of tumor growth.[271] By using a nonimmunosuppressive product, FRCNU, a furanose derivative of nitrosourea, Mathe and co-workers have obtained a potentiation of chemotherapy by immunotherapy and vice versa (Mathe, personal communication).

9. Immunoprophylaxis of Breast Cancer: Outlook for the Future

Any discussion regarding an immunological approach to the prevention of breast cancer must first take into account data on the host response to premalignant mammary tissue. Slemmer has pointed out that premalignant mammary tissues in mice express tumor-specific neoantigens.[272] However, the tumor-bearing host is presumably unable to mount an effective immune response, at least during early tumor growth. Similar observations have been made by Billingham and Medawar and by Billingham and co-workers using allogeneic melanocytes transplanted into the guinea pig epidermis, which appear to be incapable of immunizing the host. Slemmer and others have speculated that as long as the basement membrane remains intact, antigen may not contact the appropriate cells to stimulate a rejection phenomenon. Invasion of basement membrane function must occur for such cells to become susceptible to immune destruction. Thus, *in situ* lesions fail to immunize. Black, however, demonstrated that when premalignant tissues were made to simulate *in situ* lesions or were grown in gland-free fat pads, they were rejected by a cellular infiltration that was initiated at the site of origin of the lesion. Thus, in humans, in contrast to mice, preneoplastic cells appear to be distinguished by an antigen expression different from that of normal tissue which should be able to evoke immunological reactivity. Since the tumor load is low, there should be an opportunity to reject such cells. However, as has been summarized recently, there may be a number of immunological mechanisms which paralyze the immune response to prevent rejection at this early malignant state. In addition, a weak immune response may stimulate tumor growth. However, there are encouraging data from the prophylactic use of mycobacterial fractions, which appear to be useful in impeding the preneoplastic development in the mammary parenchyma of mice. Whether such intervention could be effective in man is open to question at the present time.

There is some evidence that BCG prophylaxis may be effective against the development of leukemia in children. For example, Davignon and co-workers tested the question of whether BCG vaccination might lower the incidence of leukemia.[273] Leukemia mortality in Quebec for all children less than 15 years of age was one-half as common among BCG-vaccinated than nonvaccinated children. These results were challenged because of statistical problems. Rosenthal and co-workers analyzed leukemia mortality among a large number of black infants in Chicago who were vaccinated at birth with BCG.[274] There was a suggestion that those infants who received BCG had a lower incidence of leukemia. Many other analyses have failed to substantiate the claim that BCG might prevent leukemia. No data are available regarding BCG vaccination in breast cancer.

In further consideration of immunoprophylaxis by nonspecific means or by viral antigens, it should be stressed that immunodeficiencies need not be present for the growth and development of experimental tumors. This correlates with the data cited above that a regular immunological defect is rarely found in patients with early breast cancer. Similarly, because the discovery of occult cancer in the human breast at autopsy is frequent, and the detection of microscopic contralateral cancer in routine biopsies made at surgery for breast cancer is excessive in comparison to the relative infrequency of second primaries in large series of breast cancer patients, it appears that subclinical neoplastic cell populations in the breast may often not only fail to progress, but theoretically may also regress spontaneously. Furthermore, the frequency of occurrence of mammary hyperplastic foci which may be preneoplastic far exceeds the successful development of neoplastic foci. Thus, more work needs to be done before large-scale programs of immunoprophylaxis are started.

10. Conclusions and Prospects

The prospects for major therapeutic activity with immunological intervention seem hopeful and exciting for patients with breast cancer. The complex host–tumor relationship must be carefully evaluated. However, the early clinical data suggest that patients have already benefited from immunotherapy. Thus, further investigation seems indicated for patients with both micrometastatic as well as widespread disease. The integration of immunotherapy into the treatment plan of the breast cancer patient will require close collaboration between the radiotherapist, the surgeon, the chemotherapist, and all others involved with the care of the patient. In addition, immunotherapy should not be the arena of the immunologist alone. Oncologists working with immunologists, biologists, pharmacologists, and chemists must incorporate immunotherapy into the total therapeutic strategy against cancer. Eventual treatment of the primary breast lesion by local immunotherapy seems to be a realistic prospect. The solutions are not all present. Progress has been slow, but as we unravel the complex pathways of the immune system, we should begin to make rapid progress.

11. References

1. R. T. Prehn, Do tumors grow because of the immune response of the host? *Transplant. Rev.* **28,** 34–42 (1976).
2. T. C. Everson, Spontaneous regression of cancer, *Ann. N.Y. Acad. Sci.* **114,** 721–735 (1964).
3. M. M. Black, S. R. Opler, and F. D. Speer, Microscopic structure of gastric carcinomas and their regional lymph nodes in relation to survival, *Surg. Gynecol. Obstet.* **98,** 725–734 (1954).

4. A. C. Allison, Immunological surveillance against tumor cells, in: *Cancer: A Comprehensive Treatise* (F. F. Becker, ed.) Vol. 4, pp. 237–258, Plenum Press, New York (1975).

5. L. Thomas, Reactions to homologous tissue antigens, in: *Cellular and Humoral Aspects of the Hypersensitive State* (H. S. Lawrence, ed.), pp. 504–534, Cassell, London (1959).

6. F. M. Burnet, Immunological surveillance in neoplasia, *Transplant. Rev.* **7**, 3–25 (1971).

7. R. T. Smith and M. Lande (eds.), *Immune Surveillance*, Academic Press, New York (1970).

8. A. C. Aisenberg, Studies on delayed hypersensitivity in Hodgkin's disease, *J. Clin. Invest.* **41**, 1964–1970 (1962).

9. A. G. Levin, E. F. McConough, D. G. Miller, and C. M. Southam, Delayed hypersensitivity responses to DNCB in sick and healthy persons, *Ann. N.Y. Acad. Sci.* **120**, 400–409, (1964).

10. A. K. Y. Lee, M. Rowley, and I. R. MacKay, Antibody-producing capacity in human cancer, *Br. J. Cancer* **24**, 454–463 (1970).

11. P. Alexander and J. G. Hall, The role of immunoblasts in host resistance and immunotherapy of primary sarcomata, in: *Advances in Cancer Research* (G. Klein and S. Weinhouse, eds.), Vol. 13, pp. 1–38, Academic Press, New York (1970).

12. J. Stjernsward, Immune status of the primary host towards its own methylcholanthrene-induced sarcomas, *J. Natl. Cancer Inst.* **40**, 13–22 (1968).

13. R. Virchow, *Krankhaften*, Geschwulste, Berlin (1863).

14. W. S. Handley, The pathology of melanotic growths in relation to their operative treatment, *Lancet* **1**, 927–996 (1907).

15. H. Wade, An experimental investigation of infective sarcoma in the dog with a consideration of its relationship to cancer, *J. Pathol. Bacteriol.* **12**, 384–425 (1908).

16. W. C. MacCarty, Factors which influence longevity in cancer, *Ann. Surg.* **76**, 9–12, (1922).

17. R. V. Greenough, Varying degrees of malignancy in cancer of the breast, *Cancer Res.* **9**, 453–463 (1925).

18. O. S. Moore, and F. W. Foote, The relatively favorable prognosis of medullary carcinoma of the breast, *Cancer* **2**, 635–642 (1949).

19. H. J. G. Bloom, Prognosis in carcinoma of the breast, *Br. J. Cancer* **4**, 259–288 (1950).

20. M. M. Black, S. Kerpe, and F. D. Speer, Lymph node structure in patients with cancer of the breast, *Am. J. Pathol.* **29**, 505–521 (1953).

21. M. M. Black, Structural antigenic and biological characteristics of precancerous mastopathy, *Cancer Res.* **36**, 2596–2604 (1976).

22. M. M. Black, Cellular and biologic manisfestations of immunogenicity to precancerous mastopathy, *Natl. Cancer Inst. Monogr.* **35**, 73–82 (1972).

23. M. M. Black, T. H. C. Barclay, and B. F. Hankey, Prognosis in breast cancer utilizing histological characteristics of the primary tumor, *Cancer* **36**, 2048–2055 (1975).

24. I. M. E. Hamlin, Possible host resistance in carcinoma of the breast: A histological study, *Br. J. Cancer* **22**, 383–401 (1968).

25. J. W. Berg, Inflammation and prognosis in breast cancer: A search for host resistance, *Cancer* **12**, 714–720 (1959).

26. H. R. Champion, I. W. Wallace, and R. J. Prescott, Histology in breast cancer prognosis, *Br. J. Cancer* **26**, 129–138 (1972).

27. R. Scarff and H. Torlomi, *Histologic Typing of Breast Tumors*, World Health Organization, Geneva (1968).

28. S. C. Sommers, Histologic changes in incipient carcinoma of the breast, *Cancer* **23**, 822–825 (1969).

29. S. G. Silverberg, A. R. Chitale, A. D. Hind, A. B. Frazier, and S. H. Leavitt, Sinus histiocytosis and mammary carcinoma. Study of 366 radical mastectomies and a histological review, *Cancer* **26**, 1177–1185 (1970).

30. M. Zelen, A hypothesis of the natural time history of breast cancer, *Cancer Res.* **28**, 207–216 (1968).

31. J. J. DiRe and N. Lane, The relation of sinus histiocytosis in axillary lymph nodes to surgical curability of carcinoma of breast, *Am. J. Clin. Pathol.* **40**, 508–515 (1963).

32. S. J. Kister, S. C. Sommers, C. D. Haagensen, G. H. Friedell, E. Cooley, and A. Varma, Nuclear grade in sinus histiocytosis in cancer of the breast, *Cancer* **23**, 570–574 (1969).

33. J. W. Berg, Sinus histiocytosis: A fallacious measure of host resistance to cancer, *Cancer* **9**, 935–939 (1956).

34. J. W. Berg, A. G. Houvos, L. M. Axtell, and G. F. Robbins, A new sign of favorable prognosis in mammary cancer: Hyperplastic reactive lymph nodes in the apex of the axilla, *Ann. Surg.* **177**, 8–12 (1973).

35. E. R. Fisher, R. Gregorio, C. Redmond, A. Dekker, and B. Fisher, Pathologic findings from the National Surgical Adjuvant Breast Project (Protocol #4). II. The significance of regional node histology other than sinus histiocytosis in invasive mammary cancer, *Am. J. Clin. Pathol.* **65**, 21–30 (1976).

36. E. R. Fisher, R. M. Gregorio, and B. Fisher, The pathology of invasive breast cancer, *Cancer* **36**, 1–85 (1975).

37. V. Tsakraklides, P. Olson, J. H. Kersey, and R. A. Good, Prognostic significance of the regional lymph node histology in cancer of the breast, *Cancer* **34**, 1259–1267 (1974).

38. R. L. Hunter, D. Ferguson, and L. W. Coppleson, Survival with mammary cancer related to the interaction of germinal center hyperplasia and sinus histiocytosis in axillary and internal mammary lymph nodes, *Cancer* **36**, 528–539 (1975).

39. J.L. Turk, *Frontiers of Biology: Delayed Hypersensitivity* (A. Neuberger and E. L. Tatum, eds.), Vol. 4, American Elsevier, New York (1967).

40. J.R. David and R.A. David, Cellular hypersensitivity and immunity, *Prog. Allergy* **16**, 300–499 (1972).

41. E. M. Hersh and G. P. Bodey, Leukocytic mechanism of inflammation, *Annu. Rev. Med.* **21**, 105–132 (1970).

42. E. M. Hersh, J. E. Curtis, J. E. Harris, C. McBride, R. Alexanian, and R. Rossen, Host defense mechanisms in lymphoma and leukemia, in: *Leukemia–Lymphoma* (The XIV Annual Clinical Conference on Cancer), pp. 149–168, Year Book Medical Publishers, Chicago (1970).

43. F. R. Eilber and D. L. Morton, Impaired immunologic reactivity and recurrence following cancer surgery, *Cancer* **25**, 362–367 (1970).

44. F. R. Eilber, J. A. Nizze, and D. L. Morton, Sequential evaluation of general immune competence in cancer patients: Correlation with clinical course, *Cancer* **35**, 660–665 (1975).

45. P.M. Bolton, A.M. Mander, J.M. Davidson, S.L. James, R.G. Newcombe, and L.E. Hughes, Cellular immunity in cancer: Comparison of delayed hypersensitivity skin tests in three common cancers, *Br. Med. J.* **3**, 18–20 (1975).

46. C. M. Pinsky, H. Wanebo, V. Mike, and H. Oettgen, Delayed cutaneous hypersensitivity reactions and prognosis in patients with cancer, *Ann. N.Y. Acad. Sci.* **276**, 407–410 (1976).

47. H. J. Wanebo, P. P. Rosen, T. Thaler, J. A. Urban, and H. F. Oettgen, Immunobiology of operable breast cancer: An assessment of biologic risk by immunoparameters, *Ann. Surg.* **184**, 258, 266 (1976).

48. S. Golub, T. X. O'Connell, and D. L. Morton, Correlation in *in vivo* and *in vitro* assays of immunocompetence in cancer patients, *Cancer Res.* **34**, 1833–1837 (1974).

49. T. J. Cunningham, D. Daut, P. Wolfgang, M. Mellyn, S. Maciolek, R. Sponzo, and J. Horton, A correlation of DNCB-induced delayed cutaneous hypersensiviity reactions and the course of disease in patients with recurrent breast cancer, *Cancer* **37**, 1696–1700 (1976).

50. M. M. Roberts and W. J. Williams, Delayed hypersensitivity in breast cancer, *Br. J. Surg.* **55**, 869 (1968) (abstract #53).

51. M. M. Roberts and W. J. Williams, The delayed hypersensitivity reaction in breast cancer, *Br. J. Surg.* **61**, 549–552 (1974).

52. P. M. Bolton, C. Teasdale, A. M. Mander, S. L. James, J. M. Davidson, R. H. Whitehead, R. G. Newcombe, and L. E. Hughes, Immune competence in breast cancer—Relationship of pretreatment immunologic tests to diagnosis and tumor stage, *Cancer Immunol. Immunother.* **1**, 251–258 (1976).

53. E. M. Hersh, J. U. Gutterman, G. M. Mavligit, C. W. Mountain, C. M. McBride, M. A. Burgess, P. M. Lurie, M. Zelen, H. Takita, and R. G. Vincent, Immunocompetence, immunodeficiency, and prognosis in cancer, *Ann. N.Y. Acad. Sci.* **276**, 386–406 (1976).

54. E. M. Hersh, J. U. Gutterman, and G. M. Mavligit, Immunodeficiency in cancer and the importance of immune evaluation of the cancer patient, *Med. Clin. North Am.* **60**, 623–639 (1976).

55. T. Nemoto, T. Han, J. Minowada, V. Angkur, A. Chamberlain, and T. L. Dao, Cell mediated immune status of breast cancer patients: Evaluation by skin tests, lymphocyte stimulation, and counts of rosette forming cells, *J. Natl. Cancer Inst.* **53**, 641–645 (1974).

56. M. J. Krant, G. Manskope, C. S. Brandrup, and M. A. Madoff, Immunologic alteration in bronchogenic cancer. Sequential study, *Cancer* **21**, 623–631 (1968).

57. A. Riesco, Five year cancer cure: Relation to total amount of peripheral lymphocytes and neutrophils, *Cancer* **25**, 135–140 (1970).

58. W. J. Pendergrast, O.R. Boehm, and L. J. Humphrey, Effect of immunotherapy on peripheral lymphocyte count, *Arch. Surg.* **103**, 184–188 (1971).

59. A. E. Papatestas, G. J. Lesnick, G. Genkins, and A. H. Aufses, The prognostic significance of peripheral lymphocyte counts in patients with breast cancer, *Cancer* **37**, 164–168 (1976).

60. J. Wybran and H. H. Fundenberg, Rosette formation: A test for cellular immunity, *Trans. Assoc. Am. Physicians* **84**, 239–247 (1971).

61. C. Martinez, Effect of Early thymectomy on development of mammary tumors in mice, *Nature* **203**, 1188 (1964).

62. T. Sakakura and Y. Nishizuka, Effect of thymectomy on mammary tumorigenesis, nodaligenesis, and mammogenesis in the mouse, *Gann* **58**, 441–450 (1967).

63. M. M. Roberts, Lymphocyte transformation in breast cancer, *Br. J. Surg.* **57**, 381 (1970).

64. E. Robinson, S. Sher, and T. Mekoni, Lymphocyte stimulation by phytohemagglutinin and tumor cells of malignant effusions, *Cancer Res.* **34**, 1548–1551 (1974).

65. L. A. Knight and W. M. Davidson, Reduced lymphocyte transformation in early cancer of the breast, *J. Clin. Pathol.* **28**, 372–376 (1975).

66. J. J. Miller, P. R. Gaffney, J. A. Rees, and M. O. Symes, Lymphocyte reactivity in patients with carcinoma of the breast and large bowel, *Br. J. Cancer* **32**, 16–20 (1975).

67. M. G. Whittaker, K. Rees, and C. G. Clark, Reduced lymphocyte transformation in breast cancer, *Lancet* **1**, 892–893 (1971).

68. R.H. Whitehead, J. Thatcher, C. Teasdale, G.P. Roberts, and L.H. Hughes, T- and B-Lymphocytes in breast cancer—Stage, relationship, and abrogation of T-lymphocyte depression by enzyme treatment *in vitro, Lancet* **1**, 330–333 (1976).
69. B. Fisher, E. A. Saffer, and E. R. Fisher, Studies concerning the regional lymph node in cancer. III. Response of regional lymph node cells from breast and colon cancer patients in PHA stimulation, *Cancer* **30**, 1202–1215 (1972).
70. B. Fisher, E. A. Saffer, and E. R. Fisher, Studies concerning the regional lymph node in cancer. VII. Thymidine uptake by cells from nodes of breast cancer patients relative to axillary location and histopathologic discriminants, *Cancer* **33**, 271–279 (1974).
71. U. Ambus, G. M. Mavligit, J. U. Gutterman, C. M. McBride, and E. M. Hersh, Specific and non-specific immunologic reactivity of regional lymph node lymphocytes in human malignancy, *Int. J. Cancer* **14**, 291–300 (1974).
72. A. V. Jubert, C. M. McBride, G. M. Mavligit, J. U. Gutterman, and E. M. Hersh, Immunoglobulin on the surface of human appendix lymphocytes, *Immunol. Commun.* **3**, 1–9 (1974).
73. J. A. Buda, N. Suciu-Foca, E. Blomain, S. McManus, and K. Reemtsma, Impaired cell mediated immunity in patients with cancer, *J. Surg. Oncol.* **7**, 525–529 (1975).
74. E. J. Field and E. A. Caspary, Lymphocyte sensitization in advanced malignant disease: A study of serum lymphocyte depressive factor, *Br. J. Cancer* **26**, 164–173 (1972).
75. A.M. Steward, H.Z. Kupchick, and N. Zamcheck, Circulating carcinoembryonic antigen levels and serum suppression of phytohemagglutinin-stimulated lymphocyte DNA synthesis: An inverse correlation in the cancer patient, *J. Natl. Cancer Inst.* **53**, 3–9 (1974).
76. R. H. Whitehead, P. M. Bolton, and R. G. Newcombe, Is there factor in the sera from cancer patients that inhibits lymphocyte response to phytohaemagglutinin? *Eur. J. Cancer* **10**, 815–818 (1974).
77. H. Blomgren, J. Wasserman, and U. Glas, Capacity of sera from patients with mammary carcinoma to promote PHA-stimulation of human lymphocytes, *Acta Radiol.* **14**, 127–138 (1975).
78. D. R. Burger, D. P. Lilley, M. Reid, L. Irish, and R. M. Vetto, Alpha globulin changes during the development of cellular immunity, *Cell. Immunol.* **8**,. 147–154 (1973).
79. O. H. Plescia, A. H. Smith, and K. Grinwich, Subversion of the immune system by tumor cells and role of prostaglandins, *Proc. Natl. Acad. Sci. U.S.A.* **72**, 1848–1851 (1975).
80. H. Friedman and C. Southam (eds.), *International Conference on Immunobiology of Cancer* (New York Academy of Sciences), *Ann. N.Y. Acad. Sci.* **276**, 1–591 (1976).
81. R. T. Prehn, The immune reaction as a stimulator of tumor growth, *Science* **176**, 170–171 (1972).
82. R. T. Prehn, Perspectives on oncogenesis: Does immunity stimulate or inhibit neoplasia? *J. Reticuloendothel. Soc.* **10**, 1–16 (1971).
83. G. H. Heppner, Neonatal thymectomy and mouse mammary tumorigenesis, in: *Immunity and Tolerance in Oncogenesis* (L. Severi, ed.), pp. 503–524, University of Perugia, Italy (1970).
84. E. J. Yunis, C. Martinez, J. Smith, O. Stutman, and R. A. Good, Spontaneous mammary adenocarcinoma in mice: Influence of thymectomy and reconstitution with thymus grafts or spleen cells, *Cancer Res.* **29**, 174–178 (1969).
85. M. A. Lappe and P. B. Blair, Interference with mammary tumorigenesis by antilymphocyte serum, *Proc. Amer. Assoc. Cancer Res.* **11**, 47 (1970).

86. P. B. Blair, Immunologic aspects of tumor induction by mammary tumor virus, J. Natl. Cancer Inst. 48, 1121–1124 (1972).

87. D. L. Morton, Acquired immunological tolerance and carcinogenesis by the mammary tumor virus. I. Influence of neonatal infection with the mammary tumor virus on the growth of spontaneous mammary adenocarcinoma, J. Natl. Cancer Inst. 42, 311–320 (1969).

88. D. W. Weiss, D. H. Lavrin, M. Dezfulian, J. Vaage, and P. B. Blair, Studies on the immunology of spontaneous mammary carcinomas of mice, in: Viruses Inducing Cancer (W. J. Burdette, ed.), pp. 138–168, University of Utah Press, Salt Lake City (1966).

89. R. V. P. Hutter and D. U. Kim, The problem of multiple lesions of the breast, Cancer 28, 1591–1607 (1971).

90. S. Roberts, J. Hengesh, R. McGrath, E. McGrew, J. Valaitis, and W. Cole, Five to ten year follow up studies on circulating cancer cells, Proc. Ninth Int. Cancer Congr., p. 69 (1966) (abstract).

91. J. Song, P. From, W. J. Morrissey, and J. Sams, Circulating cancer cells: Pre- and post-chemotherapy observations, Cancer 28, 553–561 (1971).

92. M. H. Edwards, M. Baum, and C. J. Magarey, Regression of axillary lymph nodes in cancer of the breast Br. J. Surg. 59, 776–779 (1972).

93. L. E. Hughes and B. Lytton, Antigenic properties of human tumors: Delayed cutaneous hypersensitivity reaction, Br. Med. J. 1, 209–212 (1964).

94. T. H. M. Stewart, The presence of delayed hypersensitivity reactions in patients toward cellular extracts of their malignant tumors. II. A correlation between the histologic picture of lymphocyte infiltration of the tumor stroma, the presence of such a reaction and a discussion of the significance of this phenomenon, Cancer 23, 1380–1387 (1969).

95. C. Alford, A. Hollinshead, and R. Herberman, Delayed cutaneous hypersensitivity reactions to extracts of malignant and normal human breast cells, Ann. Surg. 178, 20–24 (1973).

96. A.C. Hollinshead, W.T. Jaffurs, L.K. Alpert, J.E. Harris, and R.B. Herberman, Isolation and identification of soluble skin-reactive membrane antigens of malignant and normal human breast cells, Cancer Res. 34, 2961–2968 (1974).

97. G. M. Mavligit, U. Ambus, J. U. Gutterman, E. M. Hersh, and C. M. McBride, Antigen solubilized from human solide tumors: Lymphocyte stimulation and cutaneous delayed hypersensitivity, Nature (London) New Biol. 243, 188–190 (1973).

98. J. Stjernsward, L. E. Almgard, S. Franzen, T. Von Schreeb, and L. B. Wadstrom, Tumor distinctive cellular immunity to renal carcinoma, Clin. Exp. Immunol. 6, 963–968 (1970).

99. F. Vanky and J. Stjernsward, Lymphocyte stimulation tests for detection of tumor specific reactivity in humans, in: In Vitro Methods in Cell Mediated and Tumor Immunity (B.R. Bloom and J.R. David, eds.), pp. 597–606, Academic Press, New York (1976).

100. A. Richters and R. P. Sherwin, The significance of autochthonous lymphocyte interactions with human breast cancer cells in primary tissue cultures, Cancer 27, 274–277 (1971).

101. S. D. Deodhar, G. Crile, and C. B. Esselstyn, Study of the tumor cell–lymphocyte interaction in patients with breast cancer, Cancer 29, 1321–1325 (1972).

102. I. Hellstrom, K. E. Hellstrom, H. O. Sjogren, and G. A. Warner, Demonstration of cell mediated immunity to human neoplasms of various histological types, Int. J. Cancer 7, 1–16 (1971).

103. G. Fossati, S. Canevari, G. Della Porta, G. P. Balzarini, and U. Veronesi, Cellular immunity to human breast carcinoma, Int. J. Cancer 10, 391–396 (1972).

104. M. Takusugi, M. R. Mickey, and P. I. Terasaki, Reactivity of lymphocytes from normal persons on cultured tumor cells, *Cancer Res.* **33,** 2898–2902 (1973).

105. H. F. Jeejeebhoy, Immunological studies of women with primary breast carcinoma, *Int. J. Cancer* **15,** 867–878 (1975).

106. G. M. Mavligit, J. U. Gutterman, and E. M. Hersh, *In vitro* antitumor reactivity of mononuclear leukocytes from cancer patients receiving immunotherapy with BCG, In preparation (1977).

107. K. E. Hellstrom and I. Hellstrom, Lymphocyte mediated cytotoxicity and blocking serum activity to tumor antigens, *Adv. Immunol.* **18,** 209–277 (1974).

108. H. O. Sjogren, I. Hellstrom, S. C. Bansal, G. A. Warner, and K. E. Hellstrom, Elution of "blocking factors" from human tumors, capable of abrogating tumor cell destruction by specifically immune lymphocytes, *Int. J. Cancer* **9,** 274–283 (1972).

109. R. Baldwin, M. R. Price, and R. A. Robins, Significance of serum factors modifying cellular immune responses to growth of tumors, *Br. J. Cancer* **28,** 37–39 (1973).

110. I. Hellstrom, K. E. Hellstrom, and G. A. Warner, Increase of lymphocyte mediated tumor cell destruction by certain patient sera, *Int. J. Cancer* **12,** 348–353 (1973).

111. I. Hellstrom and K. Hellstrom, Microcytotoxicity assays of cell mediated tumor immunity and blocking serum factors, in: *In Vitro Methods in Cell Mediated and Tumor Immunity* (B. R. Bloom and J. R. David, eds.), pp. 533–540, Academic Press, New York (1976).

112. N. L. Levy, Use of an *in vitro* microcytotoxicity test to assess human tumor specific cell mediated immunity and its serum mediated abrogation, *Natl. Cancer Inst. Monogr.* **37,** 85–92 (1973).

113. F. Avis, I. Mosonov, and G. Haughton, Antigenic cross reactivity between benign and malignant neoplasms of the human breast. *J. Natl. Cancer Inst.* **52.** 1041–1049 (1974).

114. G. H. Heppner, Is there evidence that immunity influences tumor host balance in breast cancer? in: *Breast Cancer: A Challenging Problem* (M. L. Griem, E. V. Jensen, J. E. Ultman, and R. W. Wissler, eds.), pp. 63–72, Springer-Verlag, New York (1973).

115. S. H. Golub, Host immune response to human tumor antigens, in: *Cancer: A Comprehensive Treatise* (F. F. Becker, ed.), Vol. 4, pp. 259–302, Plenum Press, New York (1975).

116. V. S. Byers, L. LeCam. A. S. Levin, W. H. Stone, and A. J. Hackett, Identification of human populations with a high incidence of cellular immunity against breast carcinoma: Use in transfer factor immunotherapy, *Cancer Immunol. Immunother.* (1977), in press.

117. R. H. Yonemoto, T. Fujisawa, and S. R. Waldman, Selection of donors for transfer factor immunotherapy, *Proc. Am. Assoc. Cancer Res.* **17,** 150 (1976).

118. F. Avis, I. Avis, J. F. Newsome, and G. Haughton, Antigenic cross reactivity between adenocarcinoma of the breast and fibrocystic disease of the breast, *J. Natl. Cancer Inst.* **56,** 17–25 (1976).

119. V. Anderson, O. Bjerrum, G. Bendixen, T. Schiodt, and I. Dissing, Effect of autologous mammary tumor extracts on human leukocyte migration *in vitro*, *Int. J. Cancer* **5,** 357–363 (1970).

120. A. Segall, O. Weiler, J. Genin. J. Lacour, and F. Lacour, *In vitro* study of cellular immunity against autochthonous human cancer, *Int. J. Cancer* **9,** 417–425 (1972).

121. J. L. McCoy, L. F. Jerome, J. H. Dean, G. B. Cannon, T. C. Alford, T. Doering, and R. B. Herberman, Inhibition of leukocyte migration by tumor associated antigens in soluble extracts of human breast carcinoma, *J. Natl. Cancer Inst.* **53,** 11–17 (1974).

122. A. J. Cochran, R. M. Grant, W. G. Spilg, R. M. Mackie, C. E. Ross, D. E. Hoyle, and J. M. Russell, Sensitization to tumor associated antigens in human breast carcinoma, *Int. J. Cancer* **14,** 19–25 (1974).

123. M. M. Black, H. P. Leis, B. Shore, and R. E. Zachrau, Cellular hypersensitivity to breast cancer. Assessment by a leukocyte migration procedure, *Cancer* **33**, 952–958 (1974).
124. R. J. Ellis, G. Wernick, J. B. Zabriske, and L. J. Goldman, Immunologic competence of regional lymph nodes in patients with breast cancer, *Cancer* **35**, 655–659 (1975).
125. W. J. Halliday, A. Maluish, and W. H. Isbister, Detection of anti-tumor cell mediated immunity and serum blocking factors in cancer patients by the leukocyte adherence inhibition test, *Br. J. Cancer* **29**, 31–35 (1974).
126. N. Grosser and D. M. P. Thomson, Cell mediated antitumor immunity in breast cancer patients evaluated by antigen-induced leukocyte adherence inhibition in test tubes, *Cancer Res.* **35**, 2571–2579 (1975).
127. V. Holan, M. Hasek, J. Bubenik, and J. Chutna, Antigen mediated macrophage adherence inhibition, *Cell. Immunol.* **13**, 107–116 (1974).
128. E. Rowinska-Zakrewska, P. Lazar, and P. Burtin, Dosage des immunoglobulines dans le sérum des cancéreux, *Ann. Inst. Pasteur* **119**, 621–625 (1970).
129. N. R. Hughes, Serum concentration of IgG, IgA, and IgM in patients with carcinoma, melanoma, and sarcoma, *J. Natl. Cancer Inst.* **46**, 1015–1028 (1971).
130. M. M. Roberts, E. M. Bathgate, and A. Stevenson, Serum immunoglobulin levels in patients with breast cancer, *Cancer* **36**, 221–224 (1975).
131. E. M. Edynak, Y. Hirshaut, M. Bernhard, and G. Trempe, Fluorescent antibody studies of human breast cancer, *J. Natl. Cancer Inst.* **48**, 1137–1143 (1972).
132. L. J. Humphrey, N. C. Estes, P. A. Morse, W. R. Jewell, R. A. Boudet, M. J. K. Hudson, P. G. Tsolakidis, and F. A. Mantz, Serum antibody in patients with breast disease, *Ann. Surg.* **180**, 124–129 (1974).
133. M. J. K. Hudson, L. J. Humphrey, F. A. Mantz, and P. A. Morse, Correlation of circulating serum antibody to the histologic findings in breast cancer, *Am. J. Surg.* **128**, 756–762 (1974).
134. W. F. Feller, S. E. Stewart, and J. Kantor, Primary tissue culture explants of human breast cancer, *J. Natl. Cancer Inst.* **48**, 1117–1120 (1972).
135. R. E. Nordquist, D. R. Ishmael, C. A. Lovig, D. M. Hyder, and A. F. Hoge, The tissue culture and morphology of a human breast tumor cell line (BOT-2), *J. Lab. Clin. Med.* **89**, 257–261 (1977).
136. R. E. Nordquist, F. B. Schafer, N. E. Manning, D. R. Ishmael, and A. F. Hoge, Anti-tumor antibodies in human breast cancer sera as detected by fixed cell immunofluorescence and living cell membrane immunoflorescence assays, *Cancer Res.* **35**, 3100–3105 (1975).
137. R. W. Baldwin, M. J. Embleton, J. S. Jones, and M. J. S. Langman, Cell mediated and humoral immune reactions to human tumors, *Int. J. Cancer* **12**, 73–83 (1973).
138. G. F. Springer, P. R. Desai, and I. Banatwala, Blood group MN specific substances and precursors in normal and malignant human breast tissues, *Naturwissenchaften* **61**, 457–458 (1974).
139. G. F. Springer, R. P. Desai, and I. Banatwala, Blood group MN antigens and precursors in normal and malignant human breast glandular tissue, *J. Natl. Cancer Inst.* **54**, 335–339 (1975).
140. G. F. Springer, P. R. Desai, and E. F. Scanlon, Blood group MN precursors as human breast carcinoma associated antigens and "naturally" occurring humans cytotoxins against them, *Cancer* **37**, 169–176 (1976).
141. H. J. Hansen, L. J. Snyder, E. Miller, J. P. Vandevoorde, O. N. Miller, L. R. Hines, and J. J. Burns, Carcinoembryonic antigen (CEA) assay. A laboratory adjunct in the diagnosis and management of cancer, *Hum. Pathol.* **5**, 139–147 (1974).
142. M. K. Schwarz, Biochemical Markers in breast cancer: Hormone receptors and tumor associated antigen, *Breast Dis. Breast* **2**, 7–11 (1976).

143. T. M. Chu, Evaluation of carcinoembryonic antigen in human mammary carcinoma, *J. Natl. Cancer Inst.* **51**, 1119–1122 (1973).

144. A. M. Stewart, D. Nixon, N. Zamcheck, and A. Aisenberg, Carcinoembryonic antigen in breast cancer patients: Serum levels and disease progress, *Cancer* **33**, 1246–1252 (1974).

145. D. M. Marcus and N. Zinberg, Isolation of ferritin from human mammary and pancreatic carcinomas by means of antibody immunoadsorbents, *Arch. Biochem. Biophys.* **162**, 493–501 (1974).

146. A. Jacobs, B. Jones, C. Ricketts, R. D. Bulbrook, and D. Y. Wang, Serum ferritin concentrations in early breast cancer, *Br. J. Cancer* **34**, 280–290 (1976).

147. R. K. Gupta and R. Schuster, Isoantigens A, B, and H in benign and malignant lesions of breast, *Am. J. Pathol.* **72**, 253–260 (1973).

148. I. Davidson and N. Ly, Loss of isoantigens in carcinomas of lung, *Am. J. Pathol.* **57**, 307–334 (1969).

149. A. V. Richman, Immunofluorescence studies of benign and malignant human mammary tissue, *J. Natl. Cancer Inst.* **57**, 263–267 (1976).

150. K. Irie, R. F. Irie, and D. L. Morton, Detection of antibody and complement complexed *in vivo* on membranes of human cancer cells by mixed hemadsorption techniques, *Cancer Res.* **35**, 1244–1248 (1975).

151. O. Tonder and S. Thunold, Receptors for immunoglobulin Fc in human malignant tissues, *Scand. J. Immunol.* **2**, 207–215 (1973).

152. I. Witz, S. Argov, and D. Cohen, Non-specific fixation of immunoglobulin by tumor cells *in vitro*, *Isr. J. Med. Sci.* **8**, 669 (1972).

153. D. H. Moore, Mammary tumor virus, in: *Cancer: A Comprehensive Treatise; Etiology: Viral Carcinogenesis* (F. F. Becker, ed.) Vol. 2, pp. 131–167, Plenum Press, New York (1975).

154. L. Dmochowski, The importance of studies on the mammary tumor-inducing virus in the problem of breast cancer, in: *International Symposium on Mammary Cancer* (L. Severi, ed.), pp. 655–708, University of Perugia, Italy (1958).

155. D. H. Moore, J. Charney, B. Kramarsky, E. Y. Lasfargues, N. H. Sarkar, M. J. Brennan, J. H. Burrows, S. M. Sirsat, J. C. Paymaster, and A. B. Vaidya, Search for a human breast cancer virus, *Nature* **229**, 611–615 (1971).

156. J. Schlom, S. Spiegelman, and D. H. Moore, Reverse transcriptase and high molecular weight RNA in particles from mouse and human milk, *J. Natl. Cancer Inst.* **48**, 1197–1203 (1972).

157. S. Spiegelman, R. Axel, and J. Schlom, Virus-related RNA in human and mouse mammary tumors, *J. Natl. Cancer Inst.* **48**, 1205–1211 (1972).

158. E. S. Priori, G. Seman, L. Dmochowski, H. S. Gallager, and D. E. Anderson, Immunofluorescence studies on sera of patients with breast carcinoma, *Cancer* **28**, 1462–1471 (1971).

159. E. S. Priori, D. E. Anderson, W. C. Williams, and L. Dmochowski, Immunological studies on human breast carcinoma and mouse mammary tumors, *J. Natl. Cancer Inst.* **48**, 1131–1135 (1972).

160. M. Muller and J. Grossmann, An antigen in human breast cancer sera related to the murine mammary tumor virus, *Nature (London) New Biol.* **237**, 116–117 (1972).

161. J. M. Bowen, L. Dmochowski, M. F. Miller, E. S. Priori, G. Seman, M. L. Dodson, and K. Maruyama, Implications of humoral antibody in mice and humans to breast tumor and mouse mammary tumor virus associated antigens, *Cancer Res.* **36**, 759–764 (1976).

162. K. W. Newgard, R. D. Cardiff, and P. B. Blair, Human antibodies binding to the mouse mammary tumor virus: A nonspecific reaction? *Cancer Res.* **36**, 765–768 (1976).

163. O. Stutman and R. B. Herberman, Immunological control of breast cancer : Discussion, *Cancer Res.* **36**, 781–782 (1976).

164. M. M. Black, R. E. Zachrau, B. Shore, and H. P. Leis, Biological considerations of tumor specific and virus associated antigens of human breast cancers, *Cancer Res.* **36**, 769–774 (1976).

165. S. Cunningham-Rundles, W. F. Feller, C. Cunningham-Rundles, B. Dupont, H. Wanebo, R. O'Reilly, and R. A. Good, Lymphocyte transformation *in vitro* to R111 mouse milk antigen among women with breast disease, *Cell. Immunol.* **25**, 322–327 (1976).

166. A. C. Hollinshead, Personal communication.

167. C. J. Magarey and M. Baum, Reticulo-endothelial activity in humans with cancer, *Br. J. Surg.* **57**, 748–752 (1970).

168. L. J. Old, B. Benacerraf, D. A. Clark, E. A. Carswell, and E. Stockert, The role of the reticuloendothelial system in the host reaction to neoplasia, *Cancer Res.* **21**, 1281–1300 (1961).

169. C. J. Magarey and M. Baum, Oestrogen as a reticuloendothelial stimulant in patients with cancer, *Br. Med. J.* **2**, 367–370 (1971).

170. C. R. Pentycross, D. Toussis, J. A. McKinna, S. D. Lawler, and W. P. Greening, Effect of Hormone therapy on mitogenic responses of lymphocytes from patients with cancer of the breast, *Lancet* **2**, 177–179 (1973).

171. B. Benacerraf, B. N. Halpern, G. Biozzi, and S. A. Bencos, Quantitative study of the granulopectic activity of the reticuloendothelial system. III. The effect of cortisone and nitrogen mustard on the regenerative capacity of the R.E.S. after saturation with carbon, *Br. J. Exp. Pathol.* **35**, 97–106 (1954).

172. T. Nicol, Female reproductive system in the guinea pig; intra-vital staining; fat production; influence of hormones, *Trans. R. Soc. Edinburgh* **58**, 449–486 (1935).

173. J. Thompson and R. Van Furth, The effect of glucocorticosteriods on the kinetics of mononuclear phagocytes, *J. Exp. Med.* **131**, 429–442 (1970).

174. H. G. Iversen, Influence of cortisone on frequency of tumor metastases, *Acta Pathol. Microbiol. Scand.* **41**, 273–280 (1957).

175. P. Sherlock and W. H. Hartmann, Adrenal steroids and the pattern of metastases of breast cancer, *J. Am. Med. Assoc.* **181**, 313–317 (1962).

176. J. A. McCredie, W. R. Inch, and R. M. Sutherland, Effect of postoperative radiotherapy on peripheral blood lymphocytes in patients with carcinoma of the breast, *Cancer* **29**, 349–356 (1972).

177. A. B. Cosimi, F. H. Brunster, W. T. Kemmerer, and B. N. Miller, Cellular immune competence of breast cancer patients receiving radiotherapy, *Arch. Surg.* **107**, 531–535 (1973).

178. J. Stjernsward, M. Jondal, F. Vanky, H. Wigzell, and R. Dealey, Lymphopenia and change in distribution of human B and T lymphocytes in peripheral blood induced by irradiation for mammary carcinoma, *Lancet* **1**, 1352–1356 (1972).

179. H. Blomgren, R. Berg, J. Wasserman, and U. Glas, Effect of radiotherapy on blood lymphocyte population in mammary carcinoma, *Int. J. Radiat. Oncol. Biol. Phys.* **1**, 177–188 (1976).

180. P. Alexander, The bogey of the immuno-suppressive action of local radiotherapy, *Int. J. Radiat. Oncol. Biol. Phys.* **1**, 369–371 (1976).

181. W. B. Coley, A report of recent cases of inoperable sarcoma successfully treated with mixed toxins of erysipelas and *Bacillus prodigiosus*, *Surg. Gynecol. Obstet.* **13**, 174–190 (1911).

182. H. C. Nauts, The apparently beneficial effects of bacterial infection on host resistance to cancer, New York Cancer Research Institute, Monograph 8 (1969).

183. E. Klein and O. A. Holterman, Immunotherapeutic approaches to the management of neoplasms, Natl. Cancer Inst. Monogr. 35, 379–499 (1972).

184. J. Stjernsward and A. Levin, Delayed hypersensitivity induced regression of human neoplasms, Cancer 28, 628–640 (1971).

185. G. V. Smith, P. A. Morse, Jr., G. D. Deraps, S. Raju, and J. D. Hardy, Immunotherapy of patients with cancer, Surgery 74, 59–68 (1973).

186. D. H. Partridge, F. C. Sparks, A. G. Wile, and D. L. Morton, Intratumor injection of BCG for chest wall recurrence of breast carcinoma, Proc. Am. Soc. Clin. Oncol. 18, 325 (1977) (abstract #C-238).

187. M. J. Mastrangelo, D. Berd, and R. E. Bellet, Critical review of previously reported clinical trials of cancer immunotherapy with nonspecific immunostimulants, Ann. N.Y. Acad. Sci. 277, 94–123 (1976).

188. N. V. Dimitrov, T. Singh, and E. Balcueva, Intralesional injections of C. parvum in local skin recurrences of breast cancer, Proc. Am. Soc. Clin. Oncol. 18, 270 (1977) (abstract # C-15).

189. P. W. A. Mansell, N. R. DiLuzio, R. McNamee, G. Rowden, and J. W. Proctor, Recognition factors and nonspecific macrophage activation in the treatment of neoplastic disease, Ann. N.Y. Acad. Sci. 277, 20–44 (1976).

190. G. Mathe, J. L. Amiel, L. Schwarzenberg, L. Schneider, A. Cattan, J. R. Schlumberger, M. Hazat, and F. DeVassal, Active immunotherapy for acute lymphoblastic leukemia, Lancet 1, 697–699 (1969).

191. J. U. Gutterman, G. M. Mavligit, J. A. Gottlieb, M. A. Burgess, C. M. McBride, L. Einhorn, E. J. Freireich, and E. M. Hersh, Chemoimmunotherapy of disseminated malignant melanoma with dimethyl triazeno carboxamide and bacillus Calmette–Guérin, N. Engl. J. Med. 291, 592–597 (1974).

192. W. R. Vogler and Y. K. Chan, Prolonging remission in myeloblastic leukemia by Tice strain bacillus Calmette–Guérin, Lancet 2, 128–131 (1974).

193. J. U. Gutterman, E. M. Hersh, V. Rodriguez, K. B. McCredie, G. Mavligit, R. Reed, M. A. Burgess, T. Smith, E. A. Gehan, G. P. Bodey, Sr., and E. J. Freireich, Chemoimmunotherapy of adult acute leukemia: Prolongation of remission in myeloblastic leukemia with BCG, Lancet 2 1405–1409 (1974).

194. J. A. Whittaker and A. J. Slater, The immunotherapy of acute myelogenous leukemia using intravenous BCG, in: Immunotherapy of Cancer: Present Status of Trials in Man (W. D. Terry and D. Windhorst, eds.), Raven Press, New York (1977), in press.

195. B. Hoerni, J. Chauvergne, G. Hoerni-Simon, M. Durand, and C. Lagarde, BCG in the immunotherapy of malignant lymphomas, Cancer Immunol. Immunother. (1977), in press.

196. L. Israel, Immunochemotherapy with Corynebacterium parvum in disseminated cancer, Ann. N.Y. Acad. Sci. 277, 241–251 (1976).

197. J. A. Gottlieb, G. R. Blumenschein, J. U. Gutterman, E. J. Freireich, and J. O. Cardenas, Adriamycin in the treatment of breast cancer, in: Adriamycin Review (M. Staquert, ed.), pp. 249–256, European Press, Medikon (1975).

198. J. U. Gutterman, J. O. Cardenas, G. R. Blumenschein, G. Hortobagyi, R. B. Livingston, G. M. Mavligit, E. J. Freireich, J. A. Gottlieb, and E. M. Hersh, Chemoimmunotherapy of disseminated breast cancer: Prolongation of remission and survival, Br. Med. J. 2, 1222–1225 (1976).

199. J. U. Gutterman, G. M. Mavligit, G. Hortobagyi, G. R. Blumenschein, M. A. Burgess, A. V. Jubert, and E. M. Hersh, BCG immunotherapy of disseminated breast cancer and colorectal cancer: Prolongation of remission and survival, in: BCG in Cancer Immunotherapy (G. Lamoureux, R. Turcotte, and V. Portelance, eds.), pp. 227–238, Grune and Stratton, New York (1976).

200. G. Hortobagyi, J. U. Gutterman, G. R. Blumenschein, C. K. Tashima, M. Schwarz,

M. A. Burgess, and E. M. Hersh, The use of BCG and MER plus combination chemotherapy in the management of patients with disseminated breast carcinoma, in: *Immunotherapy of Cancer: Present Status of Trials in Man* (W. D. Terry and D. Windhorst, eds.), Raven Press, New York (1977), in press.

201. C. M. Pinsky, Y. Hirshaut, H. J. Wanebo, J. Fortner, V. Mike, D. Schottenfeld, and H. Oettgen, Surgical adjuvant immunotherapy with BCG in patients with malignant melanoma. Results of a prospective, randomized trial, in: *Immunotherapy of Cancer: Present Status of Trials in Man* (W. D. Terry and D. Windhorst, eds.), Raven Press, New York (1977), in press.

202. J. U. Gutterman, G. Mavligit, C. McBride, E. Frei, III, E. J. Freireich, and E. M. Hersh, Active immunotherapy with BCG for recurrent malignant melanoma, *Lancet* **1**, 1208–1212 (1973).

203. D. L. Morton, F. R. Eilber, E. C. Holmes, J. S. Hunt, A. S. Ketcham, M. F. Silverstein, and F. C. Sparks, BCG immunotherapy of malignant melanoma: Summary of a seven year experience, *Ann. Surg.* **180**, 635–643 (1974).

204. J. U. Gutterman, G. M. Mavligit, M. A. Burgess, J. O. Cardenas, G. R. Blumenschein, J. A. Gottlieb, C. M. McBride, E. M. Hersh, K. B. McCredie, G. P. Bodey, Sr., V. Rodriguez, and E. J. Freireich, Immunotherapy of human solid tumors and acute leukemia with BCG: Prolongation of disease free interval and survival, *Cancer Immunol. Immunother.* **1**, 99–107 (1976).

205. F. R. Eilber, D. L. Morton, E. C. Holmes, F. C. Sparks, and K. P. Ramming, Adjuvant immunotherapy with BCG in treatment of regional lymph node metastases from malignant melanoma, *N. Engl. J. Med.* **294**, 237–240 (1976).

206. G. Beretta, Controlled study for prolonged chemotherapy, immunotherapy, and chemotherapy plus immunotherapy as an adjuvant to surgery, in: *Immunotherapy of Cancer: Present Status of Trials in Man* (W. D. Terry and D. Windhorst, eds.), Raven Press, New York (1977), in press.

207. G. M. Mavligit, J. U. Gutterman, M. A. Burgess, N. Khankhanian, G. B. Seibert, J. F. Speer, A. V. Jubert, R. C. Martin, C. M. McBride, E. M. Copeland, E. A. Gehan, and E. M. Hersh, Prolongation of postoperative disease free interval and survival in human colorectal cancer by bacillus Calmette–Guérin (BCG) or BCG plus 5-fluorouracil, *Lancet* **1**, 871–875 (1976).

208. M. F. McKneally, C. Maver, and H. W. Kausel, Regional immunotherapy of lung cancer with intrapleural BCG, *Lancet* **1**, 377–382 (1976).

209. J. E. Sokal, C. W. Aungst, and M. Snyderman, Delay in progression of malignant lymphoma after BCG vaccination, *N. Engl. J. Med.* **291**, 1226–1230 (1974).

210. A. Buzdar, J. Gutterman, G. Blumenschein, E. Hersh, C. Tashima, E. Gehan, and E. Freireich, An intensive new adjuvant chemoimmunotherapy program containing 5-fluorouracil (5-FU), adriamycin (AD), cyclophosphamide (CYT), and BCG (FAC–BCG) for operable breast cancer, *Proc. Am. Soc. Clin. Oncol.* **18**, 313 (1977) (abstract #C-187).

211. E. Ribi, K. C. Milner, D. L. Granger, M. T. Kelly, K. I. Yamamoto, W. Grehmer, R. Parker, R. F. Smith, and S. M. Strain, Immunotherapy with nonviable microbial components, *Ann. N.Y. Acad. Sci.* **277**, 228–238 (1976).

212. E. Lederer, A. Adam, R. Clorbaru, J.-F. Petit, and J. Wietzerbin, Cell walls of mycobacteria and related organisms. Chemistry and immunostimulant properties, *Mol. Cell. Biochem.* **7**, 87–104 (1975).

213. Y. Yamamura, I. Azuma, T. Taniyama, E. Ribi, and B. Zbar, Suppression of tumor growth and regression of established tumor with oil-attached mycobacterial fractions, *Gann* **65**, 179–181 (1974).

214. D. W. Weiss, MER and other mycobacterial fractions in the immunotherapy of cancer, *Med. Clin. North Am.* **60**, 473–497 (1976).

215. D. W. Weiss, Y. Stupp, N. Many, and G. Izak, Treatment of acute myelocytic leukemia (AML) patients with the MER tubercle bacillus fraction. A preliminary report, *Transplant. Proc.* **7**, 545–548 (1975).

216. J. Cuttner, J. G. Bekesi, and J. F. Holland, Chemoimmunotherapy of acute leukemia using MER, *Proc. Am. Assoc. Cancer Res.* **17**, 196 (1976).

217. M. Perloff, J. F. Holland, and J. G. Bekesi, Chemoimmunotherapy of breast cancer, *Proc. Am. Soc. Clin. Oncol.* **17**, 308 (1976) (abstract #C-288).

218. C. K. Tashima, G. R. Blumenschein, and J. U. Gutterman, Comparison of adriamycin combination drug program with BCG immunotherapy versus MER immunotherapy for metastatic breast cancer, *Proc. Am. Soc. Clin. Oncol.* **17**, 288 (1976) (abstract #C-207).

219. L. Milas, J. U. Gutterman, I. Basic, N. Hunter, G. Mavligit, E. M. Hersh, and H. R. Withers, Immunoprophylaxis and immunotherapy for a murine fibrosarcoma with C. *granulosum* and C. *parvum*, *Int. J. Cancer* **14**, 493–504 (1974).

220. R. W. Baldwin and M. V. Pimm, BCG immunotherapy of pulmonary growths from intravenously transferred rat tumor cells, *Br. J. Cancer* **27**, 48–54 (1973).

221. R. C. Reed, J. U. Gutterman, G. M. Mavligit, M. A. Burgess, and E. M. Hersh, *Corynebacterium parvum:* Preliminary report of a phase 1 clinical and immunological study in cancer patients, in: *Corynebacterium parvum* (B. Halpern, ed.), pp. 349–366, Plenum Press, New York (1975).

222. L. Israel, R. Edelstein, A. DePierre, and N. Dimitrov, Brief communication: Daily intravenous infusion of *Corynebacterium parvum* in twenty patients with disseminated cancer. A preliminary report of clinical and biological findings, *J. Natl. Cancer Inst.* **55**, 29–33 (1975).

223. P. R. Band, C. Jao-King, and R. C. Urtasun, Phase 1 study of *Corynebacterium parvum* in patients with solid tumors, *Cancer Chemother. Rep.* **59**, 1139–1145 (1975).

224. J. Gutterman, E. Hersh, R. Benjamin, G. Mavligit, M. Burgess, and G. P. Bodey, An effective new chemoimmunotherapy regimen for disseminated malignant melanoma, *Proc. Am. Soc. Clin. Oncol.* **18**, 300 (1977) (abstract #C-135).

225. K. Oyama, Y. Takagaki, R. Niki, T. Sato, and T. Akiba, Studies on the interrelation between clinical effects and immune response of a streptococcal antitumor agent, OK432. I. Immunological findings in animals sensitized with OK432, *Jpn. J. Clin. Cancer* **21**, 253–256 (1975).

226. E. Ribi, D. L. Granger, K. C. Milner, and S. M. Strain, Tumor regression caused by endotoxins and mycobacterial fractions, *J. Natl. Cancer Inst.* **55**, 1253–1257 (1975).

227. E. A. Carswell, L. J. Old, R. L. Kassel, S. Green, N. Fiore, and B. Williamson, an endotoxin-induced serum factor that causes necrosis of tumors, *Proc. Natl. Acad. Sci. U.S.A.* **72**, 3666–3670 (1975).

228. I. Hunter-Craig, K. A. Newton, G. Westbury, and B. W. Lacey, Use of vaccinia virus in the treatment of malignant melanoma, *Br. Med. J.* **2**, 512–515 (1970).

229. J. Lindemann, Viruses as immunological adjuvants in cancer, *Biochem. Biophys. Acta* **355**, 49–75 (1974).

230. D. S. Martin, P. Hayworth, R. A. Fugmann, R. English, and H. W. McNeill, Combination therapy with cyclophosphamide and zymosan on a spontaneous mammary cancer in mice, *Cancer Res.* **24**, 652–654 (1964).

231. W. K. Amery, Double-blind levamisole trial in resectable lung cancer, *Ann. N.Y. Acad. Sci.* **277**, 260–268 (1976).

232. A. Rojas, J. Feierstein, E. Mickiewicz, and H. Glait, Levamisole in advanced human breast cancer, *Lancet* **1**, 211–214 (1976).

233. G. N. Hortobagyi, J. U. Gutterman, G. R. Blumenschein, C. K. Tashima, A. U. Buzdar, and E. M. Hersh, Levamisole in the treatment of breast cancer, *Natl. Cancer Inst. Monogr.* (1977), in press.

234. S. E. Grossberg, The interferons and their inducers. Molecular and therapeutic considerations, *N. Engl. J. Med.* **287**, 122–128 (1972).

235. W. Regelson, Clinical immunoadjuvant studies with tilorone, *Ann. N.Y. Acad. Sci.* **277**, 269–287 (1976).

236. H. Strander, K. Cantell, G. Carlstrom, and P. A. Jakobsson, Clinical and laboratory investigations in man: Systemic administration of potent interferon to man, *J. Natl. Cancer Inst.* **51**, 733–742 (1975).

237. D. Habis, Report summary, in: *Proc. Int. Workshop on Interferon in the Treatment of Cancer*, pp. 49–50 (1974).

238. M. D. Prager and F. S. Baechtel, Methods for modification of cancer cells to enhance their antigenicity, in: *Methods in Cancer Research* (H. Busch, Ed.) Vol. IX, pp. 339–400, Academic Press, New York (1973).

239. G. A. Currie and T. J. McElwain, Active immunotherapy as an adjunct to chemotherapy in the treatment of disseminated malignant melanoma. A pilot study, *Br. J. Cancer* **31**, 143–156 (1975).

240. R. Powles, D. Crowther, C. T. J. Bateman, M. E. J. Beard, T. J. McElwain, J. Russell, T. A. Lister, M. A. Whitehouse, P. F. M. Wrigley, M. Pike, P. Alexander, and G. Hamilton-Fairley, Immunotherapy for acute myelogenous leukemia, *Br. J. Cancer* **28**, 365–376 (1973).

241. J. F. Holland and J. G. Bekesi, Immunotherapy of human leukemia with neuraminidase modified cells, *Med. Clin. North Am.* **60**, 539–549 (1976).

242. C. M. Southam, B. C. Marcove, A. G. Levin, H. J. Buchsbaum, and V. Mike, Clinical trials of autogenous tumor vaccine for treatment of osteogenic sarcoma, in: *Proc. 7th Natl. Cancer Conf.*, pp. 91–100, J. B. Lippincott Co., Philadelphia (1972).

243. R. L. Ikonopisov, M. G. Lewis, I. D. Hunter-Craig, D. C. Bodenham, T. M. Phillips, C. I. Cooling, J. Proctor, G. Hamilton-Fairley, and P. Alexander, Autoimmunization with irradiated tumor cells in human malignant melanoma, *Br. Med. J.* **2**, 752–754 (1970).

244. R. L. Powles, L. A. Balchin, G. Hamilton-Fairley, and P. Alexander, Recognition of leukemia cells as foreign before and after autoimmunization, *Br. Med. J.* **1**, 486–489 (1971).

245. J. U. Gutterman, G. M. Mavligit, E. M. Hersh, K. B. McCredie, and E. J. Freireich, Auto-immunization with acute leukemia cells: Demonstration of increased lymphocyte responsiveness, *Int. J. Cancer* **11**, 521–526 (1973).

246. T. H. M. Stewart, A. C. Hollinshead, J. E. Harris, R. Belanger, A. Crepeau, G. D. Hooper, H. J. Sacks, D. J. Klaassen, W. Hirte, E. Rapp, A. F. Crook, M. Orizaga, D. P. S. Singar, and S. Raman, Immunochemotherapy of lung cancer, *Ann. N.Y. Acad. Sci* **277**, 436–466 (1976).

247. N. P. Czajkowski, M. Rosenblatt, P. L. Wolfe, and J. Vazquez, A new method of active immunization to autologous human tumor tissue, *Lancet* **2**, 905–909 (1967).

248. T. J. Cunningham, K. B. Olson, R. Laffin, J. Horton, and J. Sullivan, Treatment of advanced cancer with active immunization, *Cancer* **24**, 932–937 (1969).

249. J. M. Anderson, Prolonged survival after autograft immunotherapy of mammary cancer, *Proc. Am. Assoc. Cancer Res.* **17**, 186 (1976) (abstract #744).

250. L. J. Humphrey, O. R. Boehm, B. J. Boehm, and W. R. Jewell, Adoptive and passive immunotherapy, in: *Proc. 7th Natl. Cancer Conf.*, pp. 85–89, J. B. Lippincott Co., Philadelphia (1973).

251. P. Alexander, E. J. Delorme, L. D. G. Hamilton, and J. D. Hall, Effect of nucleic acids from immune lymphocytes on rat sarcomata, *Nature* **213**, 569–572 (1967).

252. Y. H. Pilch, D. Fritze, and D. H. Kern, Immune RNA in the immunotherapy of cancer, *Med. Clin. North Am.* **60**, 567–583 (1976).

253. H. S. Lawrence, Transfer factor, in: *Advances in Immunology* (F. J. Dixon and H. G. Kunkel, eds.), Vol. 11, pp. 195–266, Academic Press, New York (1969).

254. L. J. Brandes and G. J. Goldenberg, Peripheral leukocyte migration inhibition reactivity to breast cancer antigens in patients with breast cancer and normal control, *Cancer Res.* **36**, 3707–3710 (1976).

255. H. F. Oettgen, L. J. Old, J. H. Farrow, F. T. Valentine, H. S. Lawrence, and L. Thomas, Effect of dialyzable transfer factor in patients with breast cancer, *Proc. Natl. Acad. Sci. U.S.A.* **71**, 2319–2323 (1974).

256. B. W. Papermaster, O. A. Holterman, E. Klein, I. Djerassi, D. Rosner, T. Dao, and J. J. Costanzi, Preliminary observations on tumor regressions induced by local administration of a lymphoid cell culture supernatant fraction in patients with cutaneous metastatic lesions, *Clin. Immunol. Immunopathol.* **5**, 31–47 (1976).

257. A. L. Goldstein, G. H. Cohen, J. L. Rossio, G. B. Thurman, C. N. Brown, and J. T. Ulrich, Use of thymosin in the treatment of primary immunodeficiency diseases and cancer, *Med. Clin. North Am.* **60**, 591–606 (1976).

258. L. Israel, P. Mannoni, E. Radot, and E. Greenspan, Réactions immunitaires et tumorales à l'échange de plasma dans les cancers avancés, *Nouv. Presse Med.* **5**, 433 (1976).

259. E. M. Hersh, Modification of host defense mechanisms, in: *Cancer Medicine* (J. F. Holland and E. Frei, eds.), pp. 681–699, Lea and Febiger, Philadelphia (1973).

260. H. W. Bruckner, M. B. Mokyr, and M. S. Mitchell, Effect of DTIC on immunity in patients with malignant melanoma, *Cancer Res.* **34**, 181–183 (1974).

261. J. A. DiLorenzo, D. E. Griswold, C. R. Bareham, and P. Calabresi, Selective alteration of immunocompetence with methotrexate and 5-fluorouracil, *Cancer Res.* **34**, 124–128 (1974).

262. J. L. Turk and L. W. Poulter, Selective depletion of lymphoid tissue by cyclophosphamide, *Clin. Exp. Immunol.* **10**, 285–296 (1972).

263. G. B. Mackaness, P. H. Lagrange, and T. Ishibashi, The modifying effect of BCG on the immunological induction of T cells, *J. Exp. Med.* **139**, 1540–1552 (1974).

264. A. R. Cheema and E. M. Hersh, Patient survival After chemotherapy and its relationship to *in vitro* lymphocyte blastogenesis, *Cancer* **28**, 851–855 (1971).

265. L. Borella and R. G. Webster, The immunosuppressive effects of long-term combination chemotherapy in children with acute leukemia in remission, *Cancer Res.* **31**, 420–427 (1971).

266. D. Farquhar, T. L. Loo, J. U. Gutterman, E. M. Hersh, and M. A. Luna, Inhibition of drug metabolizing enzymes in the rat after bacillus Calmette–Guérin treatment, *Biochem. Pharmacol.* **25**, 1529–1535 (1976).

267. B. Fisher, N. Wolmark, and H. Rubin, Further observation on the inhibition of tumor growth by *Corynebacterium parvum* with cyclophosphamide. Effect of *Corynebacterium parvum* on cyclophosphamide metabolism, *J. Natl. Cancer Inst.* **57**, 225–229 (1976).

268. G. M. Hahn, J. Braun, and I. Har-Keder, Thermochemotherapy: Synergism between hyperthermia (42–43°) and adriamycin (or bleomycin) in mammalian cell inactivation, *Proc. Natl. Acad. Sci. U.S.A.* **72**, 937–940 (1975).

269. B. Fisher, H. Rubin, E. Saffer, and N. Wolmark, Effect of *Corynebacterium parvum* in combination with 5-FU, L-phenylalanine mustard or methotrexate on the inhibition of tumor growth, *Cancer Res.* **36**, 2714–2719 (1976).

270. J. U. Gutterman, G. M. Mavligit, R. C. Reed, and E. M. Hersh, Immunochemotherapy of human cancer, *Semin. Oncol.* **1**, 409–423 (1974).

271. G. Mathe, L. Schwarzenberg, O. H. Halle-Pannenko, and M. C. Simmler, Discussion paper: Experimental and clinical immunopharmacology data applicable to cancer immunotherapy, *Ann. N.Y. Acad. Sci.* **277**, 467–491 (1976).

272. G. L. Slemmer, Host response to premalignant mammary tissues, *Natl. Cancer Inst. Monogr.* **35,** 57–71 (1972).
273. L. Davignon, P. Lemode, P. Robillard, and A. Frappier, BCG vaccination and leukemia mortality, *Lancet* **2,** 638 (1970).
274. S. R. Rosenthal, R. G. Crispen, M. G. Thorne, N. Piekarski, N. Raisys, and P. G. Rettig, BCG vaccination and leukemia mortality, *J. Am. Med. Assoc.* **222,** 1543–1544 (1972).

Subject Index